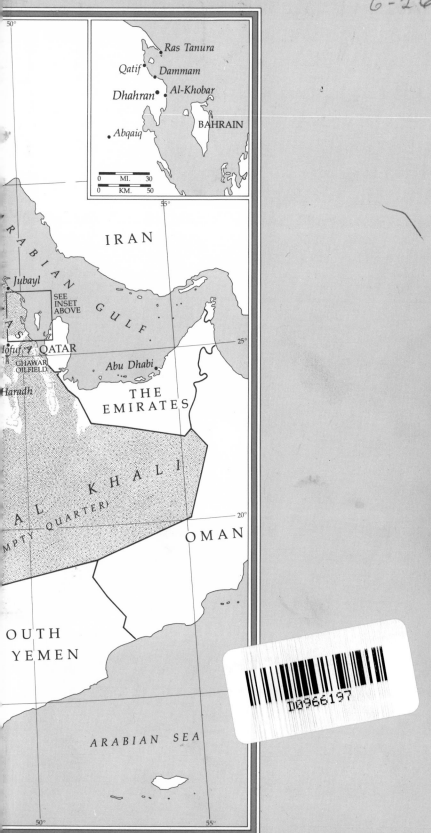

50°

Ras Tanura

Qatif • • Dammam

Dhahran • Al-Khobar

• Abqaiq

BAHRAIN

| 0 | MI. | 30 |
| 0 | KM. | 50 |

55°

IRAN

A R A B I A N

G U L F

Jubayl •

SEE
INSET
ABOVE

QATAR

Hofuf •

GHAWAR
OILFIELD

Abu Dhabi •

THE
EMIRATES

Haradh •

25°

A L   K H A L I

EMPTY QUARTER)

20°

OMAN

OUTH

YEMEN

ARABIAN   SEA

50°

55°

SEYMOUR GRAY

BEYOND *the* VEIL

the adventures of an American doctor in Saudi Arabia

A Cornelia & Michael Bessie Book

HARPER & ROW, PUBLISHERS, New York
Cambridge, Philadelphia, San Francisco,
London, Mexico City, São Paulo, Sydney

1817

610
Gray

FIRST EDITION

Designed by Ruth Bornschlegel

This book is set in 10-point Autologic Electra. It was composed by TriStar Graphics, Minneapolis, and printed and bound by R. R. Donnelley and Sons Company, the Lakeside Press, Chicago.

Map by George Colbert

Library of Congress Cataloging in Publication Data

Gray, Seymour Jerome, date
  Beyond the veil.

  "A Cornelia & Michael Bessie Book."
  Includes index.
  1. Gray, Seymour Jerome, date. 2. Physicians—United States—Biography. 3. Saudi Arabia—Social life and customs. I. Title.
R154.G766A33 1982   610'.92'4 [B]   82–47523
ISBN 0-06-039014-X   AACR2

---

86 87 10 9 8 7

2519

899

To Those Who Minister to the Sick in Distant Lands

CONTENTS

ACKNOWLEDGMENTS

FIRST AND FOREMOST, I would like to thank the Saudi Arabian people for opening their hearts and minds to me during the three years I spent in their country. Many expressed themselves freely before a tape recorder, not without personal risk, and to these I am particularly beholden.

I owe a deep debt of gratitude to my friends Melvin and Marcia Lafrenz, who had spent most of their lives in Saudi Arabia and were an invaluable source of knowledge and insight into the human scene.

I am also grateful to Joseph B. Darby III, Debbie Danielpour, and Pamela Painter for their editorial expertise, and to Margaret Cheney for her copyediting contributions. Similarly, I am indebted to Elizabeth M. McCabe, who read and commented on the manuscript.

Special thanks are due to my editor, Simon Michael Bessie, for his encouragement and enthusiasm, and to my old friend, Garson Kanin, who originally brought us together.

My wife, Ruth, shared many of my experiences in Saudi Arabia and accepted the hardships and challenges with good cheer. She has been adviser, critic, and contributor and, as always, my inspiration.

He was conscious, while it lasted, that he saw deeper into the beauty, the sadness of things, the very heart of them, and their pathetic evanescence, as with a new inner eye—even into eternity itself, beyond the veil.

GEORGE DU MAURIER

Beyond the Veil is a true story. However, with the exception of certain prominent figures the names have been changed and individual traits and locales have been altered.

◇ *1* ◇

FLIGHT INTO THE PAST

ON A CRISP October morning in 1975, I boarded a Saudia Airlines jet at London's Heathrow Airport, destined for Riyadh, the capital of Saudi Arabia. An attractive Lebanese stewardess greeted me at the door of the plane and led me to a comfortable, swivel-type seat in the first-class section. As I sat down, I noticed the baggage identification label which was attached to my brown leather carrying case. It read: *"King Faisal Specialist Hospital, Riyadh, Saudi Arabia."*

Somehow the tag brought home the reality of the situation: I was on my way to Saudi Arabia, the home of Mecca and Islam, the land of the Bedouin nomad, the camel, and the boundless desert. It seemed so strange! I felt like Alice in Wonderland about to walk through the looking glass into the tenth century.

In my pocket was a two-year contract to serve as physician and medical specialist at the new King Faisal Specialist Hospital, an appointment that promised to be both professionally rewarding and personally fascinating. I would be working in one of the newest and best-equipped medical facilities in the world. The personal satisfaction would come from taking care of Saudis in all walks of life, including important members of the royal family. Actually, I had treated a number of talented and world-famous people over the years and I did not expect to be overawed. But it was definitely intriguing to think that the King himself or the Crown Prince might be one of my patients. After all, how many people have been the physician to the richest monarch in history? The most appealing aspect of the job, however, was the intimate contact I would have with many people from all strata of society, rich and poor alike.

When my colleagues learned that I was planning to spend two or more years in Saudi Arabia they were astonished. They couldn't understand why I would interrupt my medical practice, teaching, and research, to go off to a strange desert land thousands of miles away. Most of my friends reacted in a similar fashion. Why give up a comfortable and productive life in Boston, they argued, for a primitive existence in an unknown country the other side of the world? Ruth Gordon, the actress, put it more succinctly: "What the hell you gonna do in Saudi Arabia? It's so damn far away!" On the other hand, Katharine Hepburn, who was rehearsing *A Matter of Gravity,* was full of enthusiasm: "I think it's a wonderful idea! Dad and I once went to Iran and found it exciting. I'll come to visit you in Riyadh when the play closes."

My wife was equally encouraging. Her first response was: "What is the weather like in Saudi Arabia? I have to know what to pack."

Actually my interest in international medicine went back many years. It began when I persuaded an American pharmaceutical company to finance a postgraduate program at Harvard for doctors from the developing countries. The foreign doctors worked with me and others for several years and then returned to their own countries to spread the gospel of medicine as physicians or as professors at their medical schools.

Later, as a lecturer for the U.S. State Department, I had more personal contact with people in foreign lands while touring Central and South America. Finally, the State Department asked me to head a task force to evaluate medical education in Africa and Asia as well as in Latin America. This provided an added incentive for me to participate more directly in the care of people living in underdeveloped areas where the shortage of physicians was so desperate. Therefore, when the opportunity to go to Saudi Arabia presented itself I accepted with enthusiasm.

As the Tri-Star took off I leaned back and stared out the window. I felt that I had made the right decision and that there was a much greater medical need for me in Saudi Arabia than in Boston. It gave me a sense of satisfaction to feel that I might help more people there in two years than perhaps in a lifetime at home.

I was fascinated by this feudal kingdom, which had been completely cut off from the rest of the world for over a thousand years. Following the recent oil embargo and the quadrupling of oil prices, Saudi Arabia had become the center of world attention. The economic structure of the Western world depended upon oil and therefore upon Saudi Arabia. Our country, too, relied heavily upon the Saudis and was anxious to help them whenever possible. Saudi Arabia, in turn, was favorably disposed to the United States. The Saudis, for example, selected an American corporation to manage the new hospital where I would be working. This multi-million-dollar contract was granted to the Americans in the face of keen competition from England and other countries.

Most of all, I was intrigued by the Saudis' unique way of life. It was based upon the deeply rooted precepts of Wahabism, which advocated a strict ultra-puritanical religious life as practiced in the days of Mohammed. The Wahabi sect of Islam had dominated the country for more than two hundred years. Consequently, Saudi Arabia remained the most orthodox society in the Moslem world.

Crime was practically nonexistent, unbelievable as that may seem. I had been deeply disturbed by the epidemic of crime and violence which infested our society and by the vulnerability and permissiveness of our people and our courts of law. We had the highest crime rate in the world and it was slowly paralyzing our society. Our social structure was apparently coming unglued. It seemed that in this country personal freedom was being interpreted as a license for lawlessness, and individual rights were taking precedence over the rights of society. Corruption in government was equally distressing. The Watergate burglary and the subsequent televised congressional investigations were still fresh in my mind.

Now, I was leaving the tragedies and mayhem that surrounded me to taste another culture, which was ultra-conservative and backward by American standards. Yet there was a tightly-knit quality to its social fabric that, from eight thousand miles away, appeared to have many of the attributes I so deeply mourned in my own culture. I was seeking a quiet haven, free of crime, corruption, and pressing economic problems, where people felt safe and could follow their pursuits in peace and with optimism about the future. Whether I would find the sanctuary in Saudi Arabia remained to be determined. But I had no doubt that this would be an exciting and novel undertaking.

As my resolve to take the job in Saudi Arabia grew more firm, I began to educate myself about the country. I started with *Seven Pillars of Wisdom* by T. E. Lawrence; *The Arabs in History* by Bernard Lewis; *Saudi Arabia* by Harry St. John Philby, and *The Desert King* by David Hawarth. From there I began to read everything else that I could find, including *The Arab Mind* by Patai, *Arabian Sands* by Wilfred Thesiger, and an excellent *Area Handbook for Saudi Arabia* published by the United States government. Finally, before leaving, I spoke with visiting Arab scholars at Harvard and with students from Saudi Arabia.

From these varied sources I drew a strange and anomalous picture of the country to which I was about to devote two years or more of my life. There seemed to be an indefinable mystique about Saudi Arabia. Although it occupies about 80 percent of the Arabian Peninsula (the desolate knob of land at the crossroads between Africa, Europe, and Asia), few countries knew of its existence. It remained an unexplored enigma.

Saudi Arabia is roughly the size of the United States east of the Mississippi. The topography is mainly desert, including a vast expanse of sandy waste too arid to support life. The Arabs call this enormous desert wilderness Rub Al Khali, the Empty Quarter. It is the size of the state of Texas and occupies the southeast portion of the country.

For as long as recorded history, wandering nomadic tribes of Bedouins, desperately poor and often bordering on starvation, spent their lives searching for water and pastures for their camels, raiding and fighting each other for survival. Until a few decades ago Saudi Arabia consisted of a handful of mud-brick towns scattered throughout the desert in isolated oases.

Indeed, the arid characteristics and the lack of urban permanency had been Arabia's great historical shield, which it wore the way a porcupine wears its quills. Arabia offered too many obstacles and too little wealth, and so it remained throughout history as virtually the only area that was not subject to either occupation or colonization by a foreign power.

There was very little on the surface to attract the covetous eyes of foreign colonizers, who saw only the sand of this poverty-stricken desert wasteland, never dreaming of the vast treasures of oil beneath. For a while, the Turks occupied some areas but eventually they were driven out and the Arab island continued to live in a vacuum.

Until very recently, Saudi Arabia remained as remote as the lost continent of Atlantis. It was not even mentioned, for example, in Julian Huxley's book *The Middle East and Its History,* which was published in 1954.

The Kingdom of Saudi Arabia, as we know it today, came into existence in 1932, just fifty years ago. It was created single-handedly by a remarkable man, King Abdul-Aziz Al Saud, known to the Western world as Ibn Saud. He was a direct descendant of Emir Mohammed Ibn Saud, the eponymous founder of the House of Saud, who captured Riyadh in 1764 and created the first Saudi state. Ibn Saud started out as a penniless young prince, whose father had lost his throne to the rival Rashid family. In 1902, at the age of twenty-two, he led a daring raid into Riyadh and recaptured the Saud dynasty's ancestral capital. It was the first in a long string of military victories.

Over the next twenty-five years, Ibn Saud fought, married, and politicked his way into control of the Arabian Peninsula. When necessary, he fought with his enemies; when possible, he allied with them, often marrying their daughters to cement the alliance. In this way, he managed to entwine his fortunes with those of almost every leading tribal family in Arabia. By 1926, the last of his opponents was defeated, and after consolidating his conquests, Ibn Saud unified the various regions officially as the Kingdom of Saudi Arabia in 1932. It is the only nation in the world named after a clan or family. King Abdul-Aziz Al Saud is as much a legend in

Saudi Arabia today as George Washington and Abraham Lincoln are in the United States.

In conquering and unifying his realm, Ibn Saud was married over three hundred times. Most of these marriages were political alliances with important tribal families. From this multiplicity of marital unions, he produced forty-four sons and an unknown number of daughters. It is estimated that at least two thousand Saudi princes are descended from Ibn Saud. In all its branches, the Saudi royal family numbers more than four thousand male members. The extraordinary size of the royal family is one of its greatest assets; the Saudi government and armed forces are heavily infiltrated with members of the family, whose loyalty to the throne is unquestioned.

In 1932 when Saudi Arabia was first recognized as a nation, it was primitive and destitute. There was no electricity until 1960 and slavery flourished until 1962. It had no significant source of income apart from the money derived from the yearly pilgrimages to Mecca by devout Moslems. Then, in 1938, the Arabian-American Oil Company (Aramco) discovered the largest oil field in history, and Saudi Arabia was catapulted into the center of international dominance. Within a few decades, a handful of scattered, semistarved nomadic tribes had been transformed into an incredibly wealthy nation. Beneath its sands was one-third of the world's oil reserves, the greatest single petroleum treasure on earth.

At Ibn Saud's death in 1953, Saudi Arabia's oil revenues were just beginning to reach truly substantial proportions, and thus the country lost its experienced leader at a time when firm and rational guidance was most necessary. Under the dissolute rule of Ibn Saud's son and successor, King Saud, Saudi Arabia embarked on an erratic course, spending the huge oil revenues faster than they accumulated. Finally, in 1964 Saud was deposed and replaced by his half brother Faisal, who proved to be a strong and dedicated leader. King Faisal was assassinated in 1975 by a demented young member of the royal family, and the family elders appointed Crown Prince Khalid as King to lead the country. At this time they also appointed Prince Fahd, another of Ibn Saud's many sons, to become Crown Prince and heir apparent to the throne.

Today, the wealth of this small country, one-fourth the size of the United States, is mind-boggling. Saudi Arabia is the world's leading producer and exporter of oil. Its oil reserves are estimated at a staggering 300 billion barrels. The country's income from oil is $100 billion a year, or about $15,000 for every man, woman, and child.

With a population of only about six million people, the per capita income is by far the highest in the world, almost twice that of the United States. To top it off, Saudi Arabia's foreign assets are estimated at $100 billion, and its international monetary reserves exceed those of Great Britain and the United States combined.

As my plane climbed into the eastern sky, I felt a surge of excitement. Who, after all, could resist living in a fairy-tale society? Saudi Arabia is a country of enormous contrasts, with gigantic wealth that has not yet concealed a past of dire poverty, and with technical modernism that does not eliminate an almost feudal social structure. It is a meeting place of Western materialism and a strict Eastern moral code, with the potential of a head-on collision between the two. Whatever else it would prove to be— and despite my reading, I had no clear picture of what was in store for me in Saudi Arabia—I knew that I was heading east for a unique experience.

While the production and distribution of energy represent international power, the most oil-rich country on this planet remains veiled in obscurity. And I would learn that what lies beyond the veil is incredible, sometimes shocking.

"Water, fruit juice, or soft drink, sir?"

I awoke from my daydream to find the Lebanese stewardess standing next to me, pushing a drink cart down the aisle of the plane.

"I'd like some water, please," I said.

The stewardess wrapped a large white napkin around the bottle as though it were champagne, and with a flourish she filled my glass. This was my first experience with Sohat water, a Perrier-like water bottled in Lebanon and distributed throughout the Middle East. It was ice cold and delicious. At the time I was amused by this rather ceremonious handling of the water. Later, when I learned that a bottle of Sohat water was more expensive in arid Saudi Arabia than a bottle of champagne in London, the ceremony no longer seemed so inappropriate.

When the stewardess left, I opened my leather carrying case and extracted the small bottle of scotch which I had picked up at the duty-free shop at Heathrow Airport. Saudia Airlines follows strict Islamic law and forbids the serving of alcoholic beverages to the passengers. Consequently, almost every foreigner on the plane had brought along a private bottle for consumption during the flight. The Saudis are indulgent of this practice, and since any alcohol left over is confiscated when the flight arrives in Riyadh, Saudia Airlines often hosts some of the most hilariously drunken flights in the history of air travel.

The man sitting in the seat next to me watched in amusement as I poured some scotch into my Sohat water, then opened his briefcase and pulled out the ingredients for a vodka and tonic. He poured himself a generous drink, and then held up his glass in salutation. We had established a common ground.

"Where are you bound for?"

"Riyadh," I replied.

"That's where I'm going," he said, holding out his hand. He introduced himself as Bill Thompson, and explained that he was an electrical contractor from California who was working on one of the myriad construction projects then underway in Riyadh. A stocky, balding man in his mid-forties, Bill did a substantial amount of business with Saudi Arabia. This was his third visit.

"I'm planning to be in Riyadh for two years," I said.

"God!" he exclaimed. "That's an awfully long time. About the longest I can stand to be in Saudi Arabia is a month. I get a hell of a lot done in that month, though. There's nothing to do in Riyadh except work. It's like living in the desert."

The thought of Riyadh seemed to cause a parching in his throat, and he paused to sip his vodka and tonic. "You may be in for a rough time," he warned me. "There are no movies, no theaters, no alcohol, and no women. You practically never see a Saudi woman in public, not even in a restaurant. Nobody laughs, it seems. It can get really depressing."

"What's it like for foreign women?" I asked. "Do you ever bring your wife?"

"I don't have one," he answered, "but if I did, I definitely wouldn't bring her. The Saudi laws apply to foreign and Saudi women alike. Women are forbidden to drive a car, they can't hold any job that brings them into contact with men, and they can't go anywhere alone, unless they want to be harassed unmercifully.

"You should see the Saudi women! Perhaps I should say you can't see the Saudi women because they conceal their faces completely with a black veil and wear a long black cloak over their clothes. Even then, they must always be accompanied by a chaperone."

By now Bill was warming up to the topic. "You want to know how peculiar the Saudis are about women? I'll tell you a true story. A few months ago, Queen Elizabeth of Britain was supposed to visit Saudi Arabia. Naturally, it presented a terrible dilemma, because, according to Saudi tradition, women are not even supposed to attend an important ceremony, much less to be feted as the guest of honor. Finally, the Saudis found a solution. They made Queen Elizabeth an 'honorary man' so that she could visit their country!

"The segregation of the sexes is amazing," continued Bill. "The women are kept at home and are not allowed to mix socially with men. You can never meet any Saudi women, and you usually don't even see any *pictures* of women in the newspapers or magazines because they are blacked out by the censors. The Saudis confiscate or censor everything they consider offensive by Islam standards. A customs officer confiscated an art book recently because it contained the photograph of a nude statue—Venus de Milo!

"I wonder what they would think of *Playboy* magazine," pondered Bill, with a faraway look and a smile.

He drained his glass and then pointed to two attractive young women sitting across the aisle. They were slender, olive-skinned brunettes with luxuriant hair and large brown eyes, chatting and laughing as young women are wont to do. Both were dressed elegantly although casually, in the latest French fashions, crossing and uncrossing their legs with abandon and exposing well-rounded thighs. Sitting with them was a middle-aged man, presumably their father or uncle, who joined them in conversation from time to time.

"The man with them never lets them out alone, you can be sure of that," whispered Bill. "He's a member of the family and chaperones them everywhere."

Now and again, wafts of a heady, seductive perfume filled the air.

"Saudi women traditionally wear a lot of perfume," Bill explained. "They're probably royals coming home from a European holiday or they're from one of the Saudi business families. The oil boom has created a hell of a lot of Saudi millionaires these days, and the first thing they do when they make their money is to go to London or Paris and spend it."

"What's it like doing business with the Saudis?" I asked.

"Oh, it's a pain usually. They're shrewd as hell, and you have to be on your toes. What's more, they take their sweet time on every deal and keep you waiting around for weeks on end before they give you an answer. They play it like a game, according to their own rules, and they're wonderfully polite, offering you coffee and everything, but sometimes they drive me crazy."

"If that's the case, why do you do business with them?" I asked.

"Money," he replied. "They know what they want and they usually don't care how much it costs as long as you can deliver what you promise. The profit margins on these construction projects are fantastic.

"Of course," he added, "they're incredibly slow about paying their bills. They may keep you waiting a year or two before they pay up."

This observation turned out to be curiously prophetic. Six months later, the King Faisal Hospital almost closed down because the Saudis had not paid several million dollars long overdue to a hospital supply company, and as a result the company stopped shipment of crucial medical supplies.

"I suppose that we have to adapt ourselves to a foreign country's traditions and economic practices, no matter how strange they may appear to us," I said, remembering what I had learned while visiting some of the developing countries a few years ago.

Eventually, we lapsed into silence, and I began to think back over my prior experiences with the Saudi Arabian royal family. During the 1960s, many eminent people flew to Boston to consult with medical specialists at the numerous prestigious hospitals in that city. One such person was Princess Iffat, whose husband, Prince Faisal, would later become the King of Saudi Arabia. Iffat was an attractive, articulate, and powerful woman, reputedly the dominant of Faisal's wives. She had persuaded the Saudi government to open an elementary school for girls, and later a high school, despite intense opposition from the conservative religious leaders. Education for women was a heresy in Saudi Arabia at that time, but Iffat, who was of Turkish origin, stood her ground, and eventually triumphed. As we discussed her medical problems, she chain-smoked long black Turkish cigarettes. When I asked how many she smoked in a day, she replied, squinting to keep the smoke out of her eyes, "Three packs, more or less." I knew it would be useless to ask her to stop smoking. Iffat obviously had a mind of her own.

A day or two later, I had examined Iffat's fifteen-year-old son, Prince Saud bin Faisal. He was a handsome young man, who was attending prep school in New England in preparation for Princeton. Now, sixteen years later, he was the Foreign Minister of Saudi Arabia, and many people were predicting that he would one day be the King. I had both of their medical charts packed safely in my bags, just in case we should meet again in Riyadh.

My second experience with Saudi Arabian royalty took place three years later, in August 1962. While making my rounds at the hospital one day, I encountered two huge black men, about six feet four inches tall, standing guard at the end of the hall. They wore colorful turbans, long white robes, and ominous, oversized gold daggers in their belts.

"What's going on?" I asked the head nurse. "Who are your friends with the daggers?"

"The King of Saudi Arabia has just been admitted," she replied grimly. "Those are his bodyguards. They're taking over the whole floor, which means that your patients, among others, will be moved to another area."

"I don't approve of moving all the patients unnecessarily," I said.

The head nurse shrugged. "It's over and done with," she replied, scanning a paper in her hand. "By the way, your name is on the list of consultants who are being called to examine His Royal Highness. His personal physician is with him and will translate."

"Is this an emergency?" I asked.

"No, but the sooner we get started, the better."

"I'll be back later," I promised, glancing nervously at the guards and their daggers.

I soon discovered that the entire third floor of the hospital had been cleared, not only for security reasons but also to accommodate King Saud's enormous entourage. Five times daily, waiters arrived and scurried about carrying huge trays of food from a nearby restaurant. In front of the hospital, there was a continuous stream of long, shiny Cadillac limousines, shuttling his sons, their friends, and visiting dignitaries to and from the King's bedside. The King was said to have had countless wives and concubines and more than one hundred children. His traveling entourage included his four current wives, his favorite sons, and some of his advisors, aides, and servants. The total number of people in his party was between seventy-five and one hundred.

A wave of excitement passed through the hospital when his wives came to visit. They arrived together, wearing thick veils and covered completely by their black robes. They were all a bit plump and heavily perfumed. Although they made only one visit during the King's stay, their fragrance seemed to linger on for days.

King Saud was the eldest son of King Abdul-Aziz, whom he succeeded upon the death of his father in 1953. Saud was a well-meaning but simple man. He had no ability to manage the increasingly complex affairs of the Saudi Arabian government. Above all else, Saud loved luxury, and his spendthrift and sybaritic lifestyle nearly bankrupted Saudi Arabia in the 1950s, despite the massive oil revenues that were already beginning to flow into the government coffers. His incompetence was an international scandal, and within two years of his visit to Boston, he was forced to abdicate the throne in favor of his younger brother Faisal.

When I was finally asked to examine King Saud, I was appalled to discover that His Majesty was riddled with disease. All of his ailments were chronic, and most of them were irreversible. The King was virtually blind in one eye from an old trachoma infection, and he had mild diabetes, which he compounded by refusing to follow his diet. He also had cirrhosis of the liver. All of us who examined Saud gave him sound medical advice on how to take care of himself. The King followed none of it. He died in exile seven years later.

My most poignant memory was of Sanwa Al Saud, the twenty-two-year-old wife of one of King Saud's aides. Sanwa was a beautiful Egyptian woman who had married the young Saudi Arabian prince when she was eighteen. Early in their marriage she had borne him a son, who, at the time I met her, was three years old and was her pride and joy. Normally, Sanwa would have remained at home while her husband joined the King on his international jaunts. This time she had been brought along so that she could get medical treatment for a lump on her right arm.

After carefully examining her, I told Princess Sanwa, "It's only a fatty tumor. If it bothers you, we can remove it surgically under local anesthesia. However, all your tests are normal; you're in excellent physical condition."

"I must speak to my husband," she replied. "He will want to discuss it with you."

The next day, the young prince, a nephew of the King, came to my office at the hospital. He was about thirty years old. The prince wore expensive, well-tailored Western clothes and spoke excellent English, for which I complimented him.

"Thank you," he said. "I went to college in California."

I explained to him about the lipoma: "It's a common tumor that grows under the skin and is not dangerous to Princess Sanwa in any way. It can be removed surgically with ease and there is nothing to worry about. It is most certainly benign."

He hesitated. "Can I get it from her?" he asked apprehensively. He was serious. "I heard that tumors are caused by a virus and can be passed from one person to another."

"It is not contagious and it is not a cancer," I explained patiently. "In fact, it is completely harmless. If you have any doubts, then let's go ahead and have it removed. The operation is very simple, and it can be performed in the outpatient department."

The prince thanked me and left.

The next day Princess Sanwa arrived at my office accompanied by the same plump woman who had escorted her on her first visit. This woman was Sanwa's lady-in-waiting, and her name was Fahada.

When the two of them entered my office, they immediately burst into tears.

"He divorced me," sobbed Sanwa. "He divorced me." She began to weep uncontrollably.

Stunned, I turned to Fahada. "What happened?" I asked.

"Her husband divorced her last night because of the lump on her arm," replied Fahada, who was crying herself.

"How can he divorce her?" I asked. I didn't understand.

Between deep breaths, she explained. "Divorce is very easy in Saudi Arabia. All the man has to do is repeat, 'I divorce you,' three times to the woman, and the marriage is finished. The prince did this last night."

"Is that legal?" I asked, incredulous.

Fahada nodded. "Now the princess must return to her family in Egypt, and her son will remain with the prince."

"It's finished," sobbed the princess. "My baby, my baby . . ."

"That *idiot!*" I shouted angrily. "Let me talk to him. I'll get this straightened out."

"It won't do any good," said Fahada. "He is afraid that the tumor is contagious and may spread to his son or to him."

"That's absolutely ridiculous," I snorted. "I explained all that to him yesterday. I want to talk to him again. Maybe I can change his mind."

Fahada looked at the princess with pitying eyes. "It is useless," she said to me, "but thank you for trying."

When the women left my office, I gathered my papers together and drove to the hotel where the royal party had rented several floors. I was ushered into the living quarters set aside for the princes. It had the atmosphere of a bordello. Loud music was blaring from all directions, and white-coated waiters were running back and forth, carrying trays of assorted drinks and snacks. The young princes and their friends were shouting to each other through the walls. There was loud, raucous laughter coming from the rooms, punctuated at times by a female scream. Semi-clad women could be seen darting from room to room, giggling, followed by Saudi princes who were unshaven and disheveled. Everyone seemed drunk to the gills. It looked as though the bacchanal had been going on for some time.

In a central reception room that was set up as a bar, I asked to see Sanwa's husband and then sat down and waited while my request for an interview was passed on to the prince. Merchants were coming and going, carrying display cases of jewelry and clothes. Young attractive girls, all blondes, were also selling their merchandise, unabashedly entering or leaving the suites. I was soon joined by a pretty blonde American girl in her early twenties, who was very friendly and very drunk. She was carrying an Arabic-English dictionary in her hand.

"I'm going to Saudi Arabia with my prince," she announced, pausing unsteadily to sip her drink. "That's why I'm studying Arabic. As soon as I get my visa, I'm going over to join him. I am going to be a princess!"

I looked at her sadly, certain that the visa would never materialize.

When the woman wandered off, I overheard two salesmen who apparently had an appointment with one of the princes. They were drinking beer.

"The assistant manager of the hotel told me," said one, "that the King sent an aide to the cashier's desk for some 'pocket money.'

"The cashier said, 'Surely. How much would you like?' and the aide said, without blinking an eye, 'One hundred thousand dollars would do,' and then the cashier said, 'We don't keep quite that much money on hand. You might try the bank across the street.'"

They both laughed and sipped their beer.

"I heard," said the other, "that the owner of one of the women's shops on Newbury Street brought display cases full of gowns for the King's wives. She left a few hours later carrying back the cases full of hundred-dollar bills."

"I hope we're that lucky," sighed his companion.

It soon became apparent that Sanwa's husband was "not available" and had no intention of seeing me. There was something pointless and degenerate about the scene in the royal suites, and I concluded that my arguments would have been futile, as Fahada had predicted. I returned home in a bewildered state of mind.

The next day Fahada called me at the office and asked if I could possibly come over to the hotel and say goodbye. "We know what you did," she said, "and we appreciate it very much. Sanwa wants to see you before she leaves. She has a surprise for you."

That evening, I met Fahada in the lobby of the hotel. Her eyes were red, and it was clear that she had been crying.

"We are so grateful to you for coming," she said. "Sanwa has been shattered by the divorce. Having her child taken away is a terrible shock."

We rode up the elevator in silence, past the area where the royal orgy presumably was still in progress, and arrived at the floors that were reserved for the women members of the royal entourage. Princess Sanwa, ironically, was living in the presidential suite; Fahada was in a small suite down the hall.

We entered the lavishly furnished room, which was heavy with the scent of perfume, rosewater, and sandalwood. In one corner a portable record player was sitting on a table. Flower arrangements graced many of the delicately carved tables. The lights were low.

Fahada and I sat on petit-point-covered chairs, and she served me coffee and light pastries.

"Sanwa will be here shortly," she said softly.

After a few minutes, Fahada silently approached the record player and turned on the music. The music was arabesque and beautiful, with a lilting tonal splendor that reminded me of Rimsky-Korsakov.

Suddenly, out of a shadow, a thin, almost boyish figure appeared, clad in diaphanous lavender veils, revealing all of her body and yet none of it. She began to dance slowly with seductive movements, sensuous but not provocative. She danced effortlessly, with grace and eloquence.

As the music increased in tempo, she seemed transformed into a whirling dervish, as though possessed by its rhythmic excitement. Tears streamed down her face as she pirouetted faster and faster. Then tranquillity gradually returned, and the dance became slow and ecstatic. As the music came to an end, she seemed to disappear into thin air.

All was still. In the hushed silence, I meditated on what I had just seen, as one will sometimes ponder a dream. I thought of Havelock Ellis: "Dancing is the loftiest, the most moving, the most beautiful of the arts, because it is no mere translation or abstraction from life; it is life itself."

Sanwa appeared a few minutes later, dressed and more composed, although her face was still wet with tears.

"You are the only man who has ever seen me dance, except for my husband," she said quietly.

"I am honored," I said helplessly. "I will never forget your dance."

Thirteen years have passed and I have not forgotten.

Near sundown I awoke from a brief nap. We were flying over the desert now, an endless sea of sand that appeared pink in some areas and white or gray in others. Viewed from a plane five miles above, the scene conveyed a feeling of desolation and loneliness.

On board the plane, people were beginning to stir. A male flight attendant knelt on a rug at the end of the aisle, praying as the sun set.

Next to me, Bill opened his eyes, struggling to shake off the effects of several vodka-and-tonics. He looked out the window and then at his watch.

"We're passing over Egypt," he said. "We should be coming to the Red Sea pretty soon. Then we fly east of Mecca to Riyadh.

"How many more hours?" I asked.

"About two and a half," he replied. "We should get there around eight o'clock Riyadh time, or five o'clock London time. That's twelve noon Boston time," he added.

I watched the Saudi attendant praying on his rug, while the others began to set up the dinner trays.

"The Saudis are very orthodox about their religion," said Bill, indicating the kneeling figure in the aisle. "I've been on flights where half the passengers got down in the aisles to pray.

"That man is a Saudi," explained Bill. "The female attendants are all English, Lebanese, or Egyptian, because Saudi women are not allowed to do anything that will bring them in contact with men. By the way, the Saudia Airline is run by TWA, under a five-year contract. There are Saudis aboard as part of their training program."

"The pilots are American, aren't they?" I asked with apprehension.

"Yes, they are," Bill assured me, "but the Saudis will take over in five years, theoretically."

"Why theoretically?"

"Because I know the Saudis. Deep down, they really don't believe they can master all these things within a few years. Not long ago, an American management team turned a power plant over to their Saudi trainees, and within a year the whole damn plant exploded. There's no way they can run an airline independently in such a short time."

"The hospital I'm going to is run the same way," I said. "It will be managed by an American health-care company for five years, but it will take at least ten years to train enough doctors to take over, probably longer. The Saudis will have to extend the contracts."

"Amen," said Bill, raising his glass to mine. "A toast to Saudi Arabia, and to longer and bigger contracts."

"And, now," he added, "you better enjoy your scotch because it's the last good drink you'll be having for a while."

We crossed the Red Sea at dinnertime, eating and drinking as we continued our discussion of Saudi Arabia. The attendant again poured the "wine" with the traditional amenities accorded vintage Château Lafite Rothschild, 1959. The carbonated cider was cold and refreshing. Maybe the large napkin folded neatly around the bottle contributed to the illusion.

Bill and I were both a bit high, and judging from the singing behind us, we weren't the only ones. After dinner, we handed our empty liquor bottles to the stewardess. She accepted them with an understanding smile.

As we began to fly over Saudi Arabia, the two beautiful young ladies from across the aisle arose, each carrying a small traveling case. They gave us disarming smiles as they entered the aisle and made their way toward the back of the first-class section.

A few minutes later they returned, heavily veiled and covered from head to toe by a black robe called an *abeyya*. The black veil, known as a *gutwah,* covering their faces was so thick that their features were no longer discernible.

The transformation of these beautiful, elegantly dressed women into nondescript, black-veiled, black-robed figures was startling. It was as though a colorful butterfly had returned to its cocoon. The girls now appeared silent and reserved.

I could hardly believe my eyes. It seemed that we were passing through the looking glass into the cocoon of history. We were flying backward through time into the shrouds of the past. All that remained was the lingering scent of the present.

A few minutes later, the man accompanying the women followed the same routine. He exchanged his English tweeds for a white *thobe,* which is a long shirtlike garment made of cotton, the Saudi national dress for men. The collar of his thobe was decorated with braid. Over his thobe he wore a beige robe called a *bisht.* It was edged with a band of gold embroidery.

"The gold trim," explained Bill in a low voice, "indicates royalty or high office. He's a big gun for sure."

We watched in fascination as the man across the aisle prepared his headdress. First, he put an embroidered skull cap, or *kaffiya,* on his head. Then he folded a square piece of red-checkered cloth into a triangle and draped it over his skullcap so that the base of the triangle was in front. This triangle of red-checkered cloth, known as the *ghutra,* was then anchored into place by a ring which is called an *agal.*

"The color of the ghutra is usually a checkered red or orange and white in this area of Saudi Arabia, but in Mecca or Medina it is white," explained Bill. "The agal sitting on top of his head looks like two black coils, but it is actually one ring bent into a figure eight."

Spellbound, I watched the Saudi arrange and maneuver his ghutra and agal into place without the use of a mirror.

"The ghutra can come in handy on many occasions, as you can imagine," confided Bill. "It sometimes serves as a prayer rug in an emergency or as a towel in a pinch, and always as protection against the sun."

"Fasten your seatbelts, please. We are making our approach to Riyadh," announced the attendant, first in Arabic and then in English.

Excited, I looked out the window and was surprised to see a broad sprawl of electric lights. At night, it looked no different from Milwaukee. In a way I was disappointed. I was hoping for tents, campfires, and camels.

We soon landed and then taxied to an open area near the terminal, where a movable stairway was pushed up to the door of the plane. Bill and I watched as a long black Mercedes limousine drove up right next to the plane. The man in the gold-trimmed mantle and the two young ladies with him, covered in black, entered the car and were swiftly whisked away.

"Damn royals," muttered Bill, as we made our way to the terminal. "They don't even have to go through customs."

Inside, the airport was a mob scene. The new arrivals were brought into the customs area, which was separated from the rest of the airport by a glass partition. A guard in a khaki uniform stood at the only door to make sure that no one passed through until the baggage had been inspected. On the other side of the partition, hundreds of friends and relatives stood shouting to the new arrivals and waving messages written in Arabic and English. Everyone was pushing to get as close to the glass partition as possible. The noise was deafening. The airport was dimly lit and the high green walls cast an eerie light on the sea of expectant faces.

It took almost an hour to get my passport and visa inspected and stamped. There was no air conditioning, and the customs area soon grew swelteringly hot. When the baggage arrived, there was the usual mad scramble. I finally found my luggage and opened it for an inspector, who examined it very carefully, while warning me about the penalties for possession of drugs, alcohol, or pork. When he found my shaving lotion, he scrutinized it carefully before deciding that it would not make a very palatable drink. Scanning my cassettes, which consisted entirely of classical music, he chose one at random and put it aside. It was Mussorgsky's *Pictures at an Exhibition.* I protested vigorously, but the inspector spoke no English and could not explain. Maybe he thought the cassette contained Russian propaganda, but then why didn't he confiscate the Tchaikovsky as well? There was no logic to it. I asked for a receipt. He gave me a blank look. I decided to let it pass.

When the inspection was finished, I shook hands with Bill and made arrangements to meet him at his hotel later in the week. Then I passed through the guarded door and joined the throng on the other side of the glass partition. The crowd was composed entirely of men, most of whom were Saudi Arabians dressed in their thobes, many of which were soiled. Little Yemenis were carrying mountains of luggage on their backs, and the few Americans or Englishmen in the crowd stood out noticeably.

On a bench in a corner of the room were four little girls, sitting in a row, cross-legged with their feet tucked under them. Their faces and bodies were covered completely in black. They were absolutely immobile and reminded me of black pawns on a chessboard. Their father sat motionless beside them.

Soon a tall Saudi approached me. He was dressed in a sparkling white thobe and headdress. "Dr. Gray?" he inquired. "My name is Mashur. I'm from the hospital. Please wait here until I find the others, and then I'll take you to your hotel." He disappeared into the crowd.

I didn't know who the "others" were, but I stacked my luggage against a wall and sat down to wait. The crowds had thinned out somewhat. In one corner, a man was asleep with his belongings stuffed into a half-broken suitcase, tied with a rope. A veiled woman covered in black squatted next to him, holding a sleeping child in her arms.

Suddenly, a handsome, swashbuckling young Saudi strode by, beautifully attired in a white thobe, which was covered by a beige robe lined with gold. His headdress was white and he wore it at a rakish angle by throwing one corner of it back over the top of his head. Instead of the usual flip-flops or sandals, he wore glistening brown shoes. He was obviously a royal out on the town or more likely arriving to greet a friend.

Mashur returned with three men in tow. They introduced themselves: one was an administrator from California; the second a biomedical engineer from London; and the third a security officer from Washington. They had arrived on the same plane, in the tourist section. A Yemeni piled our luggage into Mashur's Toyota station wagon and we were on our way.

As we drove along, Mashur announced that the hospital was experiencing a "critical housing shortage," and that as a result we would all be placed in a "luxury hotel" for the time being. Our luxury hotel proved to be the Al Yamama, a shabby, brokendown hotel that had seen better days. The lobby contained some threadbare oriental carpets and some massive but faded, badly worn chairs. Over in the corner of the meagerly lit lobby, the television was featuring an Egyptian orchestra, which seemed to be playing repetitiously and out of tune. I learned later that "Al Yamama" means "turtle dove," but how the name applied to our hotel remained a mystery.

Mashur began to address the room clerk in Arabic, and their conversation soon blossomed into a loud argument. Apparently, the hotel was also experiencing a shortage of rooms. However, after a monumental debate, Mashur prevailed, and we were eventually led by the surly clerk to our accommodations. Mine proved to be a hot, dirty, musty room. I turned on both of the small lamps on either side of my narrow bed. They dimly revealed high green walls with badly cracked plaster. There was one window, however, overlooking an area with a few trees—a definite plus. The bathroom was large, but the faucets leaked and there was a uriniferous odor, indicating defective plumbing. "Well," I told myself hopefully, "it's only temporary." Somehow, I did not feel encouraged.

I took the rickety elevator three stories down to the lobby to join my new acquaintances. It was past midnight. We tried to get some coffee, but the recalcitrant room clerk shook his head sadly, pointing to his watch, indicating that it was too late. We sat down and chatted for a while. Their rooms were apparently as bad as mine. None of us really knew what to expect in the next two years. As we talked, I felt a kinship, a certain bond, developing between us, just as the early immigrants to America must have felt when they came over together to a new and different world. We were all in this together for better or for worse.

Before returning to my room, I asked the room clerk in sign language whether he could provide me with something to drink. Finally, he disappeared behind the desk and returned several minutes later with a green bottle under his arm. I took the bottle back to my room. It was Sohat water! Remembering the stewardess on the plane, I wrapped the bottle in a ragged towel and poured some water into a glass.

"Welcome to Saudi Arabia," I said, saluting myself in the mirror. I took a long drink, then undressed quickly and flung myself upon the narrow bed. Within seconds, I was sound asleep.

◇ 2 ◇

THE BLEEDING PRINCE—
THE KING COMES TO VISIT

THE NEXT MORNING at 4:30 A.M. I was awakened by a loud wailing sound outside my window. Was somebody being strangled? I dragged myself to the window and looked out, just as dawn was breaking over the city of Riyadh. I quickly identified the source of the wailing: it was emanating from a tall minaret about three hundred yards to my right.

"*La ilah illa'llah Muhammadun rasulu'llah* [There is no god but God and Mohammed is the Messenger of God]."

This was my first experience with the muezzin, the Moslem caller to prayer—part of a ritual performed five times daily, at dawn, noon, mid-afternoon, sunset, and in the evening one-and-a-half hours after sunset. I had read about it but I had never expected it to be as loud and penetrating as this well-amplified screech. How can anybody possibly sleep through this? I wondered to myself. Later, this call to prayer would become such an inexorable part of my daily life that I would be awakened only by its absence.

At 6:30 A.M. I staggered out of bed, dressed in my lightest summer suit, and then went downstairs, where I joined my companions from the evening before. Breakfast was served at a long table covered by a dirty tablecloth, flies, and bread crumbs. It consisted of tea or coffee, canned fruit juice, rolls, and butter which had turned rancid. Among our group was an English anesthesiologist named Tom, who had been in Riyadh for about a week and therefore qualified as an "expert" on Saudi Arabia. Tom was friendly and helpful in the face of our naïve questions.

"For God's sake," he told me, "take off your coat and tie and go native. You're in Saudi Arabia, my friend, not bloody Boston."

"How hot will it get today?" I asked as I loosened my tie.

"Only about 120 in the shade," he said. "In Saudi Arabia, that is considered springtime. Be sure to drink plenty of water so that you don't get dehydrated."

Following breakfast, we congregated at 7:30 in the lobby of the hotel, where we awaited the bus which was to transport us to the hospital. Presently, a Toyota bus arrived, bearing the inscription "King Faisal Specialist Hospital and Research Center" in both English and Arabic. Since the bus was designed to carry Japanese, it was extremely small, and we squeezed our way into the seats by tucking our knees up against our chests, laughing all the while at our rather foolish predicament. The mood on the bus was garrulous and festive, like that of children embarking on a field trip.

As we squirmed to find a comfortable position, a woman at the front of the bus introduced herself as Laura Ball, and announced that she was in charge of our orientation program. Ignoring some rude remarks about the size of the bus, Laura outlined our agenda for the day, which consisted mostly of orientation lectures, and tours of the hospital facilities. As she spoke, the bus lurched into gear, and I quickly found myself distracted by the sights and sounds of Riyadh passing outside the window. We were driving down a wide, modern boulevard, with large fortresslike government buildings and new skyscrapers on one side of the street and mud huts, litter, and rubbish on the other. Swiveling my head from side to side, I perused the scenery with interest, absorbed by the contrast of the very new buildings and the very old rubble.

It was obvious that massive construction programs were sprouting everywhere. Huge cranes stood like giant black fingers pointing to the morning sky, and the whole city seemed to vibrate with the sound of jackhammers. Hundreds of swarthy Yemeni and Pakistani laborers were bustling about, wearing dirty ankle-length thobes and skull caps as they pushed wheelbarrows and swung pickaxes. Some were climbing ladders with loads of heavy bricks, and occasionally the wind would billow their skirts and cause them to totter. Despite this hazard, none of them seemed to fall or drop a brick. Laura explained that menial labor is against Saudi tradition. A Saudi will drive a truck, taxi, or ambulance, but will never load or unload. They do no cleaning, digging, or hauling because they consider this type of work degrading. Consequently about 70 percent of the work force in Saudi Arabia is imported, and approximately 1.5 million laborers are brought in from Yemen, Pakistan, Egypt, South Korea, and the Sudan.

Laura went on to say that there was no adequate housing for the workers. She pointed to a cluster of tents and shacks made from crates, tin cans, paper, and cardboard, without electricity or sanitation.

"The contractors," she continued, "import the laborers in gangs, and assign them jobs to be completed in a fixed period of time. They are not permitted to bring their wives. The workers stay for a few years, save what money they can, and return home. They don't live, they just exist."

Later, I would learn that the construction boom in Saudi Arabia was unlike anything elsewhere in the world. Although the Saudis had an ostensible Five Year Plan to spend $144 billion for development, the logistics lacked central coordination. As a result, a tremendous amount of repetition and waste occurred. A street that had been dirt for two hundred years would be paved one day by a Lebanese contractor, torn up the second day by a Korean company laying telephone lines, then repaved the third day by a German contractor. A different foreign contractor carried out each job independently, and there was little guidance or consultation from the Saudis. This careless waste is perhaps inevitable in a country that acquired its immense wealth almost overnight. Consequently there was a marked and obvious shortage of managerial skills.

Our bus passed a huge white satellite saucer standing guard over an old, dilapidated post-office building, where one could place a phone call to any country in the world. Here, beneath the mammoth telemetry saucer, used to bounce signals off the satellites, the Saudi scribes gathered to sit cross-legged on small carpets, as illiterate Saudis crouching in front of them dictated their letters. What a fantastic country of contrasts this was, scribes for the illiterate gathered in front of a communications satellite saucer!

We soon passed the nearly completed Intercontinental Hotel, on a magnificent boulevard named Sharah Mathar. Here again, squalor and opulence coexisted side by side. The rush to the cities from the desert had spawned shantytowns and overcrowding. Perched on a huge hill of sand, about a half mile from the Intercontinental Hotel, was another group of shacks surrounded by a herd of goats, tended by black-shrouded Bedouin women. Across the boulevard was a partially completed elegant villa.

"Look out!" someone yelled.

Out of nowhere a Mercedes was bearing down upon us, head on, at almost seventy miles an hour, on the wrong side of the road. Our calm bus driver swerved sharply out of his way, just avoiding a head-on collision. The driver was a young Saudi, perhaps fifteen years old. He smiled at us and waved gaily as he rushed past.

This was not an isolated experience. Laura told us that the death rate from auto accidents was staggering. There were no traffic lights and no police. Youngsters drove without licenses or driving tests. The automobile was just a toy like "bump-a-car" in Disneyland.

Grotesque, abandoned wrecks of cars were strewn on the side of the road. Trucks were overturned with all four wheels pointing to the sky. Many of the graceful, curved electric light poles bordering the broad avenue were snapped in half like match sticks. On subsequent morning trips, we played a macabre game of counting overturned trucks and broken electric light poles. Civilization had come too quickly.

We soon reached the outskirts of the city, and the desert loomed ahead. My first view of the King Faisal Specialist Hospital was awesome. Here in the windswept wilderness of the Arabian desert stood a majestic, twenty-first-century hospital in a tenth-century setting. This magnificent edifice, begun by King Faisal and now a monument to his memory, dominated a vast expanse of desert.

The patterned exterior walls of the hospital were constructed of small, carved blocks of honey-colored stone. They formed long undulating expanses, broken by sharp angles, making dramatic use of light and shadow.

In the early-morning sun, the building, bathed in a haze of golden sand, appeared luminescent, like a mirage, as it stood boldly silhouetted against an azure-blue sky.

We entered the main gate, manned by three security guards and a single uniformed officer carrying a gun. Laura told us that the gun was unloaded, and was there only "for appearance's sake." Just inside the gate was an elaborate fountain, the base of which was fashioned of colorful mosaic tiles. From the center rose a geyser of water that fell gracefully from one level to another. It had taken more than a year to complete and was spectacular at night when illuminated by a spectrum of ever-changing colors, according to Laura.

A long winding driveway led to the main entrance of the hospital. We drove past spacious grounds carpeted with vast beds of colorful flowers.

There were pink and white periwinkles from Madagascar, orange and yellow gazanias from South Africa, and laurel from India. In other areas could be seen crape myrtle, oleander, bougainvillea, and white jasmine. The lawns were vast, meticulously manicured and irrigated by elaborate sprinkler systems. It was a garden paradise blooming in the desert.

The bus stopped at the main entrance. Laura led us into an elegant and spacious reception area. The floors were heavily carpeted in red, and the walls were covered with the softest textured green suède, in sharp contrast to the normally spartan furnishings of an American hospital. On a wall near the entrance was an illuminated mosaic portrait of King Faisal made of lapis lazuli, a vivid blue gemstone. The deep-set eyes contained small sparkling diamonds. Laura explained that only portraits of the King and Crown Prince may be displayed.

A broad marble staircase rose to a gracious balcony, edged with wood and Plexiglass balustrades, which surrounded the entire reception area. After our disappointment with the accommodations at the Hotel Al Yamama my friends and I couldn't believe our eyes.

Following our guide, we were led on a quick tour of the hospital facilities, which began with the elaborate computer center and ended with the water-purification system, the sewage-treatment setup, and the hospital power plant. This last facility was deemed necessary because Riyadh experienced recurrent power failures, and an independent power plant furnished emergency power for the hospital's temperature and humidity control, and the life-support systems.

The hospital complex was really a city in itself—aptly named Hospital City by the administration. It maintained its own ambulances, a fire department, and a large security force. It also ran a TV station within the hospital, and a complex electronic communications network. We were told that hospital buses criss-crossed Riyadh, bringing its personnel to and from work, and making regularly scheduled shopping trips downtown and occasional sightseeing excursions. The Recreation Center showed weekly movies, organized bridge clubs, photography competitions, tennis tournaments, cooking classes, language courses, and theatrical productions.

While on this tour, I was impressed by the quality and sophistication of the hospital facilities, which were easily the best I had ever encountered. The equipment equaled or surpassed that of any single hospital in the United States, and included a nuclear accelerator for cancer treatment, a brain scanner, and a total body scanner so recently developed that it had not yet reached the hospital-rich city of Boston. The overall cost of the hospital exceeded $300 million.

To maintain the complicated equipment, the Saudis had hired a variety of specialized technicians, most of whom were American or English and had arrived within the past month. The medical staff, including the doctors and nurses, had been recruited from all over the world and would be the nucleus of an international medical community located in the middle of the Arabian desert. All of us had been brought here as a direct result of Saudi oil wealth, and it bordered on the miraculous to see the most advanced medical technology in the world assembled by a society which less than a generation ago consisted of primitive nomadic tribes.

It all seemed very strange!

In a well-appointed classroom on the third floor of the hospital our group sat at tables and listened to Laura Ball as she lectured on the background of Saudi Arabian culture. Naturally, much of her lecture focused on Islam and the dominant role that the Moslem religion had played in shaping the values of present-day Saudi Arabia.

Islam is the world's youngest universal faith and the second largest. There are 750 million Moslems compared to 990 million Christians. The muezzin's ancient call to prayer can be heard far beyond the confines of the Middle East. It reaches into Africa, Southeast Asia, Malaysia, Indonesia, and beyond. There are fifty million Moslems in the USSR alone, counting the many who live in Mongolia.

The founder of Islam, known simply as Mohammed, was born in Mecca in A.D. 570. He was left an orphan while still a child. During his youth, he managed the caravans of a rich widow, fifteen years his senior, whom he married when he was twenty-five. Mohammed had no other wives until her death, following which he had nine wives and a number of concubines.

Mohammed remained a successful merchant until the age of forty, when he became troubled by the social inequalities and idolatrous religious practices of his people. Mecca, at the time, was a thriving trading and pilgrimage center. It owed its wealth to the Zamzam well, whose waters, according to legend, gushed forth miraculously to save Ishmael and his mother, Hagar, from death when they were lost in the desert. Abraham was said to have laid the foundation nearby for the Kaaba, a cubelike structure, to commemorate the site. Ishmael, the son of Abraham, is considered the ancestor of the Arab people. The Kaaba became the religious center and pilgrims came to drink from the Zamzam well, contributing to Mecca's prosperity.

In A.D. 610, when he was forty, Mohammed began a life of contemplation and seclusion. According to tradition, he was called by God to preach a stern, monotheistic, and egalitarian religion based in part on the teachings of Judaism and Christianity. He became a street preacher in Mecca. His message was clear and simple: "There is only one God, Allah, who is the creator, all powerful, ever-living. Mohammed is his prophet. There is a judgment day. Splendid rewards in Paradise await those who obey His commands. Terrible punishment in Hell is the lot of the unfaithful."

Mohammed's teachings were viewed as highly disruptive by the leaders in Mecca, who felt threatened by his appeal to the poorer element of their society and by his challenge to their strict system of caste and primogeniture.

Mohammed and his small band of followers were forced in 622 to flee from Mecca. They migrated to Medina at the invitation of a Jewish tribe in that city. This migration to Medina is known in history as the Hegira and marks the beginning of the Islamic calendar.

In Medina, Mohammed quickly gained a following for his new religion, which he called Islam, from the Arabic meaning "submission to the will of God." To support his followers, he sanctioned the raiding and plundering of caravans, which he justified on the basis that the caravan owners were not true believers. As his army grew in strength, he gained a virtual stranglehold over the economic life of Mecca. After eight years of conflict, the Meccans in 630 submitted to Islamic rule and to Mohammed. His followers were permitted to worship in the Kaaba, where it was said people had worshiped since the time of Ishmael and Abraham. Mecca thus became the religious center of Islam, and the Kaaba became Islam's holiest shrine, a symbol of God.

Once Mecca was in his control, Mohammed turned on the other Arabian tribes, and one by one they decided to embrace Islam rather than face the specter of annihilation by Mohammed's zealous army. When Mohammed died in 632, he had united almost the entire central and southern portions of the Arabian Peninsula into his Islamic Empire.

Following Mohammed's death, Abu Bakr, Mohammed's father-in-law, whom he had chosen as his successor, emerged as the most powerful leader of the Islamic movement, and he continued to emulate Mohammed's martial ways. Realizing that it would be difficult to subdue the fanatically independent tribes of the Arabian desert, Abu Bakr shrewdly began a series of invasions to the north, while threatening severe sanctions against any tribes that did not join the Islamic alliance. Offered the riches of conquest or the threat of extinction, the tribes naturally joined the forces of Islam. Thus, Islam was actually founded on conquests, which enabled Abu Bakr to forge alliances that would have been otherwise impossible.

Within twenty years, the Islamic armies defeated the Byzantine and Persian armies, and gained control over a vast area from Tripoli in North Africa to the eastern limits of Persia.

As the Islamic forces conquered Baghdad, Damascus, and Cairo, the Arabian Peninsula became something of a forgotten area in the Islamic empire. Although it originated in the tribal environment of Arabia, Islam was truly more suitable as an urban institution. The settled permanence of the city enabled Islamic values to take root and flourish. Thus, the government of the Islamic empire moved to Damascus and other major cities, while the Arabian Peninsula lapsed into tribal strife.

For the next thousand years, Arabia remained outside the purview of world events. With harsh deserts, no significant resources, and no major cities, Arabia was regularly bypassed by the conquering empires of the world. In the eighteenth century, both the Ottoman Empire and the British Empire claimed nominal sovereignty over peripheral parts of Arabia, but in practice this colonization was limited to the small enclaves near the coastal cities, and was never extended over the mobile tribes of the interior.

The development of Saudi Arabia from the middle of the eighteenth century, however, is intimately connected with a movement inspired by a religious zealot named Mohammed Ibn Abdul Wahab, who preached a puritanical and orthodox form of Islam which became known as Wahabism. About 1750, Wahab won the support of an emir named Mohammed Ibn Saud, who ruled a small town near Riyadh named Dariya, in central Arabia. The combination of Saud's political power and Wahab's religious fervor attracted a large and fanatical Bedouin following in support of the Wahabi movement. By Moslem precept, soldiers who fell in holy battle were promised immediate entry into Paradise. It is said that each Wahabi soldier was given a written order from his leader to the keeper of the gates of heaven to let him in. With Saud as an ally, the Wahabis began a series of conquests which soon put them in control of large portions of the Arabian Peninsula, including Riyadh (in 1764) and the holy cities of Mecca and Medina.

The Ottoman Empire felt threatened by the Saudi expansion and sent the Ottoman Viceroy of Egypt, Mohammed Ali, to crush the Saudi-Wahabi empire. The Turkish armies recaptured Mecca and Medina in 1812, and destroyed Dariya in 1818. Finally, they occupied the Nejd, the central heartland of the country, which included Riyadh.

However, within six years, the Saud family once again gained temporary control over Riyadh and the Nejd, but the area became an arena for violent warfare among the powerful, competitive tribes, and the Saud family was deposed in 1891.

It remained for the legendary Prince Abdul-Aziz Al Saud to recapture the city of Riyadh in 1902 and to extend his domination over the Arabian Peninsula. The Turks were finally driven out in 1905, and Abdul-Aziz spent the next twenty-five years unifying the country into the largest peaceful kingdom established in Arabia in the last thousand years.

Much of the unique character of Saudi Arabia stems from the influence of Wahabism upon the Saudis. They fought to rule the desert and to crusade for this austere fundamentalist sect of the Moslem world: the Wahabis. Ibn Saud, like his forefathers, remained loyal to Wahabism, and the green standard which his armies followed was its symbol.

The House of Saud does not permit public smoking, drinking alcohol, or dressing in silken robes. It opposes ostentation and the show of wealth. It does not permit the display of human figures or the worship of saints, shrines, or idols. In accordance with the Koran, it permits four wives and allows men instant divorce. Women are kept veiled, completely covered, and secluded. Mixed dancing, in the Western sense, is unthinkable. Outside their own family circles, men never mention their wives, although they may have several.

Recently, to protect old values, hotel pools have been drained to prevent mixed bathing. Dolls have been banished from toy stores as idolatrous. Saudi women are completely segregated from men in all aspects of life. In short, Wahabism preaches a return to the way of life and the practice of Islam as they existed during the days of the prophet Mohammed, a thousand years ago; and Wahabism is flourishing in Saudi Arabia.

"Dr. Gray?"

"Yes?" Slowly I emerged from the deserts of Arabia and the fascinating history and joined the twentieth century. I looked up into the concerned face of a young nurse, dressed in a white trousered hospital uniform.

"Dr. Gray, I'm sorry to disturb you, but Dr. Compton would like to speak with you immediately. It's an emergency, I'm afraid."

Reluctantly, I left the classroom and followed the nurse through an intricate maze of hallways. Soon I was walking through the door of an office belonging to Dr. Hugh Compton, the Director of Medical Affairs. He was sitting behind a beautiful hand-carved mahogany desk, which was cluttered with papers and hospital records. A handsome and well-dressed man in his early fifties, Compton looked harried. He rose to greet me.

"Welcome to the hospital," he said, shaking my hand and then motioning for me to take a seat. "I'm sorry to disturb you, but we have a serious problem here and we need your help. Have you ever heard of Prince Yusef Al Saud?"

"Not in the past hour," I replied dryly. "I only arrived this morning."

"He's one of the most powerful men in the kingdom," said Dr. Compton, ignoring my remark. "He is the first cousin of King Khalid, and they are very close companions. They go falcon hunting together, I believe. In any case, Prince Yusef was admitted early this morning with massive bleeding from the gastrointestinal tract."

Reading from his papers, Dr. Compton filled me in on the details. The prince was sixty years old, had diabetes and high blood pressure. The source of the bleeding had not yet been established, and the surgeons considered him a poor surgical risk.

"This is in your area of special interest," he said with a look of sympathy, "and I would like to put you in charge of the prince. You'll be directly responsible for his care."

My inclination was to say, "Aren't you rushing things? I have traveled halfway around the world and just arrived. I don't know the hospital, the language, the culture, or the people. It's all very strange to me." But I said nothing.

Dr. Compton handed me the report and then looked at me rather intensely.

"This case is both medical and political," he said. "As you know, this hospital is just getting started. What you don't know is that the King has some reservations about us, and therefore this is a test case. Ordinarily, the prince would have been flown to London immediately on the King's private plane, and this is still being considered by the royal family.

"We have to convince the King that this hospital will work. If the prince recovers, then it will put us in good stead. If not, we will lose the King's support and maybe the hospital."

Then, to my surprise, he asked gently, "By the way, have you unpacked?"

"Not yet."

"Good. Don't. If the prince doesn't recover, you will be asked to leave the country. It is the custom here."

I looked at him in disbelief. He was dead serious. "King Khalid will probably be coming here this evening to visit the prince," said Dr. Compton, as we stood up. "Keep me informed. And if you need anything— *anything*—just let me know. Good luck, Seymour."

He opened the door to the adjoining office and introduced me to his secretary. Janet Powers was an attractive, slender woman with gray-streaked hair, brown eyes, and a ready smile. She wore an ankle-length beige dress with long sleeves and several gold chain necklaces.

"Marhaba [hello]," she greeted me, with a smile.

"Marhabtayn [the same to you]," I replied.

We were both practicing our Arabic vocabulary, which consisted of some thirty words and routine phrases taken from page four of the orientation manual. Not to be outdone, however, I added a dash of *"Kif halak?* [How are you?]" to which she promptly gave me the routine response, *"Alhamdu lillah* [Praise God]."

"Your Arabic is flawless," I said admiringly.

"Page four," she said, laughing, "plus three hours a week of Arabic at the Recreation Center." She went on to say that she had been Dr. Compton's secretary in California and had agreed to accompany him to Saudi

Arabia. She added that she was divorced and had a daughter, but was forbidden to bring her into the country.

Janet directed me to the nurses' desk on Ward B-2 and introduced me to an English nurse named Ann Johnson, who showed me the ward and explained some of the hospital procedures. The ward was composed of twenty-five single rooms, each of which was equipped with color television and a variety of electronic gadgets, including one that controlled the window drapes.

"Are there no double rooms here?" I asked. "The Saudis must value their privacy."

"Double rooms would be impossible in this hospital," Miss Johnson said. "Wait until you see the hordes of visitors, the servants bringing in food, and the families with their twenty-four hour-vigils. Prince Yusef has an adjoining room reserved for his family and friends.

"Here we are," she said, "Rooms B-210 and B-212."

In front of the door a very black man stood guard. The guard was of Ethiopian descent, short, and wore a huge, curved dagger at his belt. I was impressed by his fine facial features and imperious expression. He recognized Miss Johnson.

"Tabeeb Gray," she announced. He nodded and opened the door for us.

"That man stands guard out here day and night. He sleeps on the floor," she explained.

We entered the partly darkened room very quietly. The prince, wearing a white embroidered skull cap over his gray hair, was dozing. He looked old and tired. A servant in his fifties hovered nervously about the bed. A young man, immaculate in his white uniform, clean-shaven except for a small mustache, was picking up the bed linen. He looked Lebanese.

"Kamal," said Miss Johnson, "this is Dr. Gray. He will need you to interpret."

That is putting it mildly, I thought. In a situation like this, the medical history is often more important than the physical examination. The appropriate choice of words and vocal inflections is crucial in establishing a rapport with the patient. History taking is an art in itself. How reliable a medical story could I obtain with a Lebanese interpreter, speaking Arabic to a Saudi Arabian and translating it into English for an American newly arrived in a strange country?

To add to the problem, my first patient was a member of the Royal Cabinet, which had selected the present King.

"I really need your help, Kamal," I said, shaking his hand. "What country are you from?"

"Lebanon," he replied. "I am a NAT—Nurse Assistant Technician."

He was one of a group of young men and women who had come to Saudi Arabia during the Lebanese war.

"Let's awaken the prince gently, Kamal. We need a more detailed history of his illness."

Kamal touched the prince's shoulder. He awakened immediately, looked first at his servant, who reassured him, and then gazed at us.

"*Moya* [water]," he said to the servant, who brought him a glass of water and supported him while he sipped the water slowly through a straw. He's probably dehydrated, I thought.

The prince was heavy-set, a distinguished-looking man in his early sixties, well over six feet tall. He had one of those prominent Arabic noses, full lips, and the usual sculptured, carefully trimmed black beard and mustache. His facial hair was speckled heavily with gray. His eyes were brown, and his skin, an olive hue, was pale, almost white, reflecting his recent loss of blood.

It was obvious that my patient was acutely ill. Beads of perspiration stood out on his forehead. His features were pinched and he breathed rapidly with his mouth open.

As I watched silently, Kamal spoke to the prince in rapid-fire Arabic, explaining who I was and what I wanted. Then we began the questioning.

With Kamal translating, I soon elicited enough information from the prince to suspect that he was suffering from a bleeding ulcer. I also learned that the prince was taking Novalgin, a drug that contains aspirin and which is known to exacerbate ulcers. Focusing on the likelihood of an ulcer, I began to question the prince about his eating habits. The answer surprised me.

"He only eats at night, of course," said Kamal. "It is Ramadan, and he has been fasting."

I remembered reading about the holy month of Ramadan during which no food or water can be taken from dawn until sunset.

"They fire a cannon to mark the beginning and the end of the fasting period each day, don't they?" I asked.

"Yes, that is right. The prince is a very religious man. He has had no food or water during the day, and then takes the Novalgin at night to relieve the pain in his stomach."

"How long has he been fasting?"

"Three weeks. There is one more week left."

"Is there any way he can be allowed to eat during the day?"

"Yes," said Kamal. "If he is ill, he can eat during the Ramadan period, and fast at a later time."

"Explain to the prince, Kamal, that I suspect that he has either an ulcer or gastritis. We will take some x-rays of the stomach to be sure. People with ulcers should eat frequently. Fasting all day during Ramadan and then taking Novalgin at night most probably produced the bleeding. Tell the prince that he will get well on treatment."

Kamal then proceeded to convey this message at considerable length and with sweeping gestures. When he had finished, the prince smiled weakly. *"Inshallah,"* he said simply, meaning "God willing."

I was soon to learn that *inshallah* is probably the most important single word in the Arabic language. It represents the absolute fatalism of the Arab mentality: all has been predetermined by Allah—all is in the hands of Allah. They don't say it automatically. They believe it. They live by it. It rules their lives.

"Please tell the prince we are scheduling an x-ray examination of his stomach and some blood tests within the hour."

"When do I get some medicine?" asked the prince. "Will I get well on needles in my arms and blood tests?"

"Inshallah," I replied with a smile. "For the present the blood transfusions are the best medicine."

After Kamal had interpreted and elaborated on the subject, I shook his hand and thanked him profusely for his help.

"It is my pleasure, Tabeeb Gray," he said with a smile, using the Arabic word for doctor.

Leaving the room, I wandered about the hospital until I found the X-ray Department and introduced myself to the two radiologists, one American and the other English. They showed me around their sophisticated new department with pride. It was the most advanced radiology unit that I had ever seen. After explaining the prince's problem and the purpose of the x-ray examination, I left.

Walking down the hallway, I glanced at my watch. It was eleven o'clock and the x-rays were scheduled for one-thirty. Abruptly, I decided to return to the lecture hall and learn more about Saudi Arabia.

In the morning, I had listened for fun. Now, after the brief interlude with the prince, I was going to listen as if lives depended on it. In a very real way, I now understood, they did.

The orientation class was still in session. A professor from the University of Riyadh, an Egyptian, was now discussing the Koran and the Sharia, the law of the land.

Koran is the Arabic word for "recitation." Mohammed's recitations, uttered while the prophet was in an inspired state, were regarded as direct revelations from God. They were compiled, after his death, into the Koran, the sacred book of Islam. The Koran forms the core of almost all phases of Moslem life. It contains detailed instructions on how man must submit to his Maker and vivid, terrifying descriptions of the fate awaiting those who do not submit to God's will.

The law of the land is the Sharia, which means "the path to follow." It is based on the Koran and embraces a code of Islamic ethics, religious duties, and morality. Justice is administered by a council of religious scholars (the Ulema) and by religious courts whose judges are appointed by the Ulema. In Saudi Arabia the chief judge of the Ulema is a Wahabi, the direct descendant of the founder of Wahabism, emphasizing again the influence of this religious sect upon the country.

As might be expected, the Sharia laws, dating back more than a thousand years, are harsh. Murder and rape are punishable by beheading, and theft by amputation of the right hand or by flogging in public. Adultery demands the death penalty for the woman, usually by stoning, but four witnesses must testify to seeing the illicit act.

"Capital punishment in Saudi Arabia is a deterrent to crime," said the professor. "Murder and rape are rare among the Saudis. The streets here are safe and there is very little thievery. Most of the crimes in this country are committed by outsiders. But the main deterrent is the religion, particularly Wahabism."

Most Saudi Arabians are Sunni Moslems, who observe the puritanical orthodox Wahabi traditions. Sunni, in Arabic, actually means "tradition." A small Shiite Moslem minority of about 100,000 live in the Eastern Province, where the oil comes from. The Shiites make up the majority in Iran, and large numbers live in Iraq, Kuwait, and Bahrain. They are also found in Egypt, Morocco and the East Asian countries.

The five pillars of faith for all Moslems are (1) confession of faith: "There is no god but God and Mohammed is the Messenger of God"; (2) prayers five times daily while facing Mecca; (3) fasting during the daylight hours of the holy month of Ramadan, a 29- to 30-day month in Islam's lunar calendar; (4) giving to charity; and (5) making the *hajj* or pilgrimage to Mecca.

The mention of Ramadan reminded me of my patient, and how fortunate it was that this subject had come up during my interview with the prince.

Finally, the professor spent a few minutes discussing the government structure. He was very brief. The government is a benign feudal monarchy without a constitution, political parties, or elections. Access to the King, however, is the right of every citizen: he may present petitions, grievances, or pleas for help. This procedure is called the *majlis* (Arabic for "sitting" or "council"), held five days a week. It is available to poor and rich alike and helps establish a rapport between the individual and his government.

We adjourned at twelve-thirty. I thanked the professor and, before leaving, explained to Laura my abrupt departure earlier that morning. She was very understanding.

After "lunch," which consisted of coffee and crackers (the kitchen was not yet open), I went back to the Radiology Department to check up on the prince's x-rays. The barium meal revealed the presence of a definite ulcer in the stomach wall, approximately one-fourth inch in diameter. The diagnosis was now confirmed.

Returning to the prince's room, I found three of his sons gathered about his bed. They had been in the adjoining room since the night before and appeared disheveled and exhausted. Kamal introduced them. Salim was the oldest, about forty, approximately six feet tall and rather stocky. He had the classical neatly clipped beard and mustache and wore a cream-colored mantle lined with gold, indicating his royal heritage.

In all, the prince had twenty-five sons, most of them by different wives. Although they were half brothers, the three sons got along quite well. Unlike their father, all three were fluent in English.

"Now please tell me, how is our father?" Salim served as spokesman for the group. "The family is extremely concerned. We have been awake most of the night."

He went on to say that King Khalid had called several times and was also very anxious about Prince Yusef. He would be coming to see him shortly.

I told them that an ulcer was the probable cause of the bleeding and that there was a reasonable possibility that it would heal without surgery, but that we could not be certain. They listened attentively.

"Meanwhile, we will give your father two more blood transfusions and start treatment with an ulcer diet and medication."

Salim smiled, slowly nodding his head.

Turning to the prince, I explained the x-ray findings, and that the medicine he had taken while fasting during Ramadan probably had caused the bleeding.

"Fasting itself is bad for an ulcer," I remarked. "We must start treatment immediately."

At the mention of treatment, the prince smiled broadly and said, "Kweyyis [good, fine, okay]."

This was the beginning of a dialogue between us which was to continue throughout the hospitalization. The word kweyyis happened to be in my very limited vocabulary.

"Kweyyis—good?" I asked, shaking his hand.

"Goood," he replied, beaming, and adding, of course, "Inshallah."

From then on, whenever I inquired after his health in Arabic, he invariably replied, "Goood" in English whether he felt good or not, always covering himself with "inshallah" just to play it safe, or "Alhamdu lillah [Praise God]."

Since an ulcer diet was an important part of the treatment, the next step was to devise a diet the prince would be willing to follow. I consulted with the dietician and recommended rice, yogurt, and camel's or goat's milk to start with. These were among the prince's favorite foods. He seemed content providing his servant prepared the food and fed him spoonful by spoonful. He was not at all abashed by being fed like a child. I watched this nursery scene for a few minutes and then left.

As soon as I entered the adjoining room, the former slave guarding the prince's room brought some cardamom coffee he had prepared. I sat down with a sigh of relief, and explained to the prince's sons that this was my first day in Saudi Arabia and that I was very pleased with the progress we had made so far. They too appeared somewhat more relaxed and asked me where I lived in the United States. They offered to help me in any way possible, and gave me their phone numbers, for which I expressed my gratitude.

"Do you like horse races?" Nasser asked eagerly, with his thick accent. He was the youngest of the three sons.

"Well, my experience is limited, but I like watching the Kentucky Derby on television. Oh, and a friend of mine had a horse which almost won it a few years ago. I also went to some magnificent races in Argentina and Chile."

"That is good." Nasser was in charge of his father's racing stables. "We have some champion Arabian horses and racing camels."

"I didn't know that camels race," I remarked.

They all laughed. Nasser promised to take me to a camel race soon.

After we had drunk one or two cups of coffee, served in very small porcelain cups without handles, we were offered tea in delicate glass cups. It was excellent and quite sweet. After waiting a few minutes ("Haste comes from the devil"—an Arab proverb), I thanked them and left.

It was late in the afternoon. I thought it would be advisable to give Dr. Compton an update on the prince's condition. He seemed relieved and asked me to dictate a brief report.

"Give it to Janet, and we'll have it translated into Arabic and sent over to the royal palace," he said. "They will want a daily medical bulletin on the prince's condition."

While I was dictating the report to Janet, Dr. Compton came into the room. "The King and Crown Prince are coming to visit Prince Yusef at six P.M. We'll greet them at the front door. I want you to brief the King on the patient's condition."

"I don't have a white coat," I protested. "I haven't even been in the country twenty-four hours, and I am absolutely exhausted."

"Never mind," he said. "Just stick your stethoscope in your coat pocket. I'll have someone bring you a fresh cup of coffee."

After dictating the rest of the report, I joined Dr. Compton, and we walked down the stairs to the front entrance of the hospital. Soon we saw the royal procession approaching. The first car was an open American jeep carrying soldiers of the Saudi Arabian National Guard. The soldiers wore khaki uniforms and brilliant red berets. They sat on each side of the jeep, facing each other, and carried submachine guns.

The second car in the procession was a tan Pontiac, and the third car was a specially designed black Cadillac, which was not as long or pretentious as the Cadillacs used by U.S. government officials. This was in deference to Moslem culture, which frowns severely on ostentation or public display of wealth. Behind the Cadillac at the end of the procession was another jeep, this one carrying a mounted machine gun manned by a gunner with his finger on the trigger in a show of readiness.

As the procession drew to a halt in front of the hospital, a middle-aged military attaché came out of the Pontiac and then opened the front door of the Cadillac to assist the King. His Royal Highness, King Khalid, had been sitting in the front seat next to the driver. From the rear door, Crown Prince Fahd emerged and quickly joined his older brother Khalid. The two of them approached us as we stood in a group in front of the hospital.

One of the hospital administrators stepped forward and greeted their royal highnesses in Arabic, and then introduced us. We shook hands and smiled. The King and Crown Prince shook hands all around, but did not return the smiles.

King Khalid and Crown Prince Fahd were surprisingly large men, both well over six feet tall. They were dressed identically, wearing beige robes trimmed in gold, which were worn over long light-colored thobes with mandarin-style collars. Their heads were covered by red-checkered ghutras topped with black coils, the standard headdress in Saudi Arabia. The gold trim on their robes was the same as that worn by all princes and high government dignitaries. Except for a slightly better quality in the cloth, there was nothing to distinguish the King or the Crown Prince from thousands of other Saudi citizens.

As we passed through the elegant reception hall and walked into the elevator, I could see no security coverage whatsoever. I stood in the elevator within inches of the two men who controlled the economic destiny of the Western world.

While the U.S. and other countries were on the brink of disaster because of the lack of oil, these two men were sitting on an ocean of oil, estimated at 300 billion barrels, the world's greatest single petroleum reserve. And here they were, certainly two of the richest men on earth, unprotected, in an elevator, with a total stranger who had been in Saudi Arabia less than twenty-four hours, and who could have easily concealed a small weapon in his coat pocket.

The King, who had recently had an operation, appeared to be frail and unsteady on his feet. His long, melancholy face was entirely devoid of expression or emotion. He seemed to look through you rather than at you. He was said to be a simple man, unread, unschooled, and unsophisticated. He was a strict adherent to the orthodox and austere fundamentalist sect of Islam and had little sympathy for "new world" ideas or "modern" thinking.

In contrast to Khalid, Crown Prince Fahd, the King's half brother, appeared to be robust, full of energy, warmth, and good humor. He was rather portly, and gave the impression of constraint and dignity. However, something in his demeanor suggested a fun-loving disposition that, though temporarily restrained, was impossible to suppress. His eyes were dark brown, keen, and penetrating, darting from side to side while he held his head motionless. His great head, curved Semitic nose, and inquisitive, piercing eyes, constantly in motion, reminded me of a huge falcon. There was a thin smile on his face as though he were about to burst into a hearty laugh. I had the gut feeling that the Prince would be very popular at a social gathering, while the King would prefer to sit in a corner storytelling with his cronies.

The relationship between the King and the Crown Prince was curious, and the fact that they were on good terms was explainable only by the dynamics of the Saudi royal family. When King Faisal was assassinated in 1975, the leading men in the House of Saud joined in a secret family meeting to select the next King. Unlike Western primogeniture systems, the throne of Saudi Arabia is not automatically awarded to the oldest living son. Rather, in keeping with Bedouin tribal traditions, responsible members of the royal family choose the King from among themselves with the sanction of the Ulema. In the case of Khalid, he was selected to become King despite the fact that he had two older brothers. At the same time, Fahd was appointed Crown Prince, which made him the heir apparent.*

Between the two of them, Khalid and Fahd had been very effective successors to King Faisal. Khalid, the conservative Bedouin, was extraordinarily popular with the tribal leaders, and faith in his leadership often kept the more conservative elements of Saudi society from openly opposing the more progressive government initiatives. Fahd, on the other hand, was very modern and Western in his orientation, and often supported changes in Saudi society, ranging from greater industrialization to liberalization of social codes and more freedom for women. Because of the King's frail health, Fahd handled most of the day-to-day affairs of government, and was considered the actual "leader" of Saudi Arabia. However, Khalid's personal popularity was often crucial to the acceptance of Fahd's ambitious plans, and Khalid also influenced much of the substance of Fahd's decisions.

The differences between the two men extended into their personal lives. Khalid, the Bedouin, loved his falconry, and often joined his Bedouin followers on camping expeditions into the desert. Fahd, on the other hand, was urbane, sophisticated, and broadly educated in the culture of the Western world as well as in Islamic tradition. He jetted to Western Europe for his frequent vacations, where he was rumored to love many of the vices that were forbidden in Saudi Arabia. French newspapers had reported incidents of Fahd and his friends losing astronomical sums of money— $5 million or more during a single evening at the gambling casinos on the French Riviera. The previous year, King Faisal had given a mild but clear rebuke to Fahd during Ramadan, asking, "Where is our brother Fahd?" after the Crown Prince had gone to Europe during the holiest of Moslem holidays. This year, Fahd remained at home, a clear reminder of the power that the King and his conservative followers had in Saudi Arabia.

Now, as I accompanied the King and the Crown Prince to visit Prince Yusef, I found myself impressed by their certitude and quiet grace. They had what can only be called a regal bearing, a quality that is as palpable in

*Fahd became king upon Khalid's death in 1982.

person as it is elusive to define. The two princes seemed to float on the balls of their feet. While lifting their floor-length robes adroitly by one hand, holding their heads high and gazing straight ahead, they walked slowly and deliberately at a fixed pace. Above all, the two princes seemed to emanate the imperturbable timelessness that is a hallmark of Saudi culture.

As we walked down the hallway, several Saudis—relatives of hospital patients—ran up and touched their lips to the left shoulder or heart region of the robes of the King and Crown Prince as a sign of fealty to the royal dynasty. The royal party moved forward at the same pace, however, without acknowledging these demonstrations of loyalty.

When we arrived at Prince Yusef's hospital room, the ever-present guard with the curved dagger opened the door and ushered us inside. Prince Yusef looked pale and wan, but at the sight of the King he seemed to 'perk up. King Khalid walked over to the bedside and greeted the prince, then solemnly kissed him on the forehead. The Crown Prince followed suit, pressing his lips to both cheeks of the prince and then over his heart. When this ritual was completed, the two royal visitors sat down and began conversing with their cousin.

Kamal, who was present at this conversation, later told me that the three of them talked at length about the prince's physical condition, and about my diagnosis. Prince Yusef was amused that I had blamed the Ramadan fast for his ulcer problem. At that point, all three of them turned to look at me briefly, an action that was rather unnerving, in view of my ignorance of Arabic. After a short conversation with the prince, the royal party rose to leave.

In the adjoining room they shook hands warmly with Prince Yusef's sons. Their royal highnesses sat down in two very ample chairs and chatted with them for a few minutes. Then, addressing me directly for the first time, they inquired about the prince's condition.

While Kamal and Salim took turns as interpreters, I quickly outlined the medical situation. When I was finished, the King asked whether the prince should be flown to London for treatment at the Wellington Hospital, as was the custom. I replied that moving the prince might aggravate the bleeding, and that, in my opinion, the medical care and laboratory facilities now available in the hospital were equal to those available in London. Behind me, I could almost hear Dr. Compton smiling at my replies.

"What if surgery is necessary?" asked the Crown Prince through an interpreter.

"Surgery should be avoided if possible," I replied, "because of the patient's high blood pressure and heart condition. However, I have already consulted an English surgeon on the staff here, and I am confident that he is as capable as any surgical specialist in London."

"Do you need a consultant flown in from England or the United States? We can arrange this easily through our embassy."

"If you wish," I said. "I have had considerable experience in treating patients with similar problems, but if you want another opinion, I will be very glad to recommend someone."

"The King has a Boeing 747 equipped for any type of medical emergency, and the plane could be sent abroad to pick up any consultant you wish," explained Salim. "If necessary, we can fly the prince to London in this manner."

I assured them again that I did not think it necessary at the moment but that I would consider it if the prince's condition deteriorated. The King and Crown Prince talked quietly for a moment between themselves and then rose, signifying that they were ready to depart. The walk back was again in a slow, deliberate, measured gait and in silence. We conducted the royal party to the front of the hospital. There, they joined their military escort, and after a perfunctory goodbye, they entered the Cadillac and the entourage drove off.

"How serious is the prince's condition?" Dr. Compton asked as we walked back through the hospital.

"It's serious," I replied. "He should respond to treatment, but there is a ten percent mortality in this kind of patient."

"Are you sure we shouldn't send the prince to London?" asked Dr. Compton.

"London won't make any difference," I said. "The facilities here are excellent. He could die in London just as easily as here."

"I know," said Dr. Compton, "but if he dies in London, then the King will blame the London hospital. If he dies here . . ." Dr. Compton left the sentence hanging, unfinished. We walked to the elevators in silence.

"'I just hope we're doing the right thing," he said as he prepared to board the elevator.

"I hope so, too."

He gave me a wan smile. *"Inshallah,"* he said fervently. "You had better go home and get some rest. It's been a long day."

"I'll see you tomorrow, Hugh."

The elevator door closed, and I walked to the staff room, where I met and briefed the physician who would be on duty that night. I left orders for some blood tests for the prince, then called Janet and asked her to arrange transportation back to the hotel. It seemed that my bus had long since left the hospital.

Outside a blast of hot air greeted me, which seemed to soothe the tensions of the day. In the driveway, a hospital driver in a green Buick was inquiring about "Tabeeb Gray," and I gratefully fell into the back of his car. The driver was a Saudi who worked in the Transportation Department. He would be available to bring me back to the hospital during the night in the event of an emergency. Janet had arranged it. But I wondered how a message from the hospital would ever reach me: no phones in the hotel room, no beepers, and an irresponsible hotel clerk. The air conditioning and the hum of the engine lulled me and I dozed on the ride to the hotel.

Back at the Al Yamama my companions of this morning were finishing their dinner. The tablecloths were still dirty and the flies as stubborn as ever. The meal consisted of lamb and rice, which were tasteless, but the cold Sohat water went down like champagne, and the dates for dessert were delicious. Although I was exhausted, the camaraderie and good fellowship at the table revived my spirits.

After dinner, I informed the desk clerk that there might be an emergency phone call from the hospital. The clerk—an Egyptian—seemed more interested in his magazine.

"Would you write down my room number, please?" I asked.

"I remember," he said.

"Please write it down."

With clear annoyance, the clerk wrote the number; he also wrote it incorrectly.

"Here," I said, taking the pen and writing it down myself. "This is my room. If there is a phone call for me, please come and get me at this room."

"Not to worry," said the clerk, tapping his forehead. "I remember."

For the second night, I dragged myself upstairs to my room, closing the door behind me. The room was hot, humid, and dreary. The dull, peeling green paint was still ugly, but now it had the virtue of familiarity. I undressed, and before falling into a deep sleep, noticed my luggage. The bags were open, but still unpacked, reminding me of Dr. Compton's ominous remarks earlier today. They stared back at me as symbols of an intriguing yet uncertain journey.

My first day in Saudi Arabia had not been uneventful. I wondered what two years would bring.

◇ 3 ◇

A ROYAL BREAK IN TRADITION

MUCH TO MY SURPRISE, I slept through the morning call to prayer. Had I missed an urgent message from the hospital? No news was good news, I concluded, as I enjoyed a good soak in the tub.

After breakfast, featuring the usual rancid butter and aggressive flies, I took the seven-thirty bus to the hospital. My eyes stared blandly at the overturned trucks, smashed cars, and broken electric light poles lining the streets. Rubble and trash were now just part of the scene. I tried to ignore the ear-shattering, honking horns of the frustrated traffic.

The desert suddenly appeared, immaculate with quiet dignity as though disdainful of the sacrilege imposed upon it by civilization. The hospital, too, glistened pure and haughty in the morning sun. I walked directly to the prince's room. He looked pale and weak but was no longer perspiring. His pulse was one hundred, as before, but his blood count and blood pressure had risen somewhat, which was encouraging.

Kamal softly entered the room, clean-shaven and immaculate in his white uniform. I asked him to tell the prince that he was improving and did not need more blood for the present.

"*Kif halak* [How are you]? *Kweyyis* [Good, okay]?" I asked, shaking the prince's limp hand.

"Goood," he replied with a brave but condescending smile.

Salim had remained with his father all night. He looked unshaven and unkempt.

"How is my father?" he asked anxiously.

"Definitely better," I assured him. "All he needs now is rest and quiet. The medicine and diet should help his ulcer heal, but it will take time."

"The King telephoned this morning," he announced with a smile. "He talked with my father, and he asked for me to make sure I was here. The King believes in family discipline."

We shook hands, and I left, advising him to get some sleep.

After wandering about, I finally found Dr. Compton's office and dictated a brief medical report to Janet, who said she would have it translated into Arabic and sent to the palace within the hour. She gave me a list of departments to visit.

"The first thing you must do," she said, "is to go to Security, have your picture taken, and pick up your identification card and the pass for the outside gate."

"Ah, yes, I remember the guard with the gun at the gate."

"Everyone knows it's not loaded," she said, laughing. "You know, there are ninety security people here. Most of them are not in uniform, so that they can keep their identity secret."

I recalled my experience in the elevator last night when I saw no evidence of security although I stood within inches of the King.

The Security Department was a beehive of activity, registering and photographing incoming personnel and preparing badges and identification cards. The head of Security was an American with world-wide experience. He told me that the men who stood guard duty were largely Saudi Arabians. The rest of the department was made up of American and English experts.

After being duly photographed and registered, I checked into Medical Records. A chubby woman in her fifties was ruling over a desk cluttered with files, papers, and books. Helen was the only department head who was a woman except for the chief of nursing. She was responsible for all medical records and all translations of documents leaving the hospital, a demanding job in itself. She also had to police and cajole the physicians into completing their hospital summaries, a task for which she was eminently suited.

"Hi there! I already know about you from the bulletins translated here. Some first day, huh?" she said, sounding very American.

"I'm still numb."

"Well, I'm prepared to translate the prince's hospital record at any time. In case he goes to London."

"Don't hold your breath."

She laughed, leaning back loosely in her chair.

Helen was from California. Since she was located on the balcony of the main reception hall, and was privy to all the hospital records and much of the foreign correspondence, she knew more than anyone else, including security, about the goings-on within the hospital. I was soon to learn that this was the place to come for news and inside information.

The office for transportation, travel, passports, and visas was my next stop. Moussa, a tall, slender, dark, and handsome Afghan was graced with this thankless job. He was quick to complain about the uncontrolled congestion in the passport office in Riyadh and how passports sent there for processing were often "mislaid."

He told me that there were 1,600 people in the hospital who needed exit visas and re-entry visas every time they left the country.

"You can imagine the panic," he added sympathetically, "when their flights have to be canceled because the passports are misplaced. It still gives me ulcers, you know what I mean?"

I left my passport with him and asked for a receipt.

"How is the prince?" he asked as I was about to leave. "Are you going to accompany him to London? Let me know as soon as possible, so I can arrange for a re-entry visa."

I thanked him.

"Patient in B-24 wants a bed pan."

I was in the telephone switchboard station. It was "manned" by three women, who spoke English, Arabic, and French.

In the same room was a huge television console, which monitored each of the 250 hospital rooms and focused in on the patients. A bilingual attendant monitored the screen twenty-four hours a day. She could communicate with the patients directly and relay their needs and demands to the proper nurse's station. Generally, only the seriously ill patients were under constant television surveillance. The intensive care and cardiac units had their own monitoring systems.

The beepers had not yet arrived, so that all communication was by telephone. The operators were Lebanese and Egyptian. As can be imagined, the telephone station sounded like a Tower of Babel, and at times approached frenzy when there was an emergency telephone call from a foreign country.

It was 11 A.M. when I returned to check on the prince. The guard outside his door greeted me in recognition. The servant sat next to the bed, spoon-feeding the prince, and Kamal was tidying the room. The prince looked comfortable and the chart indicated no change in the vital signs.

The prince said, "Goood," without any prompting, and I replied with "Praise God" in Arabic.

The prince then spoke to Kamal, who interpreted, "The prince asked when he can have more to eat."

"Tell him we will give him more food in a day or two, when the bleeding stops completely—and that his desire for more food is a very good indication that he is improving."

"Inshallah," said the prince solemnly.

There was a knock on the door.

"Janet just called," said Miss Johnson. "The King will be here in about twenty minutes. Dr. Compton would like you to join him at the front entrance—same place as yesterday."

"I thought he comes around six o'clock," I murmured.

"Sometimes at 6 P.M. before evening prayers and sometimes at 11 or 11:30 A.M. before the noon prayers. It all depends on his schedule. He won't stay long today. It's close to noon now," she replied.

Dr. Compton and another man were standing at the entrance of the hospital waiting for the King to arrive. Compton introduced me to Frank Taylor, the Executive Director. Taylor was a six-foot-three-inch, 250-pound ex-football player, who looked as though he would burst through his clothes at any moment. He was forty years old, reputedly a hard worker and a tough administrator.

"I'm glad you're here," said Taylor. "This situation with Prince Yusef is crucial to us. We have been operating for only a few months, as you know, and the King is skeptical of our ability. Although he had open heart surgery in Cleveland not long ago, he doesn't really like Americans. The Crown Prince, on the other hand, is our friend. The hospital wouldn't have survived without him."

Compton then pointed out that the King would make the final decision about flying Prince Yusef to London for medical care, according to the tradition in Saudi Arabia.

"But if the prince is kept here and doesn't do well, that may be the end of our hospital," interjected Taylor. "We won't get a second chance."

"That applies to me, too," I said, remembering Dr. Compton's admonition the day before. "My bags are still packed."

Within a few minutes the royal entourage appeared, heralded by the soldiers, their red berets glistening in the sun. I watched the ritual again. All was the same as yesterday, except that the King and the Crown Prince sat together in the rear of a black Mercedes Benz, and they wore different-colored ghutras. We all shook hands perfunctorily and proceeded to the prince's room. Little was said. The King looked straight ahead, solemnly, with eyes fixed. The Crown Prince was wearing his constant placid half-smile.

En route, Saudis appeared again, ran up to the King or Crown Prince, placing their lips over their majesties' hearts.

The distinctive royal bearing was the same as yesterday. Their slow, steady, deliberate gait continued at the same pace, unperturbed, as though to the measure of a metronome. Again, they seemed to float rather than walk. The rest of us tagged along behind. I had a strong childlike impulse either to stand still or run up ahead, but I stifled it. This was a royal procession.

They strolled into the prince's room while we nervously moved into the adjoining room.

After about twenty minutes, the King and the Crown Prince appeared with Salim. There was a wisp of a smile on the King's face, and a full smile on that of Crown Prince Fahd.

The King addressed me while Salim interpreted. "Prince Yusef appears to be better," he said in Arabic. The Crown Prince continued to smile, but said nothing.

Something unusual then took place. We all walked together as a group toward the elevator. We were not just tagging along behind. The prince's sons, at times, walked side by side with their royal highnesses, and at other times some of us did, too, almost fortuitously. The pace was slow, as before, but not so measured. As we headed toward the reception hall, I found myself next to the Crown Prince. To my amazement, he turned to me and asked in perfect English, "How long does it take to fly from Washington to Boston?"

"About one hour," I replied, returning his nonchalance. "Eastern Airlines has a shuttle which flies regularly between the two cities."

"I have never visited Boston," he said. "It is a large city?"

We talked about Boston and New England in general. He then asked about the prince, how long he would be hospitalized, might he bleed again in the future, and what precautions should be taken.

I learned later that he had been invited to the White House for a meeting with the President during the oil crisis. But how did he know that I was from Boston? I wondered.

At the front entrance, they again shook hands with each of us, and then walked away silently to rejoin the royal entourage awaiting them. No mention had been made of transferring the prince to London.

"The King is apparently satisfied with the prince's progress," said Dr. Compton cheerfully. "This is the first break in the tradition of flying all sick royals to London for treatment."

"*Inshallah*," said Taylor fervently. "Let's hope the prince continues to improve."

Later that day Kamal told me what had transpired in the prince's room during the King's visit. They spent most of the time discussing Prince Yusef's health. The prince said he was better and felt stronger. The sons agreed. "Then they talked mostly about hunting."

Tonight I'll unpack, I said to myself. It should be safe now!

EXPATRIATE LIFESTYLE IN RIYADH

I FELT ELATED after the King left and was in the mood for a celebration. The prince was improving, and we had established rapport with the royal family, which would serve the hospital well in the future. The ultra-conservative faction in Riyadh opposed the hospital because it represented a foreign threat, an institution managed by infidels with strange ideas. The religious leaders expressed their opposition to the hospital in the mosques on Fridays, and at first they were very effective. The hospital was slow in getting started. But now the King had given it his stamp of approval, and he had broken tradition to do so.

It was high noon and very hot. I decided to celebrate by a refreshing swim at the Recreation Center, which was a large, well-staffed facility with an outdoor Olympic-size swimming pool. The delight of a swim in the cool, soothing water, when the outside temperature reaches 140 degrees, is almost beyond imagination. But a cloud hung over the Center because Moslem women were not permitted to use it, and the whole area was carefully fenced off from the prying eyes of the Yemeni and other workmen in the vicinity.

About two o'clock in the afternoon, I examined the prince again and then went to the office of the Department of Medicine, which was actually a hospital room that had been converted into an office temporarily.

Manda Blake, the secretary for the department, greeted me. She had been alerted to my arrival by Dr. Compton's office, and Janet had already told her about Prince Yusef. Manda was English and spoke with a beautiful London accent. She was in her early forties, deeply tanned, had blue eyes and brown, short-cut curly hair, heavily mixed with gray. Her brown dress was ankle-length and full. She wore no stockings, and her nail-polished toes looked comfortable in the Arabian sandals. A long, black cigarette holder was perched between her teeth at a rakish angle, and she smoked incessantly.

Manda had been one of the earliest arrivals. She told me that she had been working at the hospital for more than a year. She was born and brought up in Manchester, had married a British professor and had several children. She was divorced and, like Janet, was not allowed to bring her children to Saudi Arabia.

"Well, that's enough about me," sighed Manda. "You're new here and should know what goes on."

She went on to describe some of the problems at the hospital. There was limited office space because the architects had not anticipated the large number of physicians, technicians, secretaries, and ancillary personnel. Language and communication presented understandable difficulties. The doctors alone came from twenty-three different countries. A grievous shortage in housing made it necessary to commandeer hotel space at great cost and inconvenience, not to mention discomfort because of the poor quality of the available hotels. This brought to mind my foul-smelling hotel room at the Al Yamama.

Finally, Manda touched upon the difficult lifestyle imposed upon the single women employed in Saudi Arabia.

"Life certainly isn't convenient here," she said, "and the life of a single woman is just unbearable. We can't drive a car or go out at night unless we're with a group. We can't even take a damn taxi alone! I mean, I don't dare to go out or shop during the day unless I'm with another woman. In this place, you've got to keep your legs and arms covered, no matter how hot it is."

I learned that social activities were sharply limited. Male visitors were not allowed to enter a building in which single women were living. Housing facilities for women were inadequate. Socializing with a Moslem was frowned upon. Moslem women, such as the Egyptian employees, were forbidden to go out with Christian men.

Taking a long puff from her cigarette and dangling it with a loose wrist and casual finger, she smiled at me. "But of course, my dear, social life is not all that bad because the English community in the hospital is a closely knit group." She said that they looked after her quite adequately.

"It must take time to adjust to a new way of life," I murmured, "but after all, it's only for two years."

"Some people never adjust," said Manda, "and a good number leave after one or two months."

She then gave me a schedule of the outpatient clinics and asked me to sign up for three clinics. I chose Sunday, Tuesday, and Thursday mornings. The work week was six days. Friday was the religious holiday. Saturday and Sunday were regular workdays.

"We begin at 8 A.M. and theoretically leave at 5:15 P.M. If you work late, you can hire a taxi, but they are scarce. The best way to get back to the hotel is to call transportation and they'll send you a car and a driver. But this service is only for physicians."

While we were talking, Dr. Philip Westbrook, the chairman of the department, strode into the office. He was a handsome Englishman. His sharp blue eyes and blond hair gave this man in his fifties a boyish and vibrant appearance.

Manda introduced me and then left for the secretarial office across the hall. Dr. Westbrook was most gracious in his welcome. His refined, almost musical accent, crystal-clear articulation, and modulated, mellow tone bespoke Eton, Oxford, or Cambridge.

I proceeded to bring him up to date on the progress of my patient. He already had a copy of yesterday's bulletin, which Dr. Compton's office had sent him.

Manda sailed back into the room with the cigarette holder between her teeth at its usual angle, puffing away, and carrying a sheaf of papers under her arm.

Dr. Westbrook then detailed some of my duties, which included the outpatient clinics and responsibility for a number of patients in the hospital.

"The main problem," explained Dr. Westbrook, "is the shortage of beds and supportive personnel, such as nurses, technicians, and so forth. We now have only 150 beds available for patients, and the demand is overwhelming. Our policy is to admit only patients with medical and surgical conditions which cannot be treated elsewhere in the kingdom. Hopefully, we'll have 250 beds within twelve months."

"Are there other hospitals around?" I asked.

"There's a large, terribly rundown city hospital, with archaic equipment and facilities, and very little, if any, medical expertise. There are two other, much smaller hospitals, equally inadequate. Most of the physicians come from Egypt, Syria, or Pakistan and are definitely not qualified by our standards," explained Dr. Westbrook.

"What about Saudi Arabian doctors?"

"There are very few. Most of the doctors presently in this country are imported. A few years ago there just weren't any doctors here except for those hired by the wealthy families and by Aramco. There is now a University of Riyadh Medical School, which will graduate its first class next year."

"That's where I can help out," I said eagerly. "We can develop a postgraduate training and education program for them right here. They can serve as interns and later as resident physicians, if they qualify."

"Exactly," said Philip Westbrook, enthusiastically, selecting a paper from a stack on his desk. "You are listed on a number of committees, including medical education, teaching conferences, and postgraduate medical education."

We chatted for a while. As we parted, Westbrook invited me to tea at his apartment.

"I'll meet you at the front desk at five-thirty," he said.

Dr. Westbrook appeared on time, and we went to the parking lot adjoining the hospital. His car was a Landcruiser. It was like a jeep, with four-wheel drive and a stick shift. Just to climb into it took considerable agility.

"You'll get onto it," he said, smiling at my discomfort. "It's a great car for the desert—never gets stuck in the sand and carries extra petrol and water. Best transportation there is, next to the camel." Philip drove to his suite at the Al Sharq Hotel like a maniac. He knew all the shortcuts, mostly unpaved roads. I squeezed my eyes shut, not to keep the dust out, but for fear of an accident. I expected a crash at any moment.

"Shakes you up a bit, doesn't it?" He grinned as we were thrown from side to side violently, passing over rocks and into huge holes. "You'll get onto it."

"You weren't by any chance in the armored division during the war?" I laughed nervously, holding on for dear life.

"In the navy, actually," he replied, smiling. "Love to sail."

We arrived unharmed. The Al Sharq was of the same vintage as the Al Yamama—it looked and smelled like a musty, brokendown old hotel of the 1920s. The carpets were worn and faded. The tables and chairs were like relics out of a secondhand store. Behind the desk hung the usual portraits of King Faisal with King Khalid on his right and Crown Prince Fahd on his left.

We climbed the stairs to the second floor and walked to the end of a dimly-lighted hall, where an elderly attendant was seated so that he could command a view of the entire length of the hall and all the doors opening onto it.

"*Masal khair* [Good evening]," he said, recognizing Philip.

"*Masal khair,*" replied Philip, acknowledging the greeting while knocking on the door at the end of the hall.

A tall, handsome woman in her early fifties, with gray-streaked hair, answered the door. She was warm but reserved. Philip introduced me to his wife, Doris.

"How did you enjoy your maiden voyage with Philip?" she asked, laughing. "Ghastly, wasn't it?"

"It was a memorable experience," I replied.

"Tea will be ready in a moment," said Doris, bringing a plateful of small sandwiches. "This isn't Claridge's but it will do for now."

Their living quarters consisted of two rooms—a bedroom with a bathroom, and a sitting room all furnished in "early tenement" (brokendown, archaic furniture). There was no kitchen, but a small refrigerator sat, oddly, in the sitting room. Doris had found a hotplate and some dishes in the *suqs* (shops). The bathroom sink served as the dishwasher. There were no closets. Their clothes were hung on a broomstick which had been wedged into one corner of the bedroom.

"This is luxurious, compared to my digs," I remarked. "That broomstick is very ingenious."

"We hide the hotplate when we leave in the morning," said Doris, "because it is one luxury we couldn't do without."

Philip interrupted to tell the story of the hotplate, which had disappeared one day. He asked the manager of the hotel about it and was told that all hotplates had been confiscated. Philip explained that the hotplate was really essential, but to no avail. The manager remained adamant. About a week later he called Philip and told him about a niece of his who had been a laboratory technician in Cairo and was looking for a job in Riyadh, where she recently had been married. Philip found a job for her in the chemistry laboratory of the hospital, and within twenty-four hours the hotplate reappeared, as if by magic.

"There's a lot of quid pro quo around here," he concluded. "It's part of the Saudi tradition."

Doris went on to describe the two so-called "supermarkets" nearby, which were called the "clean supermarket" and the "dirty supermarket," the difference being that the Saudi at the cash register of one always appeared clean.

"You can get eggs, cheese, canned goods, bread, and fruit, if you can fight off the flies and climb over the crates," she added. "The apples come from Lebanon and are delicious. Be sure to wash them quite well."

While we had tea, they told me that they were from London and had been in Saudi Arabia about three months. The housing shortage was critical. There were comfortable villas within the hospital compound, but they were already occupied by the doctors and their families who had arrived earlier. The prefabricated Gerrin Village quarters were "barely adequate" and lacked privacy. They were waiting for the completion of an apartment house which was scheduled for occupancy in four or five months.

I complimented them on the air conditioner.

"I'm glad you brought that up," said Philip. "There's a power failure in this area once or twice a week, and the heat becomes really unbearable. We take turns in the bathtub or try to read by the light of our hurricane lamps. Sleeping becomes impossible, but the thought that the hospital has its own power plant is very reassuring."

"I do wonder what I'm doing here at times," Doris said sighing. "You know, I was a nurse in my younger days. Now, I'm just working in that local British school. Keeps me busy."

"We have a married daughter who lives in Edinburgh, one son who works in a British bank in New Zealand, and the other has his business in Belgium. We enjoy visiting them all," she added.

"Actually, it's the damn high taxes," Philip interrupted. "The young people are moving out of England and many doctors are leaving, too."

He picked up a little sandwich and devoured it. "It's almost impossible to keep enough money at home to educate our families, regardless of how much we earn," he said.

Not wanting to pursue economic issues, I changed the subject.

"What do you do for entertainment and relaxation?" I asked.

"As you know, there are no theaters or movies, and the television is impossible," said Doris, "so we make do with our own entertainment. There is usually a party every Thursday night and we have the hi-fi to supply us with music."

Philip went on to describe the Thursday-night parties. There was plenty of *sadiki*, the Saudi equivalent of bath-tub gin, which was colorless and tasteless. Nobody knew exactly who distilled it, but there was always somebody about who would deliver it to you secretly in a grocer's bag for about $12 a bottle. Philip gave me the name of a technician in the hospital who would get me a bottle whenever I wished, but he warned me to keep it hidden, because all alcoholic beverages were illegal, and transgressors of "the law" were deported immediately or imprisoned. The Saudis never search your home, but they might check your hotel room.

Sadiki, which means "my friend" in Arabic, was quite good in fruit punch or with fruit juices, tonic, or ginger ale, according to Philip. It flowed freely at the parties given by the Americans or English who were fortunate enough to have apartments or villas, but only those who arrived six months before were that fortunate.

The Lebanese gave great parties, with plenty of good food, sadiki, and dancing. The Saudis were quite hospitable, but generally their parties were pretty quiet, with good food but no alcohol. However, a party given by the younger royals was usually something else. They often had magnificent bars on display replete with champagne, Chivas Regal scotch, Beefeater gin, and so forth. Philip said that the royals had freedom of the port and didn't have to go through customs. After all, they owned the country! I was quite certain that Prince Yusef never touched alcohol but the young royals, like his sons, were probably more liberal. I didn't know it at the time, but some unusual parties were in store for me.

Then Doris described some interesting trips they had made into the desert and neighboring towns like Dariya, the original capital of the Saudi state, which was sacked by the Turkish armies in 1818. There was also an exciting trip on the Mecca Road with a spectacular view of the escarpments. They promised to take me to a place near Riyadh where shell fossils perhaps 150 million years old can be found, and to the "petrified forest."

Philip, who loved to travel, pointed out that the physicians were granted post leaves every four months as an incentive for coming to Saudi Arabia. In addition, they were given time off twice a year to attend scientific meetings. Philip was planning post leaves and scientific meetings in England, Japan, Australia, and New Zealand. I began thinking about the U.S., East Africa, Hong Kong, and Japan. It was exciting. I had just arrived and was already thinking about future trips out of the country. Saudi Arabia was ideally located for travel to all parts of the globe.

Doris brought me back to reality. "Did you notice that man outside our door?" she asked. "He's an Egyptian. He and his alternate stick it out twenty-four hours a day. They sleep on a small cot and eat in the linen room. Can you believe that foreign visitors are under twenty-four-hour surveillance in this country so they won't bring women or liquor into the rooms!

"There is an attendant on every floor," she continued. "They are usually older men, generally from Egypt or the Sudan because the Saudis will not do menial work like cleaning up the room or changing the beds."

Doris chuckled. "They won't change the linen on the beds or leave fresh towels unless you tip them," she added. "When we first arrived, I asked for fresh towels, and they gesticulated that there were none (*mahfi*). After several days of *mahfi* I gave them five riyals, and the fresh towels appeared like magic, forthwith. We now tip them regularly and all is well."

"There is a man stationed at the end of the hall in my hotel too," I recalled. "No wonder there is only one small towel in my room and the bed hasn't been changed in a week."

"The hotel probably pays the poor things next to nothing," Doris said sympathetically.

As I was preparing to leave, Philip offered to take me to the hospital each morning in his Landcruiser.

"A quarter before eight, sharp," he said. "Your hotel is only fifteen minutes away, and the walk will do you good."

I thanked them both, although I had some second thoughts about the Landcruiser.

It was now dusk. Leaving the Hotel Sharq, I turned right for the brief walk to the Al Yamama. There was sand and rubble everywhere. About one hundred feet ahead was a huge mound of dirt obstructing the sidewalk. No problem to get around that, I thought. I'll just walk out into the street and bypass it— Suddenly, my right leg buckled under me, and I felt a severe searing pain along my leg from the knee to the ankle. In the darkness, I had walked into an open manhole situated in the middle of the sidewalk—with no markings or guard rail whatever. My first fear was that my leg had been broken, but after I pulled my leg out, I noted that weight bearing did not aggravate the pain. I limped back to the hotel, laughing at myself for my ineptitude. I had been concentrating so hard on the pile of dirt and debris ahead that, in the dim light, I did not see the manhole in front of me.

Just before arriving at the hotel I spotted a small food store. Inside, it was cluttered with half-open crates of fruits and vegetables. Broken cartons of canned meat and fish were scattered about. There was an assortment of nuts in open sacks on the floor. Stacks of bread were piled up on the shelves next to boxes of crackers and cans of coffee. Hordes of flies were buzzing about the eggs, some of which were broken and oozing. This was the "clean supermarket," as Doris had labeled it, because the owner was immaculate in white, collecting the money at the door, while standing guard over the cigarette and cigar counter behind him. I wondered what the "dirty supermarket" was like. In the rear was a refrigerator, but I didn't want to venture that far. I settled for some apples from the crate up front, paid the owner, and limped back to the hotel.

The attendant was standing guard as usual at the end of the corridor. I beckoned him to come in, pointed to my lonely towel, held up four fingers, and asked for *arba'a* (four), while handing him five riyals—about $1.65. He thanked me excessively and returned immediately with a stack of towels and some soap. For good measure, I pointed to the bed sheets, which looked yellowed and damp, and said, "*Bukra*" (tomorrow). He nodded and left quickly.

My leg was throbbing. Blood and abraded skin covered its entire length, giving the leg a raw and ugly appearance. A rare moment: I could doctor myself! Carefully removing my clothes, I proceeded to wash my leg with soap and water, an excellent disinfectant. An antiseptic might have helped, but there was none available. We had been warned not to bring alcohol into the country, including rubbing alcohol. I had no choice but to use my aftershave lotion, which had alcohol in it. It burned like hell. I then dressed the wound with gauze from my first-aid kit.

I wondered, as an afterthought, whether the alcohol was really necessary. At any rate, the aftershave lotion, Canoé, had a delightful fragrance, certainly not unwelcome in my present lodgings.

The red, shining apples looked appetizing. They went well with the cheese Doris had given me. At that moment, the sadiki Philip had talked about would have been welcome to ease the pain. I went to bed with a pillow under my bruised and aching leg.

I didn't bother to unpack.

◇ 5 ◇

THE BEDOUIN INVASION

THE NEXT MORNING I walked over to the Al Sharq Hotel, carefully avoiding the open manholes, and met Philip at the front door.

Climbing into the Landcruiser, I remembered my injured leg. The way Westbrook held the steering wheel and shifted gears reminded me of a free-spirited, almost careless twenty-year-old.

We were joined by a cancer specialist from Ohio who lived in the same hotel. He was a Syrian, who had gone to the United States to study medicine and never returned.

His name was Nayef Al-Barras. "Everyone call me Al," he said with a thick accent. "I am United States citizen and hate Syria and Commies."

It seemed as if he had just learned English and that was one of his stock sentences. Al was a bit heavy, had olive-colored skin and pitch-black hair. He was clean-shaven, had good teeth, and smiled easily.

"How you like my accent?" he asked good-naturedly. He dropped his vowels and mixed up his verbs, or forgot them altogether, but he spoke Arabic, of course, which was more important.

"Which obstacle course we take today?" queried Al, turning to Philip.

"I'll improvise," said Philip. "We don't want to fall into a routine. It's more exciting this way—exploring the city, you might say."

Charisma, that's what Philip had.

He chose a narrow, bumpy dirt road to start with. After many turns down alleys strewn with debris and cluttered passageways, we came onto a main road. Philip's sense of direction was uncanny. The overturned trucks, smashed automobiles lying on their sides, and broken electric light poles seemed to be more abundant than ever.

"Someday this happen to us," Al said.

"Never," said Philip quite confidently. We approached the hospital gate in good time.

The prince had improved. I left orders at the desk, and proceeded to the clinic. The clinic, as well as the hospital, was open to all Saudi citizens regardless of their financial status. The charge for the initial clinic visit, which included a complete detailed medical history, physical examination, and all x-ray and laboratory tests, was two hundred riyals, equivalent to about $65. The cost in the United States would have been $250 to $750 or more, depending upon the number of x-rays and tests.

The charge for pharmacy prescriptions was the cost of the medication to the hospital plus 3 riyals (ninety cents, U.S.) as a service charge. The fee for followup visits to the clinic for treatment, including services of the physician, x-ray, and laboratory procedures was 50 riyals (about $16). It was clear that, with such nominal charges, the hospital was being subsidized by the government.

Patients with cancer, tuberculosis, or other chronic disabling diseases were treated free of charge. Nobody was turned away for lack of money. There was always a prince available to pay the bill, or a special committee which met regularly to evaluate unusual cases of financial hardship. Invariably, all financial obligations were met by the government.

Yet the hospital could not offer ideal health care to everyone. There weren't enough physicians or beds available to take care of the enormous demand. A screening procedure was devised to select only those for admission who could not be treated elsewhere in the kingdom. A patient seeking admission was asked to bring a doctor's letter stating the medical condition and reason for hospitalization.

This procedure worked for a short time. Then the clinic was suddenly overwhelmed by what appeared to be an epidemic of cancer, pneumonia, and exotic diseases. The Saudis began paying their doctors to falsify their letters of referral in order to get admitted to the clinic. If the patient had a headache, the letter would read "brain tumor"; if he had a cough, the letter noted "pneumonia," and so forth.

Eventually, a Primary Care and Family Health Center was set up in a separate building adjacent to the hospital to screen the patients before admitting them to the hospital or to the clinic.

My first clinic patient was a shabbily dressed Bedouin woman who had come with her husband from an area around Mecca near the western border of Saudi Arabia, approximately five hundred miles away. According to her clinic chart, she was a member of the distinguished Quarraysh tribe, who were the rulers of Mecca at one time, and the tribe into which the Prophet Mohammed was born. The admission papers prepared in the outpatient admitting office always included the name of the tribe in addition to the other pertinent information.

The translator in the clinic, a nurse assistant technician (NAT) from Lebanon, was a young man named Nabil, who was a close friend of Kamal. With Nabil as interpreter, I introduced myself to the patient and to her husband. She remained seated without movement of any kind, as though frozen. Her face was covered by an unusually heavy black veil. She wore the traditional black robe which was threadbare and somewhat faded, and sandals. None of her features were discernible. I couldn't even detect her age. Through Nabil, I explained that the medical history was very important, and that a female nurse would come in later during the physical examination; and that nobody else except her husband would be present.

The history taking then began. She told Nabil in a thin, high-pitched, squeaky voice that she was thirty-five years old and had been suffering from abdominal pain for several years, made worse by drinking camel's milk. On further questioning the woman, who frequently turned to her husband for help, Nabil was able to figure out that the pain was in the right upper quadrant of the abdomen, and at times it would radiate to the back or to the right shoulder.

It became quite obvious that obtaining a reliable history would be a time-consuming and difficult procedure. The Saudi Arabian idioms were sometimes different from those of Lebanon; the patient's responses weren't too clear; and her husband didn't know much about her at times. I was left with a hodge-podge of information transmitted through an intermediary in a language somewhat foreign to the interpreter himself.

I thought it might be helpful to see the patient's facial expressions during the history taking.

"Nabil, please ask her to remove her veil," I said.

"*La*," she replied with vigor, shaking her head and turning to her husband for support.

"Tell the husband I must examine her eyes, nose, and throat as part of the examination," I persisted.

He assured her softly that it might be proper to remove the veil under these unusual circumstances, and she finally removed it with great hesitation and reluctance.

In her case, the veil had been an improvement, and I wondered whether her hesitation was based solely upon custom and tradition. She appeared to be in her fifties, as did her husband. Her skin was wrinkled and drawn, her teeth were bad, and she looked old and tired. The whites of her eyes were slightly yellow, indicating mild jaundice. I asked her again about her age, and again she said thirty-five. Her husband confirmed it and said she was married at fifteen. I remained incredulous. She looked twenty years older! The woman obviously had a difficult life. She recalled fourteen pregnancies and four miscarriages. Six children survived.

A Bedouin woman of thirty-five in certain tribes is called *ajuzah*—an old woman—ready to be shelved for a younger wife. Nabil pointed out that a great number of Bedouin men and women appear to be ten to fifteen years older than their stated age. But of course, in many instances, there is no record of the date of birth and no means of confirmation.

As soon as I finished examining her eyes and throat she quickly pulled her veil over her face with a sigh of relief. In a way the veil was like a security blanket.

"How will she react to removing all of her clothes for the physical?" I asked.

"No problem at all," said the American nurse, who had been summoned by Nabil, "as long as she can keep her face covered."

The nurse, who spoke no Arabic, asked Nabil to instruct the patient to undress completely, to lie down on the examining table, and to cover up with the sheets handed to her for that purpose. The husband was asked to remain in the room. Draw curtains suspended from the ceiling were then pulled around the examining table, enclosing it to give the patient complete privacy. We then withdrew, leaving the patient and her husband alone.

When the nurse and I returned ten minutes later, the patient was lying on the examining table, stark naked except for the heavy veil covering her face. She seemed relaxed and comfortable. The folded white sheets were lying undisturbed next to her on the examining table within easy reach. She had saved face, to be sure.

A Saudi woman explained later that the women don't object to exposing their bodies providing no one knows whose body is being exposed. They gladly remove all their clothes for an examination providing they can wear their veils to hide their identity.

The soles of her feet and the palms of her hands were colored reddish orange with henna used as a cosmetic to celebrate her visit to Riyadh. According to the nurse, some women "dress up" by also coloring their nails or hair with henna.

I saw five or six brown circles, up to one inch in diameter, scattered over her chest and abdomen, mostly on her right side. They were branding marks, I was told, made by applying red-hot tent pins to the chest, back, or abdomen "to relieve pain or congestion." Branding is the standard form of treatment used by the Bedouins on infants and children as well. Sometimes branding is performed with the small mouth of a bottle held over an open flame until it is white hot. Everyone in the clinic knew about these brown burn markings. No one talked about them. I just stared in astonishment.

The physical examination was otherwise normal except for evidence of premature aging, tenderness and spasm in her right, upper abdomen, and slight jaundice. The nurse covered the patient with the sheets and motioned for her to dress.

I then instructed Nabil to tell them that certain tests and x-rays would be necessary, and that gallstones were probably the cause of her symptoms. I explained that surgery might eventually be advisable. Although Nabil addressed himself to the patient, she preferred to be silent and let her husband answer for her. They were to return in ten days.

Since this was my first clinic, it was kept brief by design. I saw only four more new patients. One was a young woman with acute viral hepatitis and jaundice, a common condition in Saudi Arabia. The disease is caused by a virus which attacks the liver. It is transmitted by drinking water or food that become contaminated because of inadequate sewage disposal and poor sanitation. Cirrhosis of the liver, as a complication of viral hepatitis, and cancer of the liver, are also very common. The second patient was a sixty-year-old man with cancer of the liver who was brought in on a stretcher from a small village outside of Riyadh. I admitted him into the hospital.

Two other patients had vague abdominal complaints which they attributed to "parasites." They were typical of the many patients who want to see a doctor for reassurance. They have innumerable complaints, none of which are related to disease, and often travel from one clinic to another carrying a large dossier of papers and reports, detailing innumerable x-rays and laboratory tests, all of which are perfectly normal.

These two patients had letters from doctors in Riyadh which they obviously had paid for, merely to get into the Specialist Clinic of the King Faisal Hospital, as a sort of status symbol, so they could tell their friends. Somehow, they had deceived the screening physician in the Primary Care Center by guile or subterfuge. They were perfectly healthy women, proud of their collection of medical reports from all over the world (London, Paris, Berlin, Zurich, Cairo, etc.), all testifying in scientific terms to their superb state of health. What they needed was a good psychiatrist or psychologist to give them some insight into their problems: boredom, insecurity, unsatisfactory sex, an unhappy marriage, or the closed society in which they lived. I soon learned that there was no shortage of psychoneurotics in Saudi Arabia.

Shortly after one o'clock, there was an emergency telephone call from Frank Taylor. "Dr. Gray, have you been up to see Prince Yusef recently?"

"No. I saw him early this morning. He was getting along very well," I said.

"Well, he should have a relapse any moment," shouted Mr. Taylor, "and if he doesn't, then I will."

"What happened?" I asked innocently.

"Ward B-2 has been invaded by a horde of Bedouins, that's what happened," screamed Taylor, who was having one of his tantrums. "At least forty of them came to visit the prince, the whole damn tribe, and they brought everything with them except their camels."

"How did they all get through the front gate?"

"The prince is a very powerful man, or haven't you heard?" He groaned. "The Bedouins are celebrating his recovery and have practically taken over the whole ward."

Taylor's volatile temper and nervous outbursts fitted the stereotype of a hard-driving successful executive. Big Frank's obsessive concern was the hospital's image in the eyes of the rich Saudis. After all, his job depended upon keeping the Royal Cabinet happy, and he was good at it, but he was also dedicated to maintaining the highest possible level of health care.

"I'll see what I can do," I said, trying to be reassuring.

"The nurses are ready to quit—and so am I," he added angrily.

Ward B-2 was bedlam. The tribe had invaded and occupied the ward. They were sitting around in groups chatting or standing about in the halls. Some of them had innocently taken over the visitors' waiting room reserved for women, and another group was ensconced in the utility room. They were dressed mostly in white or slate-colored thobes and white ghutras, often worn on holidays. All wore sandals over bare feet.

Miss Johnson was in tears. "We're behind in our medications," she said, "and we just can't do a thing under these conditions."

"I'll do my best, but it may take some time," I said, trying to be helpful.

There were at least ten visitors in the prince's room. Tea and cakes were being served. Most of the men were standing and talking quietly, sipping their tea. The prince looked pleased but tired. He introduced me to his friends, and we shook hands all around. I drew Kamal aside.

"In about five minutes, tell them to please leave so that I can examine the prince and order more medicine," I said. "Meanwhile, I'll have some tea and look around."

The Bedouins were handsome people, medium to tall in stature, sinewy, and lean, with broad, muscular shoulders. Their heads and faces were long, accentuated by well-trimmed dark beards. Their skin was olive to brown, creased and weatherbeaten by the sun and wind, like that of New England fishermen. Their brown eyes were sharp, penetrating, and inquisitive. The lips were full, and the noses prominent and classically Semitic like that of the prince and the royal family. Above all, their bearing was erect, haughty, and almost defiant.

Kamal carried out his mission and the room was cleared except for the ever-present servant, sitting on his haunches in the corner. The prince had held up well under the ordeal although he looked exhausted. His blood pressure was now normal, but his pulse was still rapid. The blood count was improving.

I asked Kamal to fetch Salim and the other two sons, who were in the adjoining room entertaining another roomful of Bedouins. When they arrived, we all sat down and I tried to explain that today's events might be harmful, if not dangerous, to the prince. At the present stage of his illness he was still very anemic, and the bleeding had only diminished in the past twenty-four hours.

"My father was happy to see his friends," explained Salim, adding, "They are his hunting companions and his tribesmen."

"One or two visitors each day would be permissible, but the whole tribe is here, or so it seems," I said seriously.

"They are very concerned about him," said Salim.

"Too much excitement and stress, no matter how pleasant, might start the bleeding again," I warned. "We should restrict the number of visitors or we may have trouble. Your father needs rest."

"They have come a long way, from the northwest province of Hejaz," he argued.

"We need your help," I persisted. "Your friends are disrupting the whole ward. They are breaking all the regulations. The nurses can't get their work done, and the other patients are suffering because of it. Mr. Taylor is very disturbed."

"Mr. Taylor does not own this hospital. We do!" affirmed Salim in no uncertain terms.

"Certainly you can understand that hospital regulations must be followed, particularly when the health of your own father and of others is involved," I pleaded.

He paused and thought for a couple of seconds. "I understand," he said, rising. "Let's go into the next room and see what can be done."

We all went into the adjoining room, still full of people. Salim explained the situation to them, and we compromised by suggesting that they all stay in the large reception hall on the ground floor, where there was ample seating, and where tea and coffee would be served. In deference to the prince's health, visitors would be restricted to three at any one time for brief periods, monitored by Kamal. We shook hands. I thanked them in Arabic, and they left.

Salim and I sat down while tea was served by one of the attendants. He looked pleased.

"They are really wonderful people," he said with admiration. "They are the purest of the Arabs, the blood and guts of this country."

"How do you mean?" I asked.

"These particular Bedouins," remarked Salim proudly, "are members of the Anizah tribe, the aristocrats of the desert. They claim descent from Ishmael the son of Abraham. Our family belongs to this tribe. So does the entire family of King Abdul-Aziz, including King Khalid and Crown Prince Fahd."

He went on to explain that the Bedouins are nomadic people of the desert and oppose the ways of city life. They are hunters, herdsmen, and camel breeders, living in tents and moving periodically to find grazing grounds for their sheep, goats, and camels, usually far from civilization.

Salim pointed out that the Bedouins are proud of their heritage and their way of life, as described in poetry and legends handed down from generation to generation by word of mouth. They regard the Hedari (settled Arabs) as inferior, and the practice of agriculture or crafts as beneath their dignity.

"I thought the Bedouins were very poor, illiterate, and malnourished, robbing and pillaging other tribes and travelers," I said.

"Those are the inferior, non-Sharif tribes, who are entirely different from our tribe," said Salim. "They not only robbed everyone in sight but they also raided each other, plundered settlements and villages, and demanded payment from weaker tribes for protection."

Salim then went on to say that this situation had existed before King Abdul-Aziz unified them into one kingdom and banned the raiding and the robbing. He had great influence because he was one of them, having married into all of the principal tribes. To ensure their loyalty, he instituted grants-in-aid from the government, which are still in effect today.

"Although many of the city people still look down upon them—because of their poverty and ignorance—we were all Bedouins at one time, every one of us," said Salim quietly, as he sipped his tea and gazed out the window.

He went on to say that the Bedouin represents, somehow, the qualities of the ideal man, which are personal bravery, physical power, sexual virility, boldness in opposing outsiders, generosity within the family group and among selected friends, hospitality, and loyalty to Islam.

"And they want to retain every aspect of life exactly as it was in the days of the Prophet Mohammed," he concluded. "I believe this may eventually cause some serious problems."

"Well, how many nomadic Bedouins are there in Saudi Arabia now?" I asked.

"There are only about 400,000 left, yet they're the foundation upon which the royal dynasty stands," Salim replied. "The King and Crown Prince court the Bedouins and identify with them. They're part of our heritage."

After a second cup of tea, I thanked him and left to call Taylor to tell him of the compromise we had made with the Bedouins, and that order and tranquillity had been restored to Ward B.

"Dr. Gray," he said, with excess nervous energy, "there were times today that I wished to God we had flown the prince to London, after all. Maybe we should build a separate wing for the royals or set aside a certain area in the hospital for them."

"Terrible idea," I said, "very undemocratic. Allah will reward you, however, if you do me one favor."

"What's that?" he said with suspicion.

"Can you call off the King's visit today? The prince is really exhausted since the Bedouin invasion, and so is the nursing staff, and so are we all."

"Good idea," he said. "I'll ask Dr. Hassan, who has a direct line to the palace, to put in a word. He has been away, to Switzerland, I believe, and will want to visit the prince, a courtesy call, you know."

"*Bucra-bucra* [tomorrow]," I pleaded. "See if he can defer the royal visit for twenty-four hours."

"Yeah, yeah, I'll do what I can," promised Taylor, hanging up without saying goodbye.

Dr. Hassan was married to King Faisal's sister-in-law. King Faisal had given him the responsibility of building and developing the King Faisal Specialist Hospital. Hassan also serves as the liaison between the hospital and the palace.

Two hours later I was riding back to the hotel with Philip in his lofty Landcruiser. We were heading south from the hospital on Naseriyah Street to a circle with four connecting roads. As we came to the circle a military guard in a red beret drove up in a jeep and stopped all traffic.

"The King's coming," said Philip. "We had better get back to the hospital."

"Nothing we can do now," I replied, "until the entourage passes."

The royal procession, with the colorful red berets shimmering in the sun, approached us on Naseriyah Street coming from the south to the circle, then proceeded halfway around the circle and appeared to be heading north for the hospital. At that juncture, the military guard drove up to the lead car of the royal entourage, and the procession stopped. An attaché stepped out, spoke with the guard, and then approached the King's car. After a few minutes, the attaché returned to the lead car, and the procession changed its course, circled the roundabout an additional ninety degrees, and proceeded west on Mathar Road, leading directly to the palace. After the last car trailed away, the guard directing traffic returned to his jeep and drove off in pursuit.

The message from the hospital had been delivered to King Khalid, who canceled his visit to the prince and was now heading for his palace to retire for the day. We finally drove on, and Philip dropped me off at my shabby hotel.

Drunk with power, I picked up a can of corned beef and other delights at the dirty supermarket. It may have resembled dog food, but with the tomatoes, apples, and Sohat water it composed a sumptuous supper, which I devoured in my room without even feeling sorry for myself. After all, I was happy with my work. Nothing else really mattered.

I felt a little homesick. It was a balmy evening, and there was a full moon. I went out for a walk.

◇ 6 ◇

EAST AND WEST STROLL
HAND IN HAND

I HAD OFTEN WONDERED what it would be like to be a monk or a priest. My first week in Saudi Arabia gave me some insight into such an experience. I began to live a monastic existence. The trappings of civilization had not yet caught up with me. My trunks, books, and other paraphernalia did not arrive until a month later.

There were no newspapers, magazines, radios, or television. I never realized what a trauma the news media could be. I lived in a simple room, alone, with no friends and no diversions to dilute or interfere with my work. I arose early, spent all day at the hospital, had a simple meal at night, and went to bed exhausted and content. I found comfort and serenity in this way of life. Sadly, it only lasted a few months, but I shall never forget them. It was a cleansing experience.

My existence centered about the lives of other people. It was a simple life, unencumbered by possessions, free of the pressures to compete or to achieve, free of distant goals or money matters. My sole commitment was to help people and to heal the sick. It was a marvelous experience while it lasted and carried with it a certain indefinable peace and sense of accomplishment. A doctor friend told me later, "You always have a smile on your face," but I was unaware of the smile. It apparently came from within.

I lost all track of time and often had to consult my calendar watch to determine the day of the week. There were no weekends as such. Saturday and Sunday lost their meaning because they were work days. Friday was the only holiday, but it seemed like any other day. I often spent it taking care of the many patients in the hospital and tending to my clinics, which were fascinating. The people I attended really needed me, and this gave me a sense of fulfillment. For the first time in my life I felt indispensable.

The days not only lost their identity but at times I couldn't be sure which century we were in. Sometimes, when I delved into the lives of the desert people, I became lost in time and space as they transported me into the past. I wondered, indeed, whether this was the tenth century or the twentieth century. They seemed to fuse into one another. The external surroundings were from the twentieth century, but the people were often a thousand years behind. It was an eerie experience! This was certainly a country of contrasts and contradictions.

One Friday morning, during my daily hospital rounds, I happened upon a memorable scene in Prince Yusef's room. It was filled with the most elegant men I had ever seen. Their thobes and white mantles were of the finest cloth and, of course, trimmed in gold. Every one of them was six feet tall or more. Royals! I glanced quickly at their shoes, which, sure enough, were of the best leather, probably from England or Italy. Many wore platinum watches.

I supposed they had just arrived because they were greeting each other with kisses on the cheeks, forehead, tip of the nose, and even the lips. They were delicate, but deliberate, subtle kisses—not at all offensive. The kisses on the nose and lips were repeated. "Kissing cousins," I thought to myself.

The prince noticed me and motioned to his son to make the introductions. Some of the names were familiar, like Salman, Naif, Abdallah, and Sultan. They were between thirty-five and forty-five years old, wore beards, and looked amazingly alike—tall, slender, erect, and regal. This was the top echelon, the family of Ibn Saud, all half brothers or full brothers and cousins bound by bloodlines to each other and to their distinguished cousin, Prince Yusef.

It suddenly dawned on me that this was a singularly powerful conglomeration of royalty, many of whom controlled the destiny of Saudi Arabia. In short, this was a microcosm of the royal Saudi Arabian power structure, the nucleus of the Royal Cabinet, much more powerful in some ways than the members of the President's Cabinet in the United States, and certainly much wealthier. They chatted for a while, standing in groups around the prince's bed, some laughing, others holding hands while they talked. A few sat on chairs arranged around the periphery of the room. After a while, they went over to Prince Yusef, kissed him again on the nose, cheeks, or forehead, embraced, and bade him farewell. They shook hands with me politely as they left. Some thanked me in English.

There was a definite aura of camaraderie and warm fellowship among them which one sometimes experiences at a bachelor party among old friends or at a men's smoker at the club after the third round of drinks. The kissing and holding of hands, performed with elegance and grace, signified a true, deep, and intimate friendship, a genuine bond of loyalty, love, and respect among men. There was nothing feminine about it.

This man-to-man companionship was all the more binding and profound because of the very limited intercourse between husbands and wives. I learned that relationships with close family and friends are intimate and private but are restricted to the same sex. Men and women just do not mix socially. Men dance in groups with other men. Women dance only for each other and with each other. A man never dances with a woman. At a wedding, the celebration is held at separate sites for the men and for the women, usually many miles apart. The family unit is very strong—the segregation of sexes is probably stronger.

After they left, Kamal said they talked mostly about the prince's health and wondered why he hadn't gone to London as was the custom. Prince Yusef, in turn, was effusive in his praise of the medical care he had received. Some of the princes laughingly deplored this break in tradition, which would deprive them of their travels to London. They also swapped stories of hunting trips and falconry, favorite topics of Prince Yusef, subjects akin to golfing yarns told in the United States whenever men of substance congregate.

During the ensuing weeks, as the prince regained his strength, our talks became more frequent and more personal. He sensed my interest in him as a person, in his attitudes toward life, and in the society and culture in which he lived. He began to speak more freely. Kamal, as usual, served as the interpreter.

The prince represented the older generation of the privileged class, which inherited great wealth in addition to handsome yearly subsidies from the crown.

I learned that he had palaces in Riyadh, Jidda, Taif, and Medina for each of his four wives. A "palace" by Saudi Arabian definition is really a large villa with perhaps twenty to thirty rooms. The surrounding grounds are huge and often beautifully landscaped. The servants generally live in separate quarters within the compound. Personal servants and maids, often liberated slaves, may sleep on the floor near their master or mistress. True, the villas were not replicas of Buckingham Palace, but he had four of them, usually identical, in each city. In addition, he had a large farm eighty kilometers away where he bred his Arabian racehorses and racing camels. He also owned an unspecified amount of real estate of enormous value in the north.

One day while we were discussing financial matters he told me that he was in the construction business. "Saudi Arabia is growing fast," he said, "and we need roads and housing."

"You must have a very successful business," I remarked. "The government is spending many billions on construction."

He said that the business which he owned outright grossed about $300 million a year. There were four thousand workers in his employ, many from outside the country.

I wondered whether that was the cause of his ulcer. The prince was obviously carrying quite a burden, but it had its compensations. His personal income, he said, was roughly $60 million a year in addition to his stipend from the crown.

"That's tax free, isn't it?" I choked.

"Yes," he said patiently, "the Saudi Arabian citizens pay no income taxes. In a way, it's against our tradition."

"There are some corporations in the U.S. which earn a great deal of money, your royal highness, but their taxes are very high."

"Maybe your government should join the brotherhood of Islam," he said, half in earnest, "and cancel all taxation on income."

"The taxes in the U.S. are used to help the poor," I countered, "and giving to the poor is an important part of Islam, particularly at Ramadan."

"Taxes in the U.S. are used for many other purposes, too," interrupted Salim, who had just entered the room, "and much of the tax money is wasted." That point was beyond argument.

"You have many poor people in Saudi Arabia. What is the government doing for them?" I asked.

"Our government will spend $140 billion over the next five years for development of the country," explained Salim, "and $30 billion will go for housing, roads, schools, hospitals, and modernization of our cities. The money will come from the oil. We do not need taxes."

"And any Saudi citizen can borrow money from the government to build houses or roads," added the prince.

"How much interest does he pay on the loan?" I asked.

"He pays no interest whatever. It is against the religion," intoned the prince. "He can pay the money back to the government in twenty years, if he wishes, but the government really considers the 'loans' as gifts to the people who are developing the country and does not expect them to return the money."

"The amount he can borrow is limited to about 60,000 riyals ($20,000, U.S.), not very much, but it is a start," added Salim, "particularly for a poor man."

I sat back and tried to digest it all. This prince, in his sixties, owns outright an enormous business which nets him, personally, the equivalent of about $60 million a year, *tax free*. In addition, he has sixteen palaces, a large farm where he breeds prize racehorses and camels, and an undetermined amount of valuable real estate. His income from the crown is small by comparison, about $100 thousand a year.

I asked him about servants. After consulting with Salim, he came up with the number three hundred, who served the palaces and the wives, and took care of the children. Many were former slaves who, when liberated in 1962, chose to remain in his service.

He pointed to the man with the curved dagger standing guard outside the door. "I bought his mother when she was fifteen years old in the slave market here in Riyadh," he said. "She was from Ethiopia."

"Now," he added proudly, "her son there has four wives of his own and ten children."

I learned that the prince had married many times during his lifetime. With four wives at a time, he could account for thirty-four, not to mention innumerable concubines, all fit and proper in accordance with the Koran. He was proud of his twenty-five sons, but not certain of the number of daughters, which he approximated at twenty-two.

Many male members of the family came to visit the prince. Among them was a son who brought a little boy about seven or eight, all dressed up in an immaculate white thobe and white ghutra, to visit his father. The prince drew an absolute blank when he saw the child until Salim reminded him: "This is little Abdullah, Lulwa's boy," following which there was instant recognition, or a pretense at recognition, as the prince embraced his son, calling him now by name, "Abdullah, Abdullah." The little boy hesitated, seemingly unsure of the prince's identity, followed his brother's instructions, and approached his father respectfully, remaining silent throughout this show of paternal affection. This was a memorable encounter for little Abdullah, the son of Lulwa, the prince's youngest wife.

We never discussed his wives or other women. It would have been improper of me to inquire about them or about their health, and would have been construed as an invasion of the prince's privacy. For example, it is permissible for friends to ask: "How are you and how are the children?" No mention is ever made of the women, however. Lifelong friends may ask: "How are those behind you?" That's about as intimate as one man can get with another when inquiring about a wife or wives.

One evening, three of the prince's close friends were visiting him. It was seven-fifteen in the evening—the usual visiting hour. Suddenly, the ever-present guard stationed outside the door rushed into the room and said something to the prince very quietly. Everyone in the room including Kamal and the servant in the corner made a hurried exit as though they were about to be struck by a plague. The cause for their concern was the approach of the prince's wives. It would have been improper for the men to remain in the same room with them, since Saudi men and women do not mix outside the immediate family. I was reminded again that Saudi women outside the home must always be completely veiled and covered by a black abeyya over their clothes. They must also be chaperoned by a servant, a male member of the family, or by one or more other women. The prince had diplomatically indicated to me that, if a woman is seen outside of her home unescorted, she is automatically considered a prostitute.

Recently, a doctor's wife, an American, made the mistake of hailing a cab to take her to the Riyadh supermarket three miles away. The cab driver immediately exposed himself to her and she fled in terror. The foreign women soon learned to keep their legs and arms covered, and never to go out alone.

My thoughts drifted to Doris, the prince, and certain aspects of life in this country. . . .

Philip's wife was an individual. She had opinions, ambition, and character. She spoke her mind. But most of these Saudi women seemed unreal. They were suppressed, uninformed, maltreated, and couldn't do anything about it. What would Doris be like if she had been born in a country like this—or Madame Curie or Margaret Thatcher, the Prime Minister of England?

The gap in our social values, lifestyles, and interests was so wide perhaps we could never really know each other. The idea that cultural differences isolate people so dramatically disturbed me.

The prince made steady progress. He was now sitting up in a chair for several hours each day and walking about in his room with some help. We had many opportunities to talk quietly, but his manner was somewhat condescending. When I first arrived, he treated me like a physician hired by the government to take care of him before sending him on to London for more expert treatment. Somehow, he made me feel, in a polite way, like one of the hired hands.

There was no point, I felt, in talking more about Harvard or a Ph.D. degree, although I mentioned both. From his blank expression, I concluded that he had never heard of either. The term "professor" was equally unimpressive, since some of the Lebanese doctors in Saudi Arabia called themselves "professor" with reckless abandon. I tried to discuss some of my research, particularly with radioactive chromium, which was directly applicable to his illness in that it was used to follow the course of his bleeding. This merely meant, in his view, that I was some sort of a laboratory technician bent upon taking more of his blood "for tests."

I tried to understand his viewpoint. The royal families imported physicians from Lebanon or from Egypt. They were hired by the year and generally were not of the highest professional caliber. Most of them either had problems in their own country or were attracted primarily by money. They were at the beck and call of all members of the family, to treat minor ailments and then to transfer their patients to more skillful physicians in the event of a serious illness. It was a degrading situation for most of them, but it was a livelihood. Some of these physicians lived on the palace grounds in modest quarters, serving for many years, like family retainers.

In any event, I was frustrated by his patronizing attitude and by my inability to establish a closer rapport with him. Then one night I had an inspiration. Packed away in my luggage were some excellent colored photographs of my home, taken in the spring when the lilacs and wisteria were in full bloom and the huge copper beech tree was in its glory. It was an old, large English-type house with about an acre of lawn, typical of many old houses in New England, and the photography did it more than justice. There were similar pictures taken in October, when the foliage surrounding the house was spectacular, and still others taken after a heavy snowfall, when everything was pristinely white.

I smiled when I walked into the prince's room the following day. We talked for a minute until I felt I could introduce the pictures with an "Oh, by the way!" I took them out of my pocket and handed the photographs to him.

The effect was electrifying. Of course one picture is worth more than a thousand words.

"Is this your home?" he asked in astonishment, examining them carefully. Before I could answer, he shook his head saying, "It is more beautiful than any of my palaces."

"But you have sixteen," I protested.

"The land, the trees, the gardens—magnificent," he murmured. "And you left this to come here?"

"Our countries need each other," I said. "You have the oil, we have the technical and scientific knowledge."

"Yes," he said, "one of my sons is studying in your country."

Then, after a long pause, he added, "You must come to visit me in the palace after I leave here. Salim or Nasser will bring you."

The condescending, patronizing manner was gone. We were equals—well, almost equals. I sensed that the veil that hung between us was now lifted, enabling me to visualize his society and the whole human scene more clearly.

During the following days, we talked a great deal. Here we were, two men from different worlds, trying to span a gap of a thousand years with a bridge of understanding—one from the most technologically advanced country in the world, the other from a land completely isolated from the outside world; one man from a wide-open permissive society, the other from a tightly-closed society, desperately trying to keep it airtight, to maintain the status quo.

The prince had never been outside of Saudi Arabia, he said, except for one trip to Egypt by caravan, many years ago. The dividend of that trip was an Egyptian chef he brought back with him who was still in his service.

It was crystal clear that the most important part of his life was his faith. He had memorized the Koran in his youth. All subsequent reading matter during his lifetime pertained to the Koran and its interpretation, and to the Sharia, the Islamic code of justice based primarily on the Koran.

"Your world has no idea how important Islam is in the everyday life of the people in Saudi Arabia. Unless you understand this, you can never understand us, or our customs," he said with conviction. "Islam is in our minds and hearts every moment of the day, every moment," he added for emphasis.

"There is a difference between religion in an abstract way as it exists in the Western world, and the total dedication to Islam flourishing in Saudi Arabia," I remarked.

I told him how impressed I was to see the mechanics in the garage roll out a small prayer rug on the oil-stained floor among the buses and drop to their knees in prayer. The waiters in the hotel did the same thing on the dining-room floor, and the steward in the airplane prayed in the galley. The hotel doorman rolled out his small rug and prayed in the driveway, oblivious of the traffic and of all the foreigners. A taxi driver removed the ghutra from his head, spread it on the ground in place of a prayer rug, knelt on it to perform his prayers. Perhaps the most memorable sight was that of the guard outside the prince's room, a former slave, who took the hand of Nasser, the prince's son, and led him to the flower garden, where they both knelt and prayed together—master and servant. It was a touching scene and brought tears to my eyes.

"Our children who cannot read are taught to memorize the Koran," he explained.

"Who teaches the girls?" I asked. "Men aren't permitted to teach women in person."

"Usually blind religious teachers or the children's mothers or grandmothers," he said quietly. "Blindness is very common here because of trachoma."

"Do you know that, if the disease is discovered early enough, trachoma can be treated to prevent blindness? A number of American experts have been here for years studying the problem."

"*Inshallah*," the prince murmured.

The prince went on to say that he loved to hunt, and he promised to take me with him. They usually went into the desert in a caravan of trucks with their tents, taking a staff of servants, a cook, food, water, and supplies for ten days. Of course, the falconers and their falcons received special attention.

"Hunting with falcons began in Saudi Arabia over a thousand years ago," said the prince, "and later it was introduced into Europe."

"Sometimes, we go on safari to hunt for a beautiful large bird called the houbara bustard. It is now rare," said the prince. "A falcon can spot a houbara from one mile away. But the hunt mainly gives us a chance to return to the old traditions and to live as we saw our fathers live."

"Do you take camels with you?" I asked.

"Of course," replied the prince, forgetting himself. "The camels are sent on ahead. We must have the camels! So much of the old pre-Islamic poetry is about falconry, camels, and the chase. We like to sit around the fires at night and tell stories of the hunt, handed down from generation to generation for more than a thousand years, all by word of mouth."

Salim, always practical, said that one could buy falcons from the falconers in downtown Riyadh, and that they were very expensive to maintain because they ate a good deal of meat.

"A choice falcon may cost $5,000 to $10,000. King Khalid owns more than a hundred prize falcons. I'll call you at the hospital or at the hotel beforehand so that you can make arrangements and join us on our next hunting expedition," he said graciously.

"*Inshallah*," I replied, smiling.

Some days later, as he was preparing to leave the hospital, the prince asked me if he could have sex after he arrived at home.

"Certainly," I replied.

"How much sex?" he asked cautiously.

"As much as you like, within reason."

"How many times a day?" he persisted.

"Three or four," I said, offhand, with a smile.

"But, doctor, I have four wives!"

"That's your problem," I quipped.

We both laughed, enjoying the more personal, casual level of our relationship.

Shortly before he was discharged from the hospital, he would walk back and forth in the corridors outside his room for exercise. One afternoon I joined him.

As we walked side by side, talking, he took my hand in his. Surprised and shocked at first, I then remembered that this was the custom among close friends. In this exclusively male society, holding hands with men is an expression of true friendship. This gesture was his way of saying "thank you."

And now the East and West, a thousand years apart in our culture, knowledge, and social development—were strolling hand in hand down the corridor.

Who was the wiser man? Which of us was truly cultivated or content? I knew that these questions would never be answered with certainty, but I tried to imagine what thoughts were passing through the prince's mind at that moment.

The prince was probably thinking: I feel sorry for this poor infidel. He doesn't know God as I do—the teachings of the Koran, the glory and brotherhood of Islam, the love of Allah, the fulfillment of prayer, the peace and contentment of Mecca, and the rewards of the hereafter.

He probably pitied me for not knowing how to place my destiny completely in the hands of Allah, who would watch over me and guide me into eternity. Does this man, he wondered, know the silence and magnificence of the desert at night when one can almost reach out and touch the stars, or the sight of a falcon bringing down a bird?

I am wealthier by far, he concluded, with my twenty-five sons, and the many women to bring me pleasure, the sanctity of my family, and the virtue of my daughters.

We do not tolerate murder or adultery. Our homes and cities are safe and free from crime. Our lives are safe. We are a simple people—but we are content.

This man holding my hand, I thought to myself, has never tasted the fruits of Western civilization: the music of Beethoven and Mozart; the literature of Shakespeare, the Brownings, or Milton; the glory of the opera; the heavenly voices of Callas, Sutherland, or Caruso; the fantasy of the ballet, all brought to life by men and women who were free to develop their talents. The genius of Rembrandt and Cézanne and the philosophy of Aristotle, Plato, and Socrates are a complete blank. For him, none of these exist. He is happy or content because he does not know what he is missing. A sound is not a sound unless there is someone present to hear it. Must one have knowledge to be free? Must one experience all the arts to be lofty?

We continued to walk in silence, hand in hand. We of the Western world are pioneers in technology, I mused: electricity, the automobile, radio, telephone, air conditioning, television, the airplane, and flight into space. We are leaders in the medical sciences. We are concerned with public health, longevity, low infant mortality, preventive medicine, and molecular biology. We have produced the great physicists, pioneered in radioactivity, nuclear medicine, and the laser beam. We split the atom, created the atomic bomb; developed nuclear energy, the electron microscope, cloning.

Our people are free, our women are free. We have the highest standard of living in the world. We are Superman! But in the United States we have race riots, murder in the streets, desecration of churches and synagogues, mugging, arson, and rape. Our women are free but sexually permissive. We have drug addiction, alcoholism, and the highest crime rate in the world. We still have areas of poverty. We have free elections, Watergate, sleazy, corrupt politicians in high places, widespread neuroses, poor mental health, and sexual perversion.

Yes, I felt sorry for the prince but not too sorry. Who was the happier man, the more complete man? I was uncertain.

He looked at me, smiled, squeezed my hand, and asked, "Goood?"

"*Kweyyis,*" I replied, with a wan smile.

THE CAMEL RACE

THE PRINCE was discharged from the hospital shortly afterward. Several weeks later Nasser called as he had promised, to invite me to the camel races. He picked me up at the hospital one afternoon in his Mercedes.

The racetrack and sports stadium were located in the northeast section of Riyadh not far from Airport Road. The stadium had only recently been built, and was large and impressive. The spectators' stand was rather small but elaborate. Its steeply slanted roof was supported by white pillars. There were two rows of large, deep leather chairs down front, presumably for the royalty. The total seating capacity was only about five hundred.

Prince Nasser wore a white thobe and a beautiful royal-blue mantel lined with gold. He brought along two of his younger brothers. The youngest, about sixteen, had no facial hair; the other brother, who was a few years older, had a fine wisp of a mustache. In Saudi Arabia, there seemed to be a universal progression from clean-shaven at fifteen to a suggestion of a mustache at eighteen, which appeared full blown at twenty, and was accompanied by a beard at thirty.

We sat in the front row, reserved for royalty, but not in the center section, which was obviously reserved for the King and Crown Prince. This area was distinguished by several large, brilliant-colored carpets, upon which stood two huge blue suède chairs.

The racetrack was enclosed by white picket fencing. In the center was a cluster of camels of the one-humped dromedary variety, attended to by their grooms.

We were given four mimeographed sheets listing the details of each race. There were two camel races to be followed by four horse races. The distance and the prize money were noted for each race. The prize money for the first race was a paltry 2,500 riyals ($800). There were no prizes for second place or show. The distance was 2,800 meters, a little over one mile and a half.

Our conversation naturally turned to the camels and to the Bedouins who were racing them.

"In a way," said Nasser, "the Bedouins were like your American Indians. They were fierce fighters and hunters, constantly battling the elements. They could survive for long periods of time on camel's milk and a few dates in spite of the intense heat of the desert and the shortage of water."

"I read somewhere that the Bedouin, like the Indian, developed a sixth sense, an instinct for navigation by the shadows of the sun on the sand, and by the stars and the wind."

"No doubt about that," said Nasser. "They navigated the desert without a compass. If they got lost that was the end. Their life depended on the camel. The camel was more important to the Bedouin than the horse was to the Indian."

Nasser proceeded to give me a discourse on the camel: The camel was the Bedouins' only means of transportation in the desert and frequently their only source of food. It was indispensable because it could convert brackish water into rich milk, and desert vegetation into meat. Their hides were used for shelter and for clothing, their dung was burned for cooking or heat in the cold desert nights. They also served, of course, as beasts of burden.

"You see," he concluded, "the camel was their main means of livelihood for hundreds of years, and the replacement of the camel by the truck was a catastrophe for them."

The grooms began to walk the camels around to "warm them up." They certainly were peculiar-looking, I thought. How could anyone race them without falling off? They looked so clumsy!

"Do you know," Nasser said, "that a camel can store forty gallons of water in the stomach at one time? Its hump is an accumulation of fat, which shrinks if the camel is worked too hard. It's like a fuel gauge to the camel driver. The hump stores fat for energy. It's a sort of a natural gas tank."

"With the camel supplying its own gasoline," I remarked with a smile.

The first race began at 5 P.M. There was no starting gate. The seven camels were lined up, and at a given signal they strutted off. It looked pretty funny, at first. A rider, with his long thobe flapping in the breeze, sat on a blanket just behind the hump. There were no stirrups. Each camel wore a colored collar to which the reins were attached. Racing camels can run fourteen miles per hour, and the riders are flung about violently. It was an amusing spectacle. That they avoided being thrown off seemed little short of a miracle.

Close to the finish line two camels were in a dead heat. One of them belonged to Nasser. I stood up and was about to yell encouragement for "our" camel when I realized that the stands had been in utter silence from the beginning, and now, at this critical moment, there was not a murmur. Nasser and his brother watched in detached silence, not a flicker from any of them, not one display of emotion, not the slightest show of excitement. The prince's camel finished second in an extremely close race. Nasser remained poker-faced. I could discern no sign of disappointment whatever.

The second camel race was 1,400 meters, much shorter than the first, and carried a prize of 3,500 riyals ($1,200). Again, the race was shrouded in silence.

I asked Nasser about betting. "It is against the custom," he said.

Maybe that's why it was so quiet, I thought. There was no real excitement and there were only 150 people instead of thousands, as in the States.

"We're all friends here," explained Nasser, "and we are interested mainly in breeding. The prize money is given to the riders and to the attendants. But the last race today is for the King's Cup."

The two camel races were preliminaries to the main events—the horse races. These prizes varied from 4,300 riyals ($1,400) to 13,500 riyals ($4,500), and the number of horses running in each race varied from eight to ten.

The Arabian horses were stunning. They were impeccably groomed, their manes braided with multicolored ribbons and tassels, pink, red, white, or green. They stood from fourteen to fifteen hands in height. Their gallop was long and low, a beautiful sight to behold.

Cardamom coffee in small flowered glass cups was served before the first race and was followed later by tea poured into round, short glasses with handles, placed on gold saucers. As the races progressed, more people dribbled in. By the final cup race, there were some two hundred Saudis present, all men, with a sprinkling of Americans, English, and other foreigners.

Just before the race for the King's Cup, the King and the Crown Prince arrived with the military attachés in tow and took their seats front and center. The King, as usual, looked uncomfortable, and the Crown Prince put on his best, fixed smile. While preparations were underway for the start of the race, the King and Crown Prince were served coffee and then tea. The Crown Prince, seated some twenty feet away, to my left, became a bit restless and began drumming his fingers on the arm of his chair, still maintaining his perpetual smile. This was the end of a long day and he was probably anxious to get home, but in this instance public relations were doubly important because the royal family owned most of the horses in this race. Prince Yusef, for example, had horse No. 2 carrying his colors.

There was a stir of excitement that seemed to build.

"I hope to win this one," Nasser said eagerly, seeming not to think of anything else. I told him I'd be happy to photograph his receiving the cup from the King.

"*Inshallah*," he said fervently.

An attendant brought a huge ornate silver cup and placed it on the table in front of the King. The Crown Prince kept drumming his fingers on the arm of the chair, smiling pleasantly all the while. The horses, glistening in the late-afternoon sun, were paraded before the royal stand and slowly led to the starting line on the opposite side of the track. There were eight horses. The distance was 2,000 meters, a little over a mile.

At a given signal they were off. Nobody stood up; nobody cheered.

The stands were heavy with silence. I looked at Nasser. He was calmly drinking his tea, showing no sign of emotion or tension. A few spectators were following the horses with binoculars. It was quiet, almost hushed. Nasser's horse broke third at the start, then took the lead at the half, and gradually drew ahead. At this point, I arose and cheered him loudly. It was a spontaneous reaction.

I wasn't really conscious of what I was doing. I just wanted the prince's horse to win. As they approached the last turn another horse, suddenly appearing from nowhere, drew up to challenge the leader. As our horse drifted out a bit around the last turn into the stretch, I screamed, "Keep inside—keep inside—don't let him through," but it was too late. The challenger cut in on the inside and won the race by a nose.

I soon became aware of all the noise I had made, and besides, the jockey wouldn't have understood even if he had heard me.

"It was the jockey's fault," I announced to Nasser. "He should've stayed close to the rail on the inside. I'm terribly sorry we lost—it was so close."

Nasser just sat there drinking his tea. He looked at me with a hint of a smile. There was no expression of disappointment, frustration, anger, or remorse. He showed no emotion whatever. His brothers were similarly poker-faced.

Maybe it was their religious upbringing to accept the will of Allah, to believe that all is divine plan, that all is predetermined. In a way, it makes life a lot easier, I thought to myself.

The owner of the winning horse approached the royal area. The King handed him the silver cup without a word as the cameras clicked. They shook hands. Then the Crown Prince shook the winner's hand, and he returned to his seat nearby. Nasser and the brothers immediately approached the winner, offered their congratulations, shook hands, and returned to their seats. Several friends came up and congratulated Nasser on a close race. He just nodded and smiled. The royal party departed immediately. Their total stay was approximately thirty minutes.

I learned something about Saudi Arabian character that day. They probably learned something about crazy Americans who yell at horses in a strange language.

Nasser told me of a colorful event which I should attend, if possible. It was the annual camel marathon, always held on a Friday, at which more than six hundred camels took part. The distance was twenty-five miles and it was open to any Bedouin with a camel. There was prize money for the first three camels, but the main incentive for the others was a reward of 200 riyals (about $60) for anyone who finished the race. I was reminded of the jogging marathons at home, where hundreds of joggers run merely for the satisfaction of crossing the finish line. The vast majority know full well they can't win. It seemed that every Bedouin who owned a camel entered the marathon just to get across the finish line for the $60 awaiting them.

Westbrook enthusiastically endorsed the idea of going to the marathon and organized a caravan of four cars. I rode with Philip, Manda, Doris, and Al in the mighty Landcruiser. The only directions to the event had been published in the *Sand Script*, the hospital news bulletin. At that time there were no street signs. Directions were usually given in terms of familiar landmarks, such as the Pepsi-Cola bottling plant, the Toyota building, or an overturned truck. The directions read: "Take the road to Dhahran for 5 miles past the Toyota building then left for three miles to a large mound of sand, then right on a dirt road for four miles until you come to an overturned truck. Take a left at the first road past the truck" . . . and so forth.

The finish line of the marathon was located at an oasis about thirty miles east of Riyadh. Philip found it without difficulty. As we approached we saw a semicircle of bright green flags fluttering in the breeze, each bearing the golden emblem of Saudi Arabia. It was a clear, sunny morning and pleasantly mild. Several hundred Saudi men in thobes and some foreigners in Western clothes were milling about in an effort to get the best view.

The royals sat on large pillowed armchairs placed upon colorful carpets in front of the finish line. Among them were Prince Abdullah, the commander of the National Guard, rumored to be next in line as Crown Prince, and Prince Sultan, the Minister of Defense and commander of the army. The King and Crown Prince sat in the center upon special throne-like chairs which were taller and more impressive than the others.

The finish line was designated by two small flags. On each side stood two long lines of the National Guard dressed in khaki.

The marathon was already in progress. Every few minutes there was an announcement over the loudspeaker in a subdued monotone. Al told us that the lead camel belonged to one of King Khalid's sons.

"Anybody want bet?" he asked, dropping his vowels, as usual.

"I'll bet you ten riyals," I offered, to make things interesting.

"You crazy," he said. "Nobody try beat King's camel."

"You never can tell. His camel may break down," I replied.

He looked at me with a smile of superiority.

A half hour later a camel could be seen in the distance. It was the King's camel. As soon as he crossed the finish line, the rider, completely exhausted, flung himself to the ground.

One of the soldiers grasped the camel's reins. Nobody cheered. The next two camels were not far behind. They belonged to royals too, according to Al, who pocketed my ten riyals with glee as the announcer congratulated the three winners. One of the judges, I noticed, recorded the names of the winning riders, given to them by the soldiers at the finish line.

A few minutes later there was an avalanche of camels, the "also rans." There were hundreds of them crossing the finish line in groups of five to ten or more. There was no way of identifying rider or camel. They wore no numbers or distinguishing colors. A rider in a skull cap merely tied his long thobe into a knot above his knees, crouched just behind the camel's hump, and held on to the reins for dear life.

As soon as they crossed the line they handed the reins to the soldiers and then gave their names to the judges for the record. Eventually each would collect two hundred riyals.

As time went on there were fewer and fewer camels left. They were the stragglers, yet they would receive the same reward as the others, providing they finished the race and crossed the line.

Suddenly a figure appeared a hundred yards from the finish line. A Bedouin had fallen off his camel and was walking his animal, reins in hand, to finish the race by foot. It was a pathetic sight. His thobe was dirty and torn. One of his sandals was missing. Matted blood and dirt covered his face and knees. His arms were deeply gouged and bloody. He limped across the finish line, holding on to the reins of his camel, which also looked the worse for wear.

He held his head high and walked with pride. There was an air of arrogance about him. When he went to give his name to the judges, they refused to accept it. He became angry. His eyes sparkled with rage.

"I want to see the King," he shouted. "I know my rights." A small crowd gathered, including a few soldiers and a newspaper reporter who spoke English and interpreted for me. Someone from the King's entourage appeared with a pad of paper in his hand. He was in uniform.

"I demand to see the King," said the Bedouin with mounting fury, still holding on to his camel.

The newspaperman explained that the *majlis* is an old Bedouin tradition which allows any citizen to deliver a complaint or a request directly to the King, to the Crown Prince, or to a senior government official. The *majlis* or assembly is held at regular intervals, and anyone can attend to register his grievance.

"A *majlis* at a camel marathon will make a great story," he added with enthusiasm. "I hope they let me print it."

The King was standing some distance away, on his special carpet, chatting with some of his friends and high officials in the front row. The uniformed man carrying the pad of paper approached the King, spoke to him briefly, and returned to the Bedouin.

"The King will see you," he said.

The Bedouin turned the reins over to a soldier and hobbled over to the King. He explained that he had been thrown from the camel near the finish line, but both he and camel had completed the race together although he was not on the camel, strictly speaking, at the end of the race. He felt that he was entitled to the 200 riyals.

The King looked pensive and agreed. He instructed his aide to record the Bedouin's name on the list for payment.

The Bedouin, proud and haughty as ever, did not thank the King. He turned and walked away to collect his camel, and then disappeared into the crowd.

I imagine the King felt that $60 was not exorbitant in view of Saudi Arabia's international monetary reserves of $28.8 billion and foreign assets of $70 billion, which were increasing at the rate of $1 billion a month.

But I was impressed that this feudal elite monarchy was a benign one, and pretty much in touch with the common man. What chance would I have to arrange an interview at a moment's notice with the President of the United States at the Kentucky Derby?

◊ *8* ◊

"*YOU* DID IT!"

TWO MONTHS HAD PASSED and my monastic way of life was almost at an end. It was a gradual, almost imperceptible, but inevitable return to the ways of the world. My trunk and books had arrived from Boston and I began to read again. A tiny bookstore nearby sold the *Arab News,* the English-language paper, and the *International Herald Tribune.* I dove into both and read voraciously everything I could find in the shop. I realized, that it was an addiction. I was a social animal and could no longer remain an island unto myself.

One day soon after I had discovered the bookstore I noticed that the first *Herald Tribune* on top of the stack had a hole in the front page. That was peculiar, I thought. The second *Herald Tribune* underneath had an identical hole. All the *Herald Tribunes* had holes on their front pages, which showed a map of the Middle East. The Saudi censors had cut the State of Israel out of the map because, in the Arab view, Israel did not exist. That made me very angry and I was back to reality again.

My wife was due to leave London any day now to join me in Riyadh. I looked forward with delight to having her once again with me, and with dismay over the dreary room at the Al Yamama that would be our home. Just before she was scheduled to arrive, Philip Westbrook called with the news that an apartment similar to theirs in the Al Sharq Hotel would soon be available. He told me to stake my claim by moving several of my trunks into the apartment before the present occupant moved out. Philip assured me that this was the standard procedure. The people about to vacate the apartment were very cooperative. They had taken the same course of action previously, they assured me.

Ruth is an anglophile and the English community welcomed her with open arms, so that my life changed immediately upon her arrival. It's amazing what a woman can do, I thought. She transformed that dismal apartment by hanging brilliant-colored scarves on all the walls with Scotch tape. They fell off now and then, but we had plenty of tape and Ruth had a plethora of beautiful scarves. And because we had no closets, we hung our clothes on broomsticks which I had nailed into the corners of the bedroom as Philip had done.

Although our lifestyle at the Al Sharq was different from that in our home in Boston, Ruth adjusted wonderfully. We often laughed at our discomfort—we knew it was temporary and made the best of it.

My wife is a portrait painter and had shipped all her paints, brushes, and other equipment to Riyadh months in advance; she returned to her painting shortly after she arrived. Ruth also began to enjoy the new sights and smells of Saudi Arabia in the company of a number of women she met at the Al Sharq Hotel who were in similar circumstances.

The only real difficulties were transportation and the tradition that a woman could not leave the hotel unless she was accompanied by one or two other women. I tried to arrange for a driver and a car, but this proved impossible. I paid whatever they asked, but they would come for one or two days and then disappear. The women finally resorted to taxis, which were safe providing there were two or more women. Hospital buses came by the hotel twice a week for trips to the shopping areas, but I sympathized with the difficulties the women encountered in moving about freely in this country.

Meanwhile, Nasser and I schemed to ask Ruth to do a portrait of Prince Yusef, which we would present to him at the palace as a surprise. Nasser gave me a snapshot of his father, making me promise not to tell anyone who had given it to me. Ruth agreed that a Saudi Arabian prince would make an interesting subject, and the snapshot intrigued her. She spent several months on the portrait, and with the help of an artist friend found a gold frame which set it off beautifully.

Nasser arranged a gathering at the palace, where the painting would be unveiled. The prince was unaware of the purpose of the party, although he knew I was planning to bring my wife with me.

A few days before the unveiling the prince's secretary called me at the hospital and said the prince needed a refill of one of his medications. The secretary, a man in his fifties, discreetly broached the subject of the party when we met in the clinic.

"The prince is pleased that you will be visiting him on Friday," he said. He apparently knew nothing of the painting.

"Yes," I said, "we are looking forward to it. My wife will be with me."

He looked very uncomfortable, almost miserable. "Dr. Gray, I do not know if you understand. It would be embarrassing to have your wife at a gentlemen's social gathering."

The secretary was politely trying to tell me not to be a fool.

"I do understand, but she is not a Saudi. She's an American. It would be awkward for me not to have her come along. She has heard so much about the prince from me."

"It is against the custom," he said with emphasis. This was the real reason he had come.

I certainly wasn't going to argue by informing him that my wife had done the painting for which the surprise party was being held. So I took the risk. "Please tell the prince that I would be pleased to be his guest, but it would not be appropriate for me to come without my wife."

"It is against the custom," he said again, very firmly. "The prince, however, will see you on Friday."

We shook hands. He looked unhappy as he left.

Standing in the middle of the hall, I was dumbfounded. Of course, Ruth would go.

It was late Friday afternoon. Ruth and I were getting dressed for our royal visit. Against the wall in a corner of the bedroom the painting waited. The resemblance to the prince was uncanny.

No Saudi would ever believe a woman could be such a master at her craft.

"It's really something, Ruth," I said, staring at the penetrating eyes.

"Seymour, I feel like such an outcast already. I don't want to ruin the evening by wearing something wrong. I wonder what I should wear?"

"You must cover your arms and legs," I insisted. "What do you have?"

She tried on several dresses, to find the one most appropriate. Finally, she selected a full-length dress with long sleeves and wore a sheer golden veil on her hair.

"You look lovely," I assured her.

"I feel as though I am about to be presented at court," she said, laughing.

We had wrapped the gold-framed painting in a soft deep-blue cloth just as Nasser arrived to pick us up. Carrying the painting carefully, I placed it in his car and then introduced my wife.

"*Marhaba,*" he said respectfully and shook Ruth's extended hand. He continued, "I hope you will not be uncomfortable with my father. He is not accustomed to having women in his presence in situations like this. But, of course, in this case, you should be there."

Nasser's demonic driving had us at the palace in no time. A servant drew apart two huge gates, which opened into a large walled-off compound housing Prince Yusef's family. Nasser drove us into a vast courtyard containing four identical palatial villas, presumably one for each wife. The villas were arranged in a quadrangle, each with its own terrace and gardens. The highly manicured lawns looked too perfect to walk upon. Sculptured shrubs served as backdrops for the numerous colorful flower beds.

"I will have the servants place it in the sitting room," Nasser said, taking the painting out of the back seat.

"What do you think?" Ruth whispered to me as I opened her door.

"Don't worry. Anyway, our palace at home is much nicer. The prince said so himself. I'm sure everything is going to be just fine."

I was wrong!

We approached the villa just to the left of the entrance and proceeded through an echo-filled foyer with unusually high ceilings, designed to keep the building cool. Although the villa was palatial in size, it was utterly lacking in style, and in fact was sparsely furnished.

We were escorted into a large sitting room by two servants, and were met by the prince's secretary, who appeared stiff and uncomfortable. I sensed that this was not going to be a jolly occasion because Ruth had come with me, contrary to his admonition a few days previously.

We were shocked to find a complete absence of elegance in the home of this immensely wealthy prince. A succession of deep velvet cushioned sofas, faded violet in color, lined two sides of the room. The walls, hung with heavily textured draperies, looked drab and barren. There were no pictures or paintings to break the monotony. (Mirrors, for example, are forbidden in the orthodox home.) A gaudy Chinese carpet covered the floor. The only decoration was a gold-framed family tree adorning one wall. Even so the effect was dull and colorless.

The prince sat in one corner of the sofa wearing his full-length white thobe and red-checkered ghutra. And yet, even seated, he impressed us with his majestic bearing and dignified appearance. When he saw Ruth he looked startled and perturbed. Trying to conceal his discomfort, he stood and nodded his head when I introduced Ruth. He looked taller than ever. His smile directed toward me was forced. Forgotten was the warm bond of friendship which had grown between us, the holding of hands as we walked down the corridors, and the long discussions of our individual cultures. This was a direct East-West confrontation. I had dared to bring a woman into his house—even though she was my wife and an attractive one at that. He was furious! Women had no place here.

Nasser and his father exchanged a few words in Arabic. The whole arrangement seemed most distasteful to the prince. His eyes were sad and his pained expression betrayed his bewilderment. He could not comprehend what was going on and probably wanted to get away from it all. What was a woman doing here! It was intolerable to him. Silently he lifted the phone on the table next to him and ordered the usual cardamom coffee and tea.

Meanwhile, the servants had placed the painting, still in its blue cloth wrapping, on the table.

Coffee was served immediately.

"Nasser, what is this, please?" the prince pointed to the bulky item in blue.

"Wait, father." Nasser walked over to the table and carefully lifted the soft cloth from the painting as though he were unveiling a bride. Then he stood beside it, proudly presenting this incredible portrait to its subject.

The prince's eyes were glued to the work for a few seconds, but he expressed no emotion. He looked away in disbelief. Then the prince indulged in a more careful examination of the work. I could tell that he appreciated it. Yet he never smiled. He didn't ask any questions. But he knew it was good.

I broke the heavy silence with the coup de grâce. "Prince Yusef," I paused deliberately, leaned back, and smiled, "my wife did it." Nasser interpreted.

The prince was incredulous! His pupils dilated. Looking at me he raised his voice in anger, "No, *you* did it." He repeated for emphasis, "*You* did it!"

The secretary confronted me indignantly. "His royal highness says, '*You* did it,'" he reiterated in English.

"I had nothing to do with it," I said simply.

Nasser smiled. I asked him to explain the whole matter to the prince before things got out of hand.

"I cannot paint, your highness. My wife has been doing this for many years. She has studied this art. I could never do what she has done. Now you understand why I insisted that she come with me. It is her masterpiece for you."

The prince never looked at Ruth. He slowly sipped his coffee. "*You* did it," he said with a note of finality.

Our evening was not dull only because it was so fascinating to watch the prince's discomfort in the presence of a woman. The situation was as unbelievable to me as it was to him.

Ruth was actually pleased with his reaction. She did not need his acknowledgment to realize that she had produced an excellent likeness. It was, however, obviously incomprehensible to him that a mere woman could produce this magnificent portrait. He couldn't fathom it.

After we took our departure, Ruth asked Nasser if she could look in on another one of the villas.

"I cannot," he said with a polite smile. "I mean I should not."

"Oh, it will be just a quick look," she promised him. "I hope you will excuse my curiosity."

Nasser glanced around quickly. He walked ahead into the first villa on the right to make sure it was all clear. Then he beckoned us to follow.

It was shocking. This place was identical in every way to the other. Ruth and I tried to hide our amazement, but could not resist gaping at the mirror-image interior. The same velvet sofas were placed in the same manner. Identical Chinese carpets covered the floors, and the same dreary drapes and wallpaper adorned the plain walls.

The first floor of this miniature palace was deserted. The women were probably upstairs, I concluded. We didn't say anything; we just stared in utter amazement.

As we left I noticed the gold-framed family tree, placed on the same wall in the same location as in the prince's villa. The prince's paternal bloodline went back to the original Al Saud, the founder of the present ruling dynasty (1706–1765). The family tree listed the male ancestors only. I wondered how the women who lived here felt about it. Maybe they just took it for granted or more likely they couldn't read anyway.

I met the prince on many occasions afterward. For the next three years the ritual was always the same. Instead of greeting me with a cordial "*Marhaba,*" the prince would always smile and say pointedly, "*You* did it." He still wasn't convinced.

◇ *9* ◇

DIALOGUES WITH A PRINCESS

By THE MIDDLE of December my life in Saudi Arabia had settled into a routine that, if quite exotic by American standards, was increasingly comfortable and familiar. I found that I was growing accustomed to the sights and smells of the Middle East—the black veils on the women, the colorful ghutras on the men, and the fragrant perfumes that emanated from the members of both sexes. The weather in Riyadh was much cooler, and the noontime temperatures had dropped from a sweltering 125 degrees to a comparatively tolerable 90. In the dry plateau air these winter afternoons were exceedingly pleasant, and I often went for long walks around the city, especially near sundown, when the desert sky became a beautiful fiery orange.

At the hospital, my medical duties had likewise become patterned and predictable. The patients were no longer exotic creatures from another century, but simply Saudi Arabians, each one similar to the hundreds that had already passed through my clinic. Although I continued to have frequent contacts with the Saudi royal family, the sense of awe that had tinged my initial encounters had been replaced by a more objective appraisal. There were, I knew, approximately eight thousand people who qualified for the status of prince or princess, and the royal title soon lost its novelty and glamour. Indeed, I found that I often enjoyed treating the Bedouins more than the royalty, because there was something indecipherable and alluring about these nomadic desert dwellers who were untouched by Western ideas.

The Bedouin women were especially fascinating. Every time one of them came to the clinic I found myself involved in a confrontation of cultural norms. As I had learned earlier, much to my surprise, the Bedouin women did not object to undressing or exposing their breasts and genital areas, providing that their faces remained covered. They were adamantly opposed to removing their veils and exposing their faces, whenever they came to the clinic. I tried to convince them that it was necessary to examine their eyes, ears, and throats as part of a physical examination. Only after they had asked for and received their husbands' permission would these Bedouin women reluctantly uncover their faces, enduring an almost wrenching trauma and embarrassment in the process.

In contrast to their Bedouin counterparts, some of the women of Riyadh tended to have a more Western orientation, and were quite willing to remove their veils, at least in front of an American doctor. When they were in public—or in the presence of a Saudi male—even the modern women were scrupulous about keeping their faces covered. In the hospital, the veils were kept beside the bed, and only the more conservative women covered themselves when I entered the room. It intrigued me that the Saudi women felt more comfortable with an American doctor than with Saudi men, and I often wondered how they would react to a Saudi doctor, suspecting that they would insist on covering themselves. Unfortunately, there was no way for me to test this assumption, for at the time there were no Saudi doctors on the staff of my hospital. In a very real sense, the hospital served as a haven where Saudi women were temporarily freed from the customs and restrictions of their society.

One afternoon in December, I received a phone call from a distinguished member of the royal family, who informed me that his daughter was extremely sick and that she was being sent to the hospital by ambulance. Princess Sultana bint Musaid Al Sudairi arrived at the emergency room a short time later with what looked suspiciously like the symptoms of typhoid. I immediately started an intravenous infusion of fluids and then rushed her blood sample to the laboratory, where it was confirmed that she was dehydrated and had lost a considerable amount of salt and water. However, the blood tests and cultures revealed that the princess was not suffering from typhoid, but rather from a severe form of dysentery, probably caused by contaminated food or water.

I treated the princess with antibiotic medication and intravenous fluids to counteract the bacterial infection and to establish a more normal salt and water balance. Within several days, she began to show signs of recovery. Her fever subsided, her blood tests returned to normal, and her physical appearance began to improve. However, she was still dehydrated and very weak from her ordeal. I arranged for her to stay in the hospital, where she could recover her strength and where her condition could be monitored in the event of a relapse.

During this period of convalescence I visited the princess each day on my hospital rounds, asking her questions and keeping an eye on her medical condition. As she recovered, I gradually noticed that the princess was a beautiful young woman—stunningly beautiful, in fact. Although she was only nineteen years old, her features reflected strength and a maturity beyond her years. Her skin was fair, almost English in coloring, and it was strikingly contrasted by her glistening black hair and large brown eyes. Her facial features were flawless—smooth skin, an aristocratic nose, and a perfectly-formed mouth that smiled to reveal dazzling white teeth. She possessed the brooding sensuality of a true Middle Eastern beauty, the allure and excitement that are envisioned behind the dark, mysterious veil.

In addition to her physical beauty, the princess possessed a special elegance and grace that bespoke her aristocratic upbringing. I soon learned that Princess Sultana was a member of the Sudairi family, an ancient tribal family that formed one of the dominant wings of the House of Saud. Her father and grandfather were among the most important men in the kingdom, and she was directly related to almost every notable member of the royal family. If there was an elite within the House of Saud, it was the Sudairi family, and I knew that the princess was no ordinary patient, even by royal standards.

One day as I was making my rounds I entered the princess's private suite and found her sitting in a chair, holding a hand mirror while a servant ran a comb through her hair. The princess was clearly on the road to recovery, and for the first time I felt the full effects of her charm and beauty.

"Hello, doctor," said the princess, fixing me with her most dazzling smile.

"Hello, princess," I replied. "Are you feeling better today?"

"I feel *super!*" she said gaily. It was comforting to see her in such good spirits. Sometimes the most positive medical signs are not as encouraging as a carefree laugh.

I began to ask the princess some questions in English, which she answered with an easy, almost casual fluency. We had conversed in English on several previous occasions, but now my curiosity was aroused.

"You speak English very well," I complimented her after completing my examination. "Where did you learn it?"

"In California," she replied.

"What?" said I, looking up from my medical charts. "What were you doing in California?"

"I grew up there," she said matter-of-factly. "I lived in California until I was six years old. My mother is American."

I looked at the princess in surprise. There was nothing in her physical features that indicated an American mother; indeed, her appearance was almost classically Saudi Arabian except for her fair skin. Moreover, I knew that the royal family frowned on marriages outside the Moslem faith. Clearly, she had a very unusual background.

"How could you have an American mother? I thought the members of the royal family were forbidden to marry foreigners."

"This happened twenty years ago," she replied. "It was unusual at the time, but it was not forbidden as it is now. In those days, we Saudi Arabians still regarded the Americans with a kind of awe."

In response to my obvious interest, the princess explained that her father was the son of an important Saudi prince, and that he went to Stanford University in the late 1950s to study economics. During his second week in school he met and fell in love with an American girl, a fellow student, whom he married at the end of his first year of college. For the next seven years they lived together in California, the prince pursuing his education, including postgraduate studies, while his American wife alternated between the classroom and the maternity ward. Eventually, they had three children. Sultana was the oldest. Her brother Sultan was seventeen, and a sister was fifteen.

"You see," she said, "I was born in Palo Alto, California, and lived there until I was six. I mean, I was a real American then, you know? Then we moved to Riyadh. Of course, that didn't last long, and when I was eleven, we moved back to California. But then, after only two years, it was back to Riyadh, and I've really lived here since. Well, we take lots of vacations in Europe and the United States. . . ."

Sultana paused, lost in thought of her childhood. "Living in California was *super*," she said, with a touch of nostalgia. "I was allowed to wear miniskirts and to play the radio all day long. My father frowned on records, but my sister and I bought them anyway. My favorite group was the Beatles. I *loved* Paul McCartney!"

"Are your mother and father living in Saudi Arabia right now?"

She shook her head. "My mother asked for a divorce several years ago. She could no longer live in Saudi Arabia."

"I can understand that."

"No," said the princess, "you do not understand. My mother came to Saudi Arabia when I was six, and she made herself fit into it. She converted to Islam, and learned to speak fluent Arabic. The other women in our family did not accept her at first, partly because she was American, and partly because she married my father. You see, my father is a great man, and he is the son of a great man, and it is our custom for family members to marry cousins. Many of the women in our family hoped to marry my father one day, and instead he came back from America with three children and a wife—and an American wife at that!

"But they eventually learned to love my mother. She observed Moslem custom, and behaved like a good woman. They understood that she was American, and that she did not always do things the proper Saudi way, but they knew that she tried. They were all very sad when my mother and father were divorced."

"Why did she ask for the divorce if she fitted in so well?"

The princess shrugged. "My mother learned to accept Saudi Arabia, but she could never become a part of it. She would go to Europe and America every year, and it became harder for her to come back. One year she stayed away too long, and then she realized that she could never live here again."

"Where does she live now?"

"Los Angeles," said the princess. "Two years ago my whole family went to visit her there. My father even brought his new wife, my stepmother. My mother and stepmother had never met before. They became good friends."

"Wait a minute. Did your father have more than one wife when he married your mother?"

"No. He knew that it would hurt her, so he had only one wife. He remarried after the divorce from my mother. My stepmother is only seven years older than I am. We are very close, almost like sisters. I love my stepmother very much."

"Isn't it unusual for a prince to have only one wife at a time, particularly when he can have four?"

"My father was educated in the U.S.," replied Sultana, "and he has modern ideas, like one wife at a time."

I was about to ask another question, but, glancing at my watch, noted that I had fallen behind schedule. "I must go," I said reluctantly. "Perhaps we can talk some more this evening, princess."

"Yes!" she said with obvious enthusiasm. "I love to talk about my country. Also, it is nice to talk with a man from the outside for a change. Normally, I can only talk with the men in my family."

"Wonderful. In that case, I'll come to see you tonight after dinner."

"Groovy," replied the princess with a dazzling smile.

I walked out the door of her room, shaking my head. "Groovy?" This country seemed to grow more curious all the time.

That evening I made a return visit to the hospital room of Princess Sultana. The princess was staying in a royal suite, which consisted of a spacious bedroom and a smaller but comfortable adjoining sitting room. A female servant remained in the suite with the princess twenty-four hours a day, sleeping on the couch in the sitting room so that she could be available at all times. I remembered that Prince Yusef had had a similar arrangement, with servants at his beck and call around the clock. Sultana's servant was always there, providing a third set of ears and eyes as required by Saudi culture in a meeting between a woman and a man.

"Come in, Dr. Gray," called the princess when I knocked twice on the door. The two knocks were a signal so that the princess would not have to cover her face with a veil. I entered and found the princess lying in her bed, watching television. She immediately sat up and switched off the television set by remote control.

"I'm glad you're here," she said, pointing to the television set and grimacing. "Television in Saudi Arabia is so *awful*. I sure wish we could get some American channels."

Having watched some Saudi television myself, I knew exactly what she meant. The television programs were heavily censored, and only the most innocuous and uncontroversial subjects were presented. One of the favorite formats was a "talk show," in which religious leaders discussed and interpreted verses from the Koran. In general, the Moslem clergy were opposed to television, on the grounds that it represented a violation of the Islamic injunction against idolatry. Under Wahabism—the strict fundamentalist version of Islam practiced in Saudi Arabia—any representation of the human form was frowned upon, including even children's dolls. Portraits of royalty, however, were acceptable.

"Tell me," I said after we had finished our lament about Saudi television, "when your mother divorced your father, why did you stay in Saudi Arabia?"

"Because this is Moslem law," she replied. "When a man divorces a woman, the children stay with the man and the woman is sent back to her family."

"But did you want to go back to America?"

The princess paused. "No," she said quietly. "I am a Saudi princess and I do as my father wishes. I like going to America and visiting my mother, but this is my home. This is my country."

"If you lived the first six years of your life in California, why do you feel so strongly that you are a Saudi Arabian?"

"I don't know," she replied. "It is not something that can be explained. I like America a lot, but it is not my home. I *feel* like a Saudi Arabian."

I could sense that her nationality was a delicate issue to the princess, and so I decided to change the subject. "Let's talk about what it was like to be a woman growing up in Saudi Arabia," I suggested. "After all, it must have been very strange moving from California to Riyadh and changing from miniskirts to veils."

The princess laughed. "I was twelve or thirteen years old when I moved to Saudi Arabia, and I was very tall for my age. I remember all the Saudi men used to stare at me with guppy eyes, and I did not understand why. In California, the men would sometimes look at me, but they did not stare like the Saudi men. I found it very creepy. Later, when I had lived in Saudi Arabia for a while, I learned that it is common for girls to marry at age fifteen. For someone my age to be walking around with her face and legs bare was an extremely provocative act, almost like walking around naked in the U.S."

"Some girls do that in California," I said, laughing. "Those bikinis don't leave much to the imagination. When did you begin to cover your face and wear an *abeyya?*"

"Probably thirteen or so."

"And did your father make you wear the veil?"

"No!" she said strongly. "My father is not like that. For many months after I moved to Saudi Arabia I wore nothing except my normal Western clothing. I would go out wearing shorts and tennis shoes, and all the men would be guppy-eyed when they looked at me. But, after a while, as I became more of a Saudi, I began to feel uncomfortable in Western clothing."

"In what way did you feel uncomfortable?"

Sultana smiled. "In Saudi Arabia the old women are very direct. They would look at me and say, 'Where is your abeyya? Where is your gutwah?' They let me know that I was doing something wrong. Finally, I got tired of being harassed, and I started wearing my veil. Now I would not think to go out of the house without it."

"At what age do most Saudi women begin to wear a veil?"

"There is no special age. You are supposed to start wearing a veil when you become a woman, which is usually around fourteen or so. The point is that you are supposed to cover up when you become attractive to men. You can tell when that time comes because of the way the men leer at you."

"What do the men do?"

The princess suddenly leaned forward and opened her dazzling eyes very wide.

"The men stare at you like you are a freak," she said. "Any girl who goes around with her face uncovered will be stared at, and it's a terrible experience. You become very conscious of the stares and you begin to feel dirty. It is much easier to wear a veil and avoid these problems."

"What is it like wearing a veil?" I asked. "Is is hot? Can you see?"

The princess shrugged. "It isn't so bad. You can look at mine if you want."

She picked up the veil next to her bed and handed it to me. It was a very light gauze material, and when I held it to my face I could see through it relatively easily.

"This isn't so bad."

The princess laughed. "You are only looking through a single veil. Most women wear it doubled, so that it is much darker."

I doubled the veil and tried looking through it again. "This is terrible," I told her, peering through the two layers.

At that point I explained to the princess about my Bedouin patients, and the fact that the women would take off their clothes but would leave on their veils.

"Of course," she said contemptuously. "The Bedouin women are kept in complete ignorance. They feel safe as long as their faces are covered. It is like they are invisible—the veil prevents you from knowing who they are, so it doesn't matter if you see their body."

"Of course," she added mischievously, "some of them are so ugly that they *need* to wear a veil!"

For several minutes we talked about the segregation of men and women in Saudi society. According to the princess, it was absolutely forbidden for a woman to be alone with a man who was not her *mahrram*. *Mahrram* included the men in her immediate family—her father, her uncles, and her brothers—and also included her husband. A woman cannot leave the country without a *mahrram*.

The practice in Saudi Arabia, I had been told many times, was to keep the women as secluded as possible, preventing their contact with all men outside the immediate family.

"Women are considered personal property not to be discussed or displayed before other men," explained Sultana. "There is no social life between men and women outside the immediate family. A man, for example, never takes his wife out to dinner. And a man never dances with his wife in public or in private. It is forbidden."

The men in Saudi Arabia do not trust each other when it comes to women, according to Sultana. Even a friend might make advances toward a man's wife if she were seen in public. In this context, women are viewed as weak-willed and passive, and would be likely to succumb to advances. So, to prevent any such eventuality, women are excluded from all social activities with men, and are confined to the household.

"Princess," I said, "is it proper for you and me to be talking as friends?"

"Oh no!" she exclaimed. "It is okay for me to talk with my doctor, but only for medical reasons. Certainly I should at least be wearing my veil when I talk to a man who is not my *mahrram*. But unfortunately I cannot wear my veil right now, because I am still sick!" She burst into laughter.

"What do women do with their time?" I asked after the laughter subsided.

"Nothing, usually. Most of the women sit at home and are bored stupid. Occasionally, they visit their families, where they can gossip, play cards, and try on clothes. Those are the three main things: gossip, cards, and clothes. Sometimes there is a party for women only, of course, and everyone brings two or three dresses, just so they can change during the party and show the other women."

According to Princess Sultana, one of the ironies of Saudi Arabia is that the massive wealth brought by oil has turned women into virtual prisoners. In the nomadic days in the desert, the women at least played an important role, and had certain jobs and freedoms. They had to get water from the wells, help put up the tent, and take care of the children. Now that the material standards have improved so dramatically, the women are left with nothing to do.

She paused, stared out the window, and then spoke quietly as though to herself.

"Very strict separation of men and women, very, very puritanical—no movies, no alcohol, no dancing or music in public, women heavily veiled and kept at home—no fun at all," she reflected. "Just praying five times a day, the fast of Ramadan, the pilgrimage to Mecca, and giving alms to the poor—and that's about it!"

There was an uncomfortable pause after this deadening comment.

"It would be better for the women if we were still poor," said the princess frankly. "Some of the people, the common people who live in mud houses, can really have more fun, in their own way, than we have. Maybe something very simple makes them laugh. Like the Egyptians. They enjoy everything; they think everything's funny. Maybe they're the happy ones. We in Saudi Arabia criticize, we look at what's right. That's not funny, so hardly anything's funny the way we look at everything.

"Yeah, in this country the women really don't have anything to do. That's the truth. We cannot go anywhere in public without an escort, and we are not even allowed to drive cars. I should mention that Saudi women are very good to their chauffeurs. Sometimes I think they are more doting on their chauffeurs than on their husbands. If we want to go to a party, we must wait for the driver to take us. Without him we are stranded. To women, a driver is almost holy!"

"But what about the women who can't afford a driver? What do they do?"

The princess shrugged. "They sit inside their houses," she said simply.

"That sounds *awful*," I said. The princess looked at me, saying nothing. An awkward silence ensued.

"Is there ever a situation where you can be with other men?"

"Yes, at the family meeting, and at family parties. My family—the Sudairis—is very large. We have a family meeting regularly, and everyone goes to it, even the Crown Prince. We are all members of the Saud family, but there are families within the family, and the Sudairis are very important. We stick together, you might say."

"And the women are allowed to mix with the men at these family affairs?"

"Yes," said Sultana. "At these meetings and also at the family parties I can talk to my cousins, including the boys. The family meetings are very nice, and the women all look forward to them. Otherwise, we are always left home."

I wanted to continue my questioning, delving deeper into the fascinating puzzle of Saudi culture. However, it was late and the princess was growing tired. Reluctantly, I told her that it was time for me to leave.

"This is fun," she said, again fixing me with her dazzling smile. It occurred to me that in a different society she would probably be a renowned beauty. In Saudi Arabia, the only people who knew about it were her immediate family. And I.

"Let's do this again tomorrow," she suggested.

"I'd love to," I said. "If you like, I'll come back tomorrow night."

"I think I will have to wear a veil next time," she said. She pulled the covers up to her eyes. "How do I look?" she asked in a muffled voice.

"Like an old Bedouin woman." I teased her. I wanted to compliment her on her beauty, but I decided against it.

I said goodnight to her and then walked out the door, pondering her curious combination of Western and Saudi attributes. Sometimes she sounded entirely American, especially when she talked about the problems in Saudi Arabia and about the status of women. However, she clearly thought of herself as Saudi Arabian, and at times she showed a deep, almost fierce pride in her country. In a way, she reminded me of American expatriates I knew, people who never visited America and yet considered themselves 100 percent American. People do not really choose their country; in a way, their country chooses them.

The next day I visited Princess Sultana during my regular hospital rounds, and then returned that evening for another one of our long talks.

Her recovery was progressing nicely, and she grew healthier and more active with each passing day.

"Where is your veil?" I asked as I sat down in the chair next to her bed.

She looked at me gravely. "Unfortunately, I am still not well enough to wear it."

We laughed once more at this private joke, and again I found myself captivated by her smile. What a shame that she had to cover it up all the time!

Then I became serious, "Princess, you told me a little about your mother's divorce. What can you tell me about divorce in this country?"

My thoughts went back to Princess Sanwa and her inhumane divorce from her Saudi husband, when they were in Boston many years ago.

"A divorce is very easy under Islam," said the princess excitedly. By now, she seemed to take a perverse delight in telling me things about her culture that she knew I would find curious and exotic. "To get a divorce, the man must say, 'I divorce you,' and the woman is no longer married and must return to her family. But there is a catch: if the man changes his mind anytime within three months, he can simply take the woman back, and she must return to him. Only after three months does the divorce become permanent.

"The man can divorce his wife three times. He can say, 'I divorce you,' and then take her back three times. But if he does it again, then she is permanently free. Another way is if the man says, 'I divorce you, I divorce you, I divorce you,' three times in succession, and that's as if he had divorced her three times. She has to return home to her parents. It all depends on the words, you see? The divorce is now permanent."

Although it seemed curious that a divorce could be obtained so casually—especially after all the impediments to getting married in the first place—this was in fact the legal method for dissolving a marriage in Saudi Arabia. There was, of course, a striking injustice to the rule, because only a man could obtain a divorce simply by uttering the magic words. A woman could divorce her husband with difficulty and only in certain narrow circumstances.

"Well, what if she hates him?" I asked, posing a seemingly normal question.

"She can't do anything about it. She could tell him. Maybe he likes her. Maybe he wants to keep her, maybe he wants a harem—you know, a load of women. She can't do anything about it, unless she has a very good reason."

"Well, suppose he beats her."

"If he beats her she has a right to divorce, but it is often difficult for the woman. There are certain other reasons for a woman to ask for a divorce, like if her husband doesn't support her or doesn't have sexual relations with her for a long time.

"For instance, if the woman sees her husband completely give up his religion, anything to do with deserting the Moslem religion, if he's got anything against religion, that helps her get a divorce. Like 'My husband drinks, my husband takes drugs' . . . she must at least bring proof. There has to be proof."

When a woman is divorced from her husband, she is often sent to live with her parents. It is common for a family to have one or more "aunts" living in, some of them maidens and some of them divorced.

"But what about afterward? Will he support her?"

"He won't support her, he will support the children. Look, if she has a daughter, the child may live with her mother until she's seven and then she'll live with her father. Because for a very young girl it's not easy living with a man. When she becomes seven years old, she goes to her father. A boy stays with his mother until he is two or three, and after the breast feeding, he lives with his father."

"I thought the husband paid for his wife's support."

"No, I don't think so, unless he is very wealthy or prominent. They do it now if the man is kind enough to do it. But he is only obliged to pay the support for the children. The woman goes back to her family. I don't think she gets any support, unless her divorced husband is rich or comes from the royal family.

"I had a cousin who was married and divorced all in one month," said the princess. "She was only fifteen at the time! Her husband went away on a trip right after the marriage, and when he came back my cousin was in tears, because he went to visit one of his other wives before coming to see her. The husband became very angry and divorced her on the spot. He sent her right back to her family. But later he sent her a lot of money and twenty-five slaves."

"When was this?" I asked, startled by the reference to slaves.

"Perhaps twenty years ago," replied the princess. "My cousin is now in her thirties."

I had momentarily forgotten that Saudi Arabia was the last country in the world to outlaw slavery, and that it did not do so until 1962.

"So that's how it's done," Sultana said.

"The rich give their ex-wives houses, jewels, cars, and everything because they have money. It would be bad for their name if they left a woman in poor shape. Sometimes when an older wife feels that she will be replaced soon by a younger wife, she tries to find a young girl, say fourteen or fifteen, for her husband, and then demands a certain amount of money for finding him a new wife."

"Oh, that's just great. A trade-in deal."

"If you think that's bad," she said, "the royal women also get money from the government. My thirty-year-old cousin, you know, has received money since she was fifteen. And it's quite a bit, maybe 6,000 riyals [$2,000] a month."

"From the government?"

"You see, not everybody talks about this. I don't understand it exactly either—but there is the *mezanyah,* and it's a payment from the government to the royalty each month—a sort of government allowance."

"For everyone in the royal family? There are thousands of them!"

"Yes," the princess said. "For all of the royal family. When any of the children become fifteen, they start getting it, and it becomes more and more as they grow older."

"Would you qualify for it?" I was prying.

"But of course," she said simply, straightening the bedclothes. "We, the Sudairis, get the same thing."

"And, when you're married, will you still get it?"

"Yes, I'll still get it."

"And what does that amount to? How much do you get, if I may ask?"

"Well, right now I've only started on 150 each month [$50]," she said. "That's very little, of course, compared to the Saud family. But the older I get the more it will be. For instance, my grandfather's sisters now—some of them are still young—get around 6,000 [$2,000] a month."

"Does it come from the government directly?"

"I don't know if it's from the government directly, but I think it's from the money that belongs to the old Saud family," continued Sultana. "Nobody knows which pocket it comes from. The Saud family really owns the government and all the money in it. The government in a way is a huge corporation made up entirely of the royal family. It's part of the Saud dynasty—the House of Saud. The royal family is paid a certain amount each year as a sort of dividend."

Sultana became excited with her rhetoric.

"We all get it, and some people don't like it. The common people now complain: 'What did they do to deserve this money—how come?' . . . They complain about this. Of course, I say, it's not fair either. I agree, but we have to think about the Saud family, the ones that are related to us.

They still have to remember that we are their relatives, and there was some good in us in the past, especially in our history.

"And it would be sad to just leave us in a bad shape, especially the women who have no husbands. . . . They have no money; they'd be moving from door to door asking for help, the older women especially. And this would be embarrassing for them and for the family. You see?"

By now it had again grown late, and it was time to end this session. As I stood up, the princess gave me a look of disappointment.

"Are you leaving already?"

"Yes, you may be feeling better, but you still need your rest. I will come back tomorrow."

"Oh," she said pouting, "our next talk was going to be all about polygamy and the royal family."

This was a subject that fascinated me, and for a moment I was tempted to continue our conversation. But I decided that it was important for the princess to rest, and so I reluctantly declined her offer.

"I'm sorry, it's quite late. We can discuss royal polygamy the first thing tomorrow."

"No," she insisted, playfully, "I would rather talk about it now."

I shrugged. "You really need to get some rest, and it is almost midnight. Goodnight, Sultana."

She did not reply, and I left the room feeling guilty, like a parent forcing a child to an early bedtime. It occurred to me that for all her confidence and regal authority the princess was sometimes a remarkably immature person. At one moment she could be mature and self-assured and at another almost childlike. I attributed her childlike outbursts to the fact that she grew up pampered and sheltered by adults. She was deprived of the social interactions that help produce emotional maturity. While her swings in temperament were unsettling, I could readily understand them. After all, how would you expect a Saudi princess to act? She was, for better and for worse, exactly what I expected a Saudi princess to be.

I visited Sultana the next day during my rounds, and found her poring over a large square of white cardboard, writing furiously with colored pencils. She was in a cheerful mood, and the incident that had marred the previous evening was entirely forgotten.

"What are you writing?" I asked her.

"It's a surprise," she said, holding the board so that I could not see what she was doing. "I'll show you tonight."

When I returned that evening, Princess Sultana sat up in bed and, with a flourish, handed me the piece of cardboard.

"Thank you," I said, trying to sound grateful. The cardboard was covered with numerous names, connected by lines.

"It's a history of my family," said the princess proudly. "It is a family tree of the Sudairis."

Now I understood the significance of the gift, and I was deeply touched. Some of the names on the board were unknown to me, but others were familiar, including some of the most famous in the kingdom. I was amused to see that she had listed only the men, but suddenly realized that to include the women would have been virtually impossible, since each ancestor averaged ten or more wives during his lifetime.

Sultana began to explain how all the names were interconnected. "We of the Sudairi family are all descended from the great tribal leader Ahmed Sudairi, who had fifteen sons and eleven daughters by different wives. In the next generation the grandsons and granddaughters—all of whom were first cousins—frequently intermarried so that our family tree is extremely complicated."

"That's for sure. You would need a computer to figure out everyone's relationship at this point."

"You haven't heard anything yet," said the princess, laughing.

"The most famous of Ahmed Sudairi's children was his daughter Hussah bint Sudairi, who married King Abdul-Aziz (Ibn Saud). The King was very fond of her, but unfortunately she did not bear him any children, and so he divorced her. The King then married Hussah's sister Sultana. The King's *brother* married Hussah.

"Things now got *very* complicated because shortly after Hussah married the King's brother, she bore him a son! The King immediately wanted Hussah back, and so she was divorced from the brother and remarried to the King. She eventually bore him five daughters and seven sons."

"Are these the so-called Sudairi Seven?"

"Yes. They include Crown Prince Fahd, Minister of Defense, Sultan, and so forth."

"That's amazing," I said, shaking my head. "But what happened to. Hussah's sister Sultana when the King remarried Hussah?"

"Nothing, she remained his wife."

"So, in other words, the King was married to two sisters at the same time?"

"Yes, and he was married to one of their cousins, as well."

While the princess explained the connections between the Sudairis and the other branches of the royal family, I pondered whether to raise a question that had been bothering me for some time. Several weeks earlier, a friend had sent me a story from one of the London newspapers about a Saudi princess who was executed for adultery. I had carried the clipping in my wallet, but I had been reluctant to show it to the princess because I could not predict her response. However, I felt that this might be an appropriate time to mention it.

"A friend of mine sent me this clipping from one of the London newspapers," I began cautiously. "It is about the execution of a young Saudi princess for committing adultery. I was wondering if you knew her?"

Sultana took the clipping from me and with great interest examined it, including the now-famous photo of the execution of Princess Mishaal bint Abdul-Aziz. However, she did not make any effort to read the article itself.

"No, I do not know this girl. She is from a branch of the Saud family that lives in Jidda, and we do not see them. It is sad to hear that she was killed."

"You mean you didn't know about this?" I asked in surprise.

"No," she replied. "These things are kept secret. You hear about them sometimes, but they are not reported in our newspapers."

"Are executions like this unusual, or do they happen often?"

The princess shrugged. "It is common knowledge that these things take place. The women are usually stoned to death for adultery in front of the family, especially so that the women can see, to teach them a lesson. Adultery is a serious crime in Saudi Arabia, because it brings disgrace on the family. Family honor is a matter of life and death, especially among the royal family."

"But this was cruel and inhuman," I argued. "These laws were written a thousand years ago. Saudi Arabia can't stay in the seventh century forever!"

The princess looked at me with what seemed like sadness. "Nobody can understand how important religion and the family are in Saudi Arabia. They are more important than anything else, including life itself. I told you that everyone, even the Crown Prince, comes to the family meetings, no matter what else there is that demands his attention. Our economic and political lives are organized along family lines. The government itself is built upon the family structure. The religion and the family—that is all we have! That is all we are!"

"But then why kill only the woman? If they killed every man who committed adultery, the kingdom would be decimated. Why don't the men get stoned to death?"

"Because the honor of the family depends upon the woman! This woman had a child and was still married. Besides she was a princess. The grandfather probably made the decision."

At this point, I told Sultana the story of a Riyadh woman who had once been married to an important prince. The woman had been a slave girl from Iran, and she had been bought by her future husband when he was in his sixties and she was twelve or thirteen. She bore the prince several sons over the next few years and he eventually married her to legitimate the sons. Later, when the woman was in her twenties and her husband in his seventies, she began to take lovers. This was apparently an open secret in Riyadh, but the prince never found out about it. He died when he was in his eighties and left the woman a great fortune.

"Why wasn't she punished for committing adultery?" I asked Sultana when I was finished with the story. "If everyone knew about it, why didn't they do anything?"

"There are two explanations," replied the princess. "The woman did not bring dishonor to her family because she was a slave and did not have a family. The only family she could disgrace was her husband's, and he apparently never knew, or didn't want to acknowledge it."

"But other members of his family knew about it, including the prince's other wives. In fact, I heard that they went along because they also had things to hide."

"Remember that this Iranian woman was not a princess!" replied Sultana angrily. She was clearly distressed by the story. "This woman is called the 'mother of a prince' in Saudi Arabia because she gave the old prince several sons, and he later married her. But she was in no way a princess! She was really a slave, and she behaved like a slave."

"And she inherited several hundred million riyals."

"That means nothing," said Sultana scornfully. "She probably cannot leave the country, and she will not be able to spend the money on very much—just jewels and clothing. The money will all go to her children."

I smiled to myself as I listened to her answer. It suddenly made perfect sense: the Iranian woman had all that money, but no opportunity to spend it. I was also struck by the shrewdness of the princess, who immediately grasped the subtleties of the situation. In another era, I wondered, what would this woman be doing if she lived in the United States?

"But then answer this question for me," I said. "Do you admit that adultery takes place in Saudi Arabia?"

"Yes," she replied. "Of course, there is adultery. I will admit that. But it is not the way you think. Adultery is very rare."

"You mean that the Saudi women do not have sex before they are married?"

"Never," she said seriously. "It is crucial for a woman to be a virgin on her wedding night.

"That's the biggest thing here. The biggest deal—maybe most girls are forever thinking, 'Am I a virgin, maybe's something's wrong, maybe I did something wrong.' It's very creepy. I have my cousin who's always calling me. She tells me her problem. She says, 'I'm worried, I horseback ride a lot, I ride bicycles.' Me, myself, I'm kind of chicken; sometimes I worry. But I know my fiancé, Mahmoud. I mean he's not stupid, and I don't think he'll be foolish about it. He laughs at me about that. I don't believe he thinks about it the Saudi way."

"What is the Saudi way of looking at it?"

She paused to find the right words. "The men here are hungry for a virgin. When they get married, that is their thing. The Bedouin poets always say that a virgin is the best, that if she hasn't been married before then her mind will be clear of any other man. The men prize virginity above everything—that is why dowries are so much less the second time a woman marries."

Later I would learn a lot about the Saudi obsession with virgins, and the fact that virginity is the greatest single attribute that a woman can possess. Indeed, a Saudi man can reject his bride on their wedding night if he thinks that she is not a virgin, and this explained Sultana's extreme anxiety about the subject.

An intact hymen, of course, was the primary evidence for judging that a Saudi woman was a virgin, and this raised some interesting questions. I remembered something I thought Sultana would find amusing.

"Recently when I was in Iran, where there is a similar emphasis on virginity," I remarked, "I was told that Iranian women sometimes have their hymens repaired by surgeons prior to marriage, in order to reinstate their 'virginity.' This is a relatively simple operation that can be performed under local anesthesia."

"I'm sure I have heard of this," said Sultana, looking away.

"A young Iranian woman, born in New York but living in Iran, told me laughingly that there were as many hymen repairs in Iran as there were nose jobs in New York."

"That's pretty funny," said the princess, smiling. "There's a lesson there somewhere on moral values and the social scene."

For a while I talked to Princess Sultana about sexual values in Saudi Arabia, and the contrast with those in America. The princess was fascinated to discover that in America young people often live together, and that the prevailing attitude is "try before you buy." Then, out of curiosity, I asked her if she knew about homosexuality. I actually asked her if she knew what it was; I certainly did not expect her response.

"Oh, it's loaded," she said.

"Loaded?"

"It is so sad," she said. "There is so much of it going on around here. Among the boys and girls."

"The girls?" I blurted. I was stunned, perhaps by my own naïveté.

"Yes," said Sultana. "At my school there was so much of it going on that it scared me. The other girls even tried to approach me!"

"What did you do?"

"I told them no way. But I was nice about it, and we became friends, even though I was not like them."

"Do the girls . . . I mean, do they have long-term relationships?"

"They move around quite a bit." She smiled at the sinfulness of it all. "It's fascinating! The stories I could tell are unbelievable."

Like all Saudi girls, Sultana had gone to a school that was segregated by sex, and it was not surprising that there was an element of homosexuality present. Indeed, given the zealousness with which heterosexual activity is policed, it was probably the only feasible alternative.

"My school was terrible," recalled the princess with distaste. "We spent most of our time studying religion, because they won't teach anything else to the girls. They don't want us to learn anything about the man's world. Our teacher was a blind sheik and he did not even know how to read or write! All he knew was his religion and the Koran, and he drilled us with it until it gave us heartburn. We just memorized and threw it back up at him. We hated him!"

At that point, I told Sultana about a conversation that I had had with a doctor, a famous professor from Egypt, who was then seventy-five years old. I had mentioned to this distinguished gentleman that the teachers at the women's medical school were mostly mature men, and that I did not understand why the school forced the men to teach by television. After all, I argued, the teachers were all old men—what could happen? He looked at me with disdain, drew himself up, and bristled, "There *are* no old men in Saudi Arabia."

"It's *true*," said the princess when I finished my story. "The men never admit to old age sexually. They all want to have children when they are eighty or older. They marry young wives in their old age and keep trying. Sometimes they succeed."

"So, in other words, every man is expected to have a hunger for women. Is that why only blind men can teach the women?"

"I guess so," she replied. "It is funny, but it seems so normal for it to be this way in Saudi Arabia. I know that in America and even in Egypt the men and women go to college together, and when I am outside of Saudi Arabia that seems natural. But here it feels wrong to mix—it is part of our isolation psychology.

"It is difficult to be a Saudi Arabian right now," she continued. "We are not exactly sure who we are. Everyone is cracking up! It is a sort of schizophrenia. Men and women are coming into the country with new ideas—the airplane, radio, television. . . . These things may represent progress to you, but they are ruining our society.

"You see, now that we are threatened by outside ideas, the Wahabis are becoming stricter than ever. Veils are supposed to be thicker and sleeves longer. Pictures of women in newspapers and magazines are blacked out. They are also making a strong campaign against liquor."

"Do you think—and do the Wahabis think—that they can beat back the foreign influence?"

She shook her head sadly. "I know we cannot stop it, and it is very, very sad. The young people here are being ruined. They are changing terribly. One thing I told you about is the homosexual problem. Another thing is that every Saudi girl is now talking about how she has a boyfriend. Boyfriend! How does this happen in Saudi Arabia?

"More and more people are addicted to drugs and to liquor. There is a lot of drinking in this country, but it is kept secret because it is against the law and against the religion."

She seemed to become self-absorbed right now, and I decided to leave her to her thoughts. I stood up and walked toward the door. Before I said goodbye I paused briefly, watching her. She was a brave, intelligent, beautiful woman—and in the end she was ill prepared to grapple with the problems facing her people. As a Saudi princess, she was rich beyond the dreams of Croesus, and yet she felt insecure, perhaps intuitively.

It was difficult for her to compromise the past with the present, and she was desperately afraid of the future.

Like most Saudi Arabians, she was beginning to realize that along with the profits from oil come high costs. She did not at that very moment appear to be a member of the richest and most powerful single family in the world. More than anything, she seemed, rather, to be a victim.

"Good night, princess," I said softly.

"Good night, doctor," she replied turning toward me. "I'll see you tomorrow."

COURTSHIP: SAUDI ARABIAN STYLE

BY THE THIRD WEEK of hospitalization Princess Sultana was almost fully recovered, and the time was fast approaching for her discharge from the hospital. Having grown accustomed to our daily chats I was frankly unhappy at the prospect of her leaving. Each day we talked for an hour or two, and I would come in at night to talk some more. She was a delightful conversationalist and an astute observer of the human scene. She wanted to talk to someone who would understand, someone who would be sympathetic and compassionate. I was an eager listener. She opened a window to allow me a glimpse of the secret side of Saudi Arabian life behind the veil.

I had learned that this innocent young woman, while at times somewhat naïve, was articulate and forthright. Sultana, a unique hybrid of American and Saudi Arabian culture, seemed to have inherited the wisdom of the ages. She had a keen and analytical mind, with a bias, nevertheless, toward her royal status and her great wealth. Her English had only the slightest vestige of a foreign accent, interspersed at times with a lapse in grammar or an exclamation in the vernacular such as "wow" or "big deal" which only added to her charm. Needless to say I was captivated by her.

The princess and I had become personal friends, and I was reluctant to relinquish the warm and genuine relationship that had developed between us. Of course, we might meet again "on the outside" later on, but it would never be as free and casual as it was now. I realized that a close relationship with a woman could exist only in the cloistered world of the King Faisal Hospital. In the rigid orthodox environment of Saudi Arabia this kind of friendship would have been virtually impossible.

Happily, I soon discovered that the princess was as reluctant to leave the hospital as I was to have her go. She was enjoying the freedoms that her illness conferred, including the parade of attentive visitors, the flood of gifts from well-wishers, and—somewhere on her list of priorities—the opportunity to continue our conversations. We both wanted this interlude to last a little longer, and so we conspired to delay the date of her discharge, allowing our tête-à-têtes to continue as before.

One afternoon I entered Sultana's hospital suite to discover the adjoining room banked with flowers.

"It looks like the Garden of Eden in here," I remarked. "What's the occasion?"

"My fiancé, Mahmoud, is coming to visit," replied the princess. "The flowers are from Beirut. Aren't they beautiful?"

"They're overwhelming. I've never seen a more impressive display. I thought it was improper for your fiancé to visit you here."

The princess gave me a sly smile. "My father has given him permission. My grandfather would be very angry if he found out, but he will never know, so it's okay. He still believes that the man and woman should not see each other or be together until they are married.

"In fact," she continued, "it is common for two people to become married who have never even *seen* each other. For instance, my aunt never saw her fiancé. She had one little picture of him that was taken when he was seventeen, and he was then twenty-five. She sat around for months, wondering what he looked like, wondering what his voice was like, wondering whether he would be kind to her."

"That tradition seems medieval to me. No wonder there are so many divorces in this country."

The princess smiled sardonically. "The divorce rate in Saudi Arabia is probably no higher than that in the U.S.

"Look," Sultana said somewhat firmly. "You must understand, well, not just understand, but *feel* what these customs mean for a Moslem woman. Some Islamic women don't like the idea of having to look for a husband or to earn a living, so they're content just sticking to doing things within the family. They don't have to find a place in the work world, like in the U.S.; instead they can find a place in the family structure."

"But you yourself said they're bored stiff, and in really bad shape!" I said. "How can they be content?"

"Maybe I'm imposing my values when I make that judgment," Sultana said nobly. "But as long as these women are ignorant, no, not ignorant, but just kept closed in, they can be satisfied."

"They're prisoners that can't see their own chains, right? What they don't know can't hurt them. They don't have the freedom of choice, to do what they want in life."

She just gave me a quick glance, and paused. "Many American women," she said, "have to scheme to find a husband for themselves and worry about finding the right husband without acting like they're on a hunt.

"We can be ourselves, no acting or that kind of stuff, and literally wait for Prince Charming to fall in our laps! The father chooses the husband for his daughter, and he knows more than a seventeen-year-old about what's involved in a lifetime commitment, so we let them worry about it instead! And they take it seriously.

"Those American women don't necessarily have any more freedom. While juggling their marriages and their children, they've got to prove themselves by working in what is still a man's world. What makes you think they are so free?"

She had obviously thought about this matter before. Yet how could she, a woman aware of other freedoms, accept and insulate herself in the Saudi way of life? How could she believe that only men are capable of the responsibilities of basic freedoms? And even if it was better to be sheltered from these anxieties that come with freedom, didn't she want to be able to have some choices? I kept quiet.

"Uh huh." It was obviously hopeless to argue. "Well, what happened with your aunt?" I asked, ready to hear about her divorce.

"She was very lucky. Her husband turned out to be a wonderful man. I heard that he asked for me, but my father wanted me to finish school before I got married. In a way I am sad, because he would have been a very nice husband. He had been to college in America, and he probably would have taken me there often."

"Well, I guess your aunt is fortunate, " I said. "Just think: you might have married him instead."

"It was my father's decision!" she exclaimed. "I have no right to question him."

I shrugged and said nothing, not wanting to provoke an argument. I wondered how she could be so Western in some ways, and so completely Saudi Arabian in others.

"Do many couples get married without meeting?" I asked.

"Yes," she said. "You see, things are slow to change here in Saudi Arabia. For hundreds and even thousands of years the fathers arranged the weddings of their children, and the children obeyed. Now it is beginning to change, but very slowly. We, the children, accept it because it is crucial to the sanctity of the family. Of course, we can refuse to marry the person they select for us, but that does not happen very often."

Sultana went on to explain that the right of a father to dictate his daughter's marriage plans is deeply ingrained in Saudi tradition. For example, she cited King Ibn Saud, who married the daughters of many tribal chieftains by arrangement for political purposes. The King would visit a Bedouin tribe, and the tribal leader would offer a daughter—along with goats, camels, and gold—as a tribute to the ruler. The daughter did as she was told, and the marriage was performed and consummated the same night. The next day the King would leave, and in most cases the new wife never saw her husband again. The daughters probably knew all of this in advance yet they meekly obeyed their fathers' orders. The King later admitted that he never saw the faces of most of his three hundred wives and never conversed with them at any time.

"How did you meet your fiancé?"

"The marriage was arranged by our families," she replied.

Sultana made herself comfortable and started to tell her story. When she was eighteen years old she was asked to consider two proposals of marriage.

One was from Mahmoud Daouk's family. This had been arranged by Sultana's aunt, whose son had already married into the Daouk family. It was unusual, she stressed, for a Sudairi to initiate a proposal of marriage between a commoner and a Saudi princess.

"Maybe," she suggested, "it was because Mahmoud's father is a very wealthy man, actually a billionaire. Also, my aunt was very pleased with the Daouk family when she came to know them. Maybe she was making a trade. The Daouk family had taken her son, a Sudairi, and now she wanted the Sudairi family to take a Daouk son in return. It's very complicated."

The second proposal came from the King's brother, one of the most important princes in the kingdom, who was married to a Sudairi. He had asked for both Sultana and her younger sister Nadia for his two sons.

"The boys' mother was a Sudairi," said Sultana, "and she had had her eye on us all these years. She had been waiting for me and Nadia. We would be marrying our cousins. It was a perfect arrangement."

The marriage plans within the Saudi royal family were plotted years in advance, and other branches of the family also coveted Sultana and her sister for their sons. Indeed, Sultana would learn later that this particular royal alignment had first been proposed when she was five years old.

In his reply to the Daouk family, Sultana's father, negotiating from strength, cagily noted that, while Mahmoud might be an uncommon commoner, he was a commoner nonetheless, and that the matter would have to be carefully considered.

Although Sultana was aware of a visit by her aunt, she was not immediately informed of the marriage proposal. Shortly afterward the entire family went for a vacation to Rome, and on the plane Sultana learned of the proposal from her stepmother. The stepmother swore Sultana to secrecy, and then explained that Mahmoud Daouk was being considered as a possible husband for her. Sultana's reaction was strongly negative—she did not want to be married, to a Daouk or to anyone else. However, she hid her emotions and acted suitably surprised when, several days later, she "learned" of the marriage proposal from her father.

Sultana's father then informed her of the second marriage proposal, and indicated that the choice was up to her. Although her father did not make his feeling explicitly known, Sultana soon realized that he was fending off the royal relatives far more vigorously than the Daouk family. When the royal uncle pressed his case, Sultana's father argued that the girls were too young, that they had to finish school first. On the other hand, the father was less adamant to the entreaties made by Mahmoud's family.

For the remainder of the summer Sultana mulled over her options. Both offers were excellent, and also represented a clear choice. On the one hand, the royal cousin was from a distinguished branch of the family, and he could be expected to play a major role in the Saudi government in coming years. Marriage to him would be considered a remarkable and advantageous alliance and would guarantee an important and honorable place within the royal family.

On the other hand Mahmoud offered freedom—freedom from the burdensome role of being a royal princess, freedom from the formal life that leading members of the family were expected to live.

"Although I had never seen either of them, I was told that both were good-looking, both educated, and both likely to treat me well. But it was really a choice of lifestyles. Did I want to be married to a prince or to a commoner? It is an enormous difference, you know. When you marry a prince, you are actually married to the whole royal family. Their life is very formal; it is not a normal life. There will always be formal functions, always be parties, never a nice, quiet life with your husband and children. That is why I favored Mahmoud—he meant that I could live a simple life."

Finally, Sultana made a long-distance call to her mother in America. She began to tell her mother about the situation, that there were two men, one of them a prince and one of them a commoner. Both men were twenty-three, both good-looking, and both very rich. As she spoke with her mother, Sultana suddenly realized that she was answering her own question. She wanted the simple life; she wanted to marry outside of the family.

Having eliminated the royal cousin from consideration, Sultana began to question whether she wanted to be married at all. People began congratulating her on the marriage prospect, and she found herself uncertain, confused. Did she want to marry Mahmoud? She didn't know. She had never seen him or talked to him. Worse, her grandfather had been overheard to say that Sultana was going to marry a Daouk and that he approved. The grandfather could easily order her to marry Mahmoud, and she would have no choice but to obey.

"Oh, my God," she said, "my grandfather is making all the arrangements and I don't even know anything about it. They are doing it the old way! Everything is being settled and my father has nothing to say. Doesn't my father have a tongue?"

Seeking advice, Sultana went to her father and explained her situation. Her father answered that he had made inquiries about the young man and his family, and that the reports were very good.

A week later her father told Sultana, "They are going to be here tonight. Do you want me to tell them 'no' and finish it? What did you decide?"

Now the decision was hers. On the one hand she understood that Mahmoud presented an exceptionally good marriage opportunity. On the other hand, she had never met him, and she was unsure of her feelings.

Sultana secretly wanted to meet Mahmoud but she was too shy to use the word "meet" with her father. Instead, she said, "Dad, if you think he is a good person and if they are a good family, as you say, then I don't mind, but I would like to get to know him before I agree to the marriage."

Taking the hint, Sultana's father arranged for Mahmoud to come to their house for a visit. At this initial interview Sultana was not present, and the meeting was between Sultana's father, Mahmoud's father, and Mahmoud. In keeping with the custom, the fathers did the bulk of the talking. Sultana's father began by voicing his reservations: Sultana was too young, perhaps it would be better to wait. She would like to study in Switzerland for a year. Mahmoud's father replied by mentioning that Sultana was almost twenty, an incredibly advanced age for marriage by traditional Saudi standards, and that soon she might be too old. Both sides, of course, were bargaining in true Saudi fashion, hoping to obtain the optimal marriage contract.

At length, Mahmoud's father suggested that perhaps it was wrong to handle this matter in the old way. Perhaps, he said, Mahmoud and Sultana should meet, and if they liked each other then everything would be worked out later. This proposed meeting was heretical to Saudi traditions—letting the children make the decision—but at least it had been arrived at in true Saudi fashion. After all, the two families had negotiated for several hours in order to reach an agreement that both sides knew they wanted from the beginning.

Two days later, dressed in a simple thobe, Mahmoud came to pay his first visit. He was accompanied by his sister and her Sudairi husband. The three of them were greeted at the gate by a servant and led into the family compound. Because of the dampening effect that parents might have on the

Courtship: Saudi Arabian Style ◊ *115*

meeting, it was decided that Mahmoud and Sultana would be more comfortable if chaperoned only by the sister and brother-in-law, who were approximately the same age. This was about as close to a "private" meeting as modern Saudi etiquette could possibly allow.

The three visitors were led into the courtyard of the villa, where they sat down in chairs beside the pool to await Sultana. Meanwhile, she was nervously preparing for the first meeting with a man who would probably be her future husband. She had decided against wearing either a veil or a traditional robe, and instead chose conservative Western clothing that included a turtleneck sweater and a modest gray skirt. Her hair was hanging loose around her shoulders, and she did not have on either jewelry or makeup. "Oh well," she thought to herself as she gave her hair a final brushing, "either he likes me the way I am or *balesh,* forget it."

Walking into the courtyard where the three visitors were waiting, Sultana assumed a jaunty walk that was designed to cover up her anxiety. The guests stood up as she approached, and for the first time she saw Mahmoud Daouk. He was an incredibly large man, much larger than she had imagined, and his appearance made her feel dizzy and frightened. She offered him her hand, but she avoided his eyes. Noting her nervousness, Mahmoud squeezed her hand very hard. The sharp pain startled the princess, and she immediately glanced into his face.

"Hello, Sultana," he said, smiling. He slowly eased the pressure on her hand, but did not let go of it.

"Hello, Mahmoud," she replied weakly. Mahmoud held her hand for several more seconds, then gently released it. Shaken, she sat down in the chair beside him.

For several minutes the four young Saudis talked about every topic that they could think of, avoiding the most obvious topic of all, namely the purpose of the visit. It would seem funny later, but at the moment everyone was concerned with the outcome of their meeting. Mahmoud's sister felt that Sultana would make a good wife for her brother. Her husband was worried that Sultana, a Sudairi, would insult his wife's family by turning down the marriage. Mahmoud thought that Sultana was the most beautiful woman that he had ever seen, and he was shy and nervous in her presence.

As for Sultana, she was surprised by Mahmoud's toughness, and especially by the fact that he had squeezed her hand when she seemed to avoid him. Watching him now, she was growing more and more impressed. He was bigger and older-looking than she had expected, and he carried himself like a "real man." She could not bring herself to talk with him—she was too shy— but she watched him converse with his sister and she decided that Mahmoud was really very "nice."

The meeting lasted for two hours, and at various times the four of them were joined by Sultana's father, who was curious to find out how things were progressing. Later, he would say that he thought the marriage was off because Sultana did not seem to talk or even look at Mahmoud. When the visit ended, the five of them walked to the gate of the family compound, and Mahmoud's brother-in-law told Sultana's father that Mahmoud would be calling the next day for Sultana's decision. Sultana felt a deep resentment at this statement: they were giving her an ultimatum, forcing her to decide within a time limit. It all seemed so cool. A business transaction with a deadline!

Suddenly, Mahmoud turned and walked over to join her. "Good night, Sultana," he said, shaking her hand.

It was a small gesture, but to Sultana it had enormous significance. He had not forgotten her, had not just walked away as she had expected, as a typical Saudi man would have done. For the first time, she felt a genuine affection for Mahmoud. She was happy.

The next day there was no phone call. Instead, the aunt who had made the initial contact called Sultana's father, saying that Mahmoud did not want to pressure Sultana by forcing her to decide so quickly. In typical Saudi fashion, the aunt wanted to learn of Sultana's decision in advance, so that an embarrassing confrontation could be avoided, and everyone could save face. Sultana had not reached a final decision until that moment, but now, delighted by the fact that Mahmoud had given her the option of saying a tactful "no," she chose to give him an emphatic "yes." She thus made a commitment to Mahmoud Daouk, a man that she had met just once in her entire life, and a man that she had not yet spoken to in any meaningful way. And it was all based on one small gesture. He had given her a choice.

Several days later Mahmoud called Sultana on the telephone and they had their first real conversation. He was very bashful at first, but gradually he became more comfortable as he talked about his business, his trips to the desert, his criticism of life in Saudi Arabia, and his dealings with the Bedouins. Sultana was pleased by how easily they conversed. Like most Saudi women, she had never had a phone conversation with a boyfriend. Somehow she had expected him to recite epic love poems, which might have embarrassed her. She was happy and relieved to have such a relaxed, friendly conversation. Mahmoud phoned daily and their conversations became longer and longer.

Then he came to see her, and they talked some more. Her stepmother or her father was always there with them.

"It would be improper for us to be alone," she emphasized. "The Saudis never close the door on two people who are not married."

After several weeks had passed they made the *khotbah*, the announcement of their intention to marry.

"Our *khotbah* was different from most," said Sultana. "The two families got together and had a party to announce our engagement to be married. Mahmoud bought me this beautiful diamond necklace, a bracelet, and a ring. Ordinarily this is not done."

The diamond necklace was magnificent. It must have cost a king's ransom, I thought.

Sultana went on to say that the traditional *khotbah* involves only the bridal couple and the two fathers. Often it is the groom's only chance to see his future wife before the wedding. The bride must be completely covered except for her face. The basic purpose of the *khotbah* is to let a man see what he is getting before he commits himself to the marriage.

"He can then see that she is not lame and is not blind, just to see that she's perfect before he buys her," explained Sultana.

"By the way," she added, "in Saudi Arabia it is expected that the man will pay a dowry to his wife. My mother said it used to be common to pay dowries in America a long time ago. Here, we still do it."

"I think that in the old days the *wife's* family paid the dowry," I said. "In the United States, anyway."

"That's funny," mused the princess. "Here it's the other way around. One of the big complaints now is that the dowries are going up so quickly that some men cannot afford to marry."

"How much is the average dowry?"

The princess shrugged. "It depends, of course, on who the woman is and how much the man can afford to pay. Sometimes it is 10,000 riyals, sometimes 30,000. My dowry is 100,000 riyals, but that is because I am a princess, and because my husband's family is very wealthy."

"I see. And will your father use the dowry to pay for your wedding?"

"No!" she exclaimed. "Under the law, the dowry belongs exclusively to the wife, to do with as she pleases."

"So the 100,000 riyals [$33,000] is entirely yours?" I asked.

"Yes."

"That sounds like . . . you are selling yourself."

She smiled and shrugged. "It is our custom. Women are treated as property most of the time anyway, so it is nice that at least we are allowed to keep the dowry. It is only fair."

For several minutes the princess talked about Saudi marriage, peppering her discussion with examples of how badly women were treated.

"Oh, I've got a great story!" Sultana said with her animated voice and gestures. "I don't know who told me, but I think Mahmoud did. Anyway there was this woman who was abruptly divorced by her husband one day, and was sent back to her family. Months went by, and then someone made inquiries about her. Without informing his daughter, the father met with the prospective husband, and after several hours they negotiated a marriage agreement. Then the father returned home and told his daughter to get her belongings together, because she was now married. The father walked his daughter over to the house of her new husband, introduced them at the door, wished them good luck and left. The woman fainted dead away at the door."

About a month after they first met Mahmoud asked about the *mulka*. Sultana explained that this was the official religious act: in the presence of members of both families, a religious sheik recorded the marriage contract and joined the couple according to Moslem law. The *mulka* is not a ceremonial occasion. The bride and groom simply sign a book. The marriage, however, is not consummated until after the wedding celebration.

In discussing the *mulka* the family decided to put it off until just before the wedding. To make the *mulka* early appeared unseemly, because it implied haste and hinted at a sexual peccadillo.

"My stepmother told me that if we have the *mulka* early people might say that I want to kiss him or to have an affair with him or I don't know what," explained Sultana.

During the waiting period they were in a curious social limbo. They were not supposed to be alone together, and by traditional Saudi standards they were not supposed to be together at all. Sultana's father was an enlightened Saudi and allowed them to see each other at home, properly chaperoned. Sultana, however, was concerned that her grandfather might find out and interfere with their wedding plans.

Although Sultana and Mahmoud were comfortable seeing each other before the wedding, they were prohibited by tradition from having "sexual" contacts of even the most trivial sort. Kissing, holding hands, or being together without an escort were not considered proper. Of course, these restrictions were less burdensome than they appeared precisely because they were so clearly accepted by the young couple. For Mahmoud to propose, or for Sultana to entertain, the possibility of sexual activity would have been degrading, almost on a level with prostitution. The two of them behaved decorously throughout, going to great lengths to ensure that Sultana's reputation was protected. The most intimate contact between them, was a handshake, and then not in private.

"My father has been remarkable," said Sultana when she finished her story. "He doesn't worry about the traditional rules at all. For example, Mahmoud's mother came to our house and said that it would be good to have the *mulka* right away, so that I would not have my reputation injured by seeing Mahmoud. But there were also other reasons. You see a girl could change her mind at the last minute, you know, and Mahmoud wanted to make sure I was his. Anyway my father rejected this idea completely. He said, "I am ready to let Sultana go with him in a car, and let her go to your house, and let him stay at our house until after midnight. I don't care about any of that stuff. But I don't want to rush the *mulka*."

"Isn't this an unusual attitude for a Saudi father?" I asked.

Sultana shook her head in amazement. "It is unbelievable. To say that Mahmoud could stay at our house until after midnight? To say that I could go with him alone in a *car?* His parents could not believe it and I was shocked."

"Have you ever gone with Mahmoud for a ride in the car?"

"Oh, no!" she exclaimed. "I would be too embarrassed and ashamed. My father is very liberal, but he is not a woman, and he does not understand how bad that would be. All the rest of my life people would know about it, and would gossip about me. I would not do that until after my wedding."

It was curious that Sultana could be more conservative than her father, but in a way it was not surprising. After all, the punishment and responsibility for loose behavior fall entirely on the woman, and so Sultana would naturally be more sensitive to the sexual prohibitions than a man. Then too, it seemed that Sultana was always trying to be more Saudi than the Saudis, perhaps because of her American background. Her father had grown up in Arabia and could reject certain customs that were unacceptable; Sultana as a woman felt that she had to embrace the old ways in order to qualify as a Saudi. After all, she was only half Saudi.

"When is your *mulka* going to take place?" I asked.

"Probably a day or two before the wedding," she replied. "It would be too much of a fuss if it was on the wedding day, because so much else is going on, you know. Probably, we will get the sheik, the little old man running around, you know, with his book, and the family together and just do it. I will wear a pretty dress, someone will probably take pictures, and that will be it."

"And after the *mulka* you have the wedding party."

"Right," she said. "The bride and the groom go to their own separate wedding parties, and then the man goes to the woman, and their marriage begins."

At a Saudi wedding, as with almost every other aspect of Saudi life, the sexes are strictly segregated. The men go to one party, the women to another, and often these parties are many miles apart.

"Mahmoud is looking forward to meeting you," said Princess Sultana. "I hope you'll come tonight."

"Of course," I assured her. "I'd love to meet him."

"I've told him all about you," she said with a smile. "I think that he is a little jealous of all the time I spend with you. I'm anxious to know what you think of him."

"I feel that I know him already, because of our discussions," I remarked as I left. "I'll see you this evening after my rounds."

At seven o'clock I arrived at Sultana's suite and met Mahmoud Daouk. Sultana's attendant was very much in evidence, as a chaperone, and retired to the other room with a sigh of relief when she saw me.

Sultana introduced us and beamed as we shook hands. Mahmoud was a tall, heavy-set man of twenty-four. He wore a mustache but no beard. There was nothing particularly distinguished about him, although he had an appealing smile.

"I am very pleased to meet you," he said in good English. "I have heard a lot about you."

I thanked him and complimented him on his English. He told me he had gone to a small college in California, the name of which was unrecognizable to me. He had taken some business courses, but did not graduate.

"I was there for a good time," he explained. "I loved America. Football was my favorite sport, but now that I'm back in Saudi Arabia there is a lot of work for me to do. There's not much football around here."

"What kind of work are you in?" I knew his father was immensely wealthy, in the billionaire category, but I didn't know the source.

"We're in the water-drilling business," he said. Mahmoud went on to explain that his father had a contract from the government to drill for water. Since the country has no permanent rivers and very little annual rainfall, this is a crucial method for obtaining the water needed for drinking and other uses. Saudi Arabia has large underground water reservoirs, known as aquifers, and water could be drilled for just like oil.

"Since we have more oil than we have water," said Mahmoud, "the price of water in this country is much more than gasoline or oil."

"How much more?"

"A gallon of gasoline is 18 cents, and a gallon of drinking water costs $2.40 in Saudi Arabia," he replied.

Sultana had told me previously that she had seen Mahmoud's father on TV discussing a contract for drilling twelve wells.

Courtship: Saudi Arabian Style ◊ *121*

"Not everybody knows it, but they will make a profit of about 40 million riyals [$13 million] just for drilling these wells," she had said.

This is all tax free, too, I thought.

In the course of our conversation I learned that Mahmoud's father was a self-made man and that he owned the drilling company outright, the machinery, drilling equipment, trucking—everything.

"Drilling for water is different from drilling for oil," he said. "We don't have to drill down so far."

Mahmoud told me that they had a lot of trouble and expense with this. Sometimes they made a mistake and struck oil rather than water.

"And that is too bad," he said, "because we have no contract for oil, so we must cap the oil well at our own expense and drill elsewhere."

"Sometimes we strike an oil field and hit nothing but oil. It is one of the risks of our business." He sighed, shaking his head.

It was pretty hard to commiserate. "I wish we had such a problem in the U.S.," I said, laughing. "We work hard to drill for oil and we often strike water."

Mahmoud explained that the water business was so lucrative that a driller could suffer any number of oil wells as long as there was an occasional water well in between.

We chatted for a while about their impressions of America and about my impressions of Saudi Arabia. Mahmoud loved the desert and promised to take me on a trip to an area where there was a petrified forest millions of years old.

He was a pleasant enough person, but there was nothing remarkable about him except his father's enormous wealth. I did not understand how Sultana could find him attractive. She should have chosen the prince, I concluded. On the other hand, from all appearances Mahmoud was in love with her, and probably would make her happy.

Then, glancing at Sultana, he gave me a wide smile.

"Dr. Gray," he said in a very formal voice, "we would like to invite you to our wedding."

I looked at Sultana. She was beaming. They had apparently discussed this beforehand.

"I'm flattered," I finally managed to say. "Of course, I'll come. I would consider it an honor."

For several minutes the three of us discussed the wedding plans. The men's party was scheduled to be an elaborate affair at the Daouk family compound. The women's party, on the other hand, would be at the new and very plush Intercontinental Hotel in Riyadh. The distance between the two parties was almost fifty miles. Mahmoud would spend the evening at the men's party. When the celebration was in full swing, probably after midnight, he would leave and drive to the Intercontinental to claim his bride.

In the course of this discussion, Mahmoud offered to arrange for me to go to the Intercontinental Hotel so that I could have a glimpse of the women's wedding party. He looked at Sultana as he said this, and it was clear that she had asked him to make this offer.

"Men are forbidden to attend the women's wedding party," said Mahmoud, "but Sultana wants you to have a look, if possible."

This was a chance of a lifetime, to be at the center of a formal Saudi wedding, and the wedding of a royal princess at that! I was excited at the prospect, and both Sultana and Mahmoud teased me about my enthusiasm.

"My brother Sultan and Mahmoud's brother Monsoor will bring you to the wedding," said Sultana.

"After the wedding we are going to California to see my mother!" announced the princess gaily. "I want her to meet my husband. This will only be part of our trip, however. We will first go to Switzerland, Paris, and Cannes. After we visit California, we will fly to Hawaii."

"Wonderful!" I said, positively ebullient.

"After that, we aren't sure. We will probably return to America for a while and then we may go again to Europe on the way back home. I don't think we will go to London. There are too many Arabs there."

I burst into laughter.

"It's true!" she said. "Too many Arabs. I mean, it's disgusting. It looks just like Riyadh these days."

"Well, what will you do when you finally get back to Saudi Arabia?" I asked. "I hope you'll come to see me."

"Of course," she said. She glanced at Mahmoud, who seemed amused and not at all offended by our banter. "After we return, we'll live in the compound of Mahmoud's father. It's a beautiful place, lots of palm trees, you know—just like an oasis. It's located down in the valley, at the back of Shimasi."

"We have built a cute little prefab house on the compound," she said, "and we will stay there until our own home is built. We are planning a villa, which will be the most beautiful in Riyadh. We have already selected much of the furniture."

"I will be very happy in the valley," she continued. "It's so beautiful. We don't wear our veils there, and we even take walks up and down the road at night. But the most important thing is to see all that green. Everything in Saudi Arabia is so brown, and I love to see something green."

For several minutes Mahmoud and Sultana discussed the people who would be coming to their wedding, talking mainly to each other, while I watched. That he worshiped her was clear to even the most cursory observer. His eyes seemed to sparkle every time she spoke.

At length I excused myself. Mahmoud shook my hand—very firmly, I noted, reminding me of the story of their first meeting—and then I left them under the careful scrutiny of Sultana's servant.

Two days later Sultana was finally discharged from the hospital. She was anxious to get started on her wedding plans. Naturally, I dropped by to see her off, and while we filled out the discharge papers she asked me for my impressions of Mahmoud.

"Isn't he wonderful!" she said. "He is incredibly thoughtful. I'm sure that the two of us will be happy together."

"I'm sure you will be too," I said. Somehow, I wanted Sultana to marry a dashing young man who looked like a leader, not this plump, soft billionaire. However, I realized that I was projecting my values onto Sultana, and that my concept of a perfect husband had little to do with the reality of Saudi Arabia. In a country where wealth and family background are paramount, Mahmoud was an excellent match, and even if Sultana had been allowed to "date" many men she might well have selected him anyway. The billion dollars was hardly a drawback, but I would like to think that Sultana loved him for himself as well.

"Mahmoud called me yesterday," she said excitedly. "He just received a telegram from a hotel in Switzerland, and it was addressed to Mr. and Mrs. Mahmoud Daouk. When he read it he could hardly believe his eyes. It made him so happy that he called me up immediately. Isn't he wonderful?"

"Yes," I agreed. "I know he loves you, and I think that it will be a good marriage."

"I hope I can be a good wife to him," she confided. "I am not used to giving anyone my special attention. I will have to learn what pleases him."

I smiled at her concern. "You'll be a perfect wife," I said.

I walked her down the corridor of the hospital, and bade her goodbye in the lobby. She was wearing a veil now—the first time that I had seen it on her—and in a very symbolic way I realized that she was forever lost to me. I could go to her wedding, and perhaps even see her on occasion, but it would never again be as open and friendly as it had been these past three weeks. Always the veil would be between us, as it had to be.

◊ 11 ◊

A MOST UNUSUAL WEDDING

THE WEDDING of Princess Sultana bint Musaid Al Sudairi and Mahmoud Daouk took place on a clear, balmy evening in April. Although a minor social event by international standards, the marriage sparked a great deal of interest in Saudi Arabia, where watching the rich and the royalty is virtually the national pastime. According to my Saudi friends, the wedding was the foremost topic of conversation in Riyadh for most of the preceding week. Even the expatriate community—not known for either understanding or caring about the internal affairs of Saudi Arabia—seemed to sense that there was something special in this alliance between the beautiful Saudi princess and her billionaire fiancé.

I was particularly intrigued because with Sultana's consent I had arranged to watch the women celebrate the marriage, from a concealed vantage point at the Intercontinental Hotel. The fact that it was absolutely forbidden to men made it all the more enticing.

At 8 P.M. on the wedding night, Sultan and Monsoor, the brothers of the bride and groom respectively, picked me up in a Mercedes 450 SL to drive me to the men's half of the wedding party. The two young men were approximately seventeen years old, tall and slender, with light skin and jet-black hair. Both were trying to grow the standard Saudi mustache with a marked lack of progress. Both spoke English with substantially more success.

"Have you ever been to a Saudi wedding?" asked Sultan.

"Never," I replied.

"It's very different from anything in the States," he said with a laugh. "It'll blow your mind."

I nodded, amused by his American slang. Like Sultana, Sultan had spent his formative years in California, and seemed to revel in the use of American slang.

Sultan, Monsoor, and I got into the Mercedes, and the two young men soon exhibited another familiar Saudi trait: the compulsion to risk life and limb by driving at breakneck speed. This was no longer a unique experience after my conditioning by Westbrook and the taxi drivers of Riyadh.

As we careened down the King Abdul Aziz Road, heading for the Shimasi area, I was alarmed to see a half-pint bottle lying on its side on the ledge in front of the windshield. "My God," I wondered, "have they been drinking?"

I took the bottle, removed the cork, and sniffed the contents. It was cologne. I sighed with relief.

The two young men burst into laughter.

"You thought it was whiskey," said Monsoor accusingly.

I admitted my suspicions, adding, "The way you guys drive, I could use a drink right now." They beamed, as if this were a great compliment.

About half an hour later, we arrived at an oasis southwest of Riyadh known as Shimasi. Here, in a startlingly lush valley, lived some of the leading people in Saudi Arabia. Although the area had not yet been developed, there were several opulent villas and "palaces," surrounded by trees, bushes, and well-kept lawns. The greenness of the valley was not unusual by American standards, but in arid Saudi Arabia it was a stunning sight.

"That is Prince Abdullah's palace," said Monsoor, pointing to a palatial white villa glistening in the moonlight. It was surrounded by vast illuminated gardens, which could be seen through the gates as we passed.

"My father's compound is the next place down the road," he added with a grin. "It's very comforting to have the commander of the national guard as your next-door neighbor."

"Next door" turned out to be five miles down the road, where we arrived at a huge compound—almost a small city—composed of several smaller buildings and dwellings that were dominated by a large villa. At the gate of the compound we were greeted by the two fathers of the bridal couple. Sultana's father, who had been my patient, greeted me with a warm handshake, and then introduced me to Mr. Daouk. Although the two fathers were almost the same age, I immediately sensed that they represented different cultures and ideologies.

Sultana's father was a royal of ancient lineage, articulate, urbane, and sophisticated. He belonged to the modern faction of Saudi Arabian society, and was Western-educated. Although generally observing Saudi traditions, he was always willing to stretch a point. Mr. Daouk seemed to be straight out of Saudi Arabia's past. A commoner, he was a short, corpulent man, strictly orthodox, isolationist, and traditional. He wore sandals, spoke no English, and seemed distinctly nonplused by my appearance at the wedding. Sultana's father introduced me by explaining that I was his doctor and that I had also helped Sultana through her recent illness. Monsoor also tried to put in a good word on my behalf, but to no avail. Mr. Daouk, clutching his prayer beads, shook my hand with indifference. He was probably wondering what the hell I was doing at the wedding. The same thought passed through my mind. It was impossible to bridge the gap of a thousand years within a few minutes.

Feeling self-conscious now, I walked with Sultan and Monsoor into the family compound. There, an area larger than a football field had been set aside for the wedding party. Multicolored lights were strung in all directions, and both sides of the field were lined with the huge trucks and mechanical equipment used in the Daouk drilling operations. Although the area was not very attractive, it was enormously impressive. I wondered whether the display of sophisticated machinery was a deliberate attempt to flaunt the Daouk wealth.

About one hundred large colorful oriental rugs had been laid on the hard ground. Chairs had been placed on the rugs in the middle of the field to form a large rectangle. There were two kinds of chairs: conventional chairs for the common people and, for the royalty, large cushioned chairs which were placed at both ends of the rectangle. People began drifting in, shaking hands with their friends. Monsoor and Sultan at my side cued me in on the various royals coming in. I had learned to identify them by the gold braid on their mantles and, of course, by their shoes. Idly, I took a quick survey to test my theory that only royalty wore shoes. The evidence indicated that, while all the royals wore shoes, some of the wealthy commoners were also beginning to adopt Western footwear. Thus my system for identifying royalty—though good—was not infallible.

For perhaps a half hour, I watched the people around me, waiting for the wedding party to get started. The chairs filled up rapidly. The guests were sitting or standing in small groups while servants in long robes moved gracefully among them, serving cardamom coffee. The men sat and talked or walked about on the carpets, greeting friends and family. Gradually, it dawned on me that the wedding party had already started. Apparently, this was how the Saudis celebrated a marriage. Although Sultan and Monsoor were still with me, they were conversing excitedly in Arabic, enjoying the party at a level that I could not appreciate. Bored, I began to count the number of chairs on the rugs. There were 250.

Suddenly, I spotted two doctors from the hospital, and I eagerly walked over to greet them. One was an American gynecologist. He told me that he had prescribed birth-control pills for many Saudi women and that the pill was used by the more educated women in Saudi Arabia, but never by the Bedouin or orthodox women. The other doctor was an Egyptian surgeon who was an old friend of the Daouk family. Our host, he said, was a self-made man of enormous wealth, but had no idea what to do with all his money.

"He is fat and occasionally drinks too much, considering his diabetes," asserted the Egyptian doctor, who was also fat and looked as though he too drank too much.

"The doctor is a drinking partner of my father's," confided Monsoor as we walked away. "They will probably get drunk together tonight after everybody leaves."

"That's their privilege," I said. "I still can't believe that no one is drinking at a wedding, especially an all-male wedding."

"It's against our religion," said Monsoor solemnly. I glanced at him to see if he was being facetious, but he was dead serious. Like most Saudis, he saw nothing strange or inconsistent about having a "dry" wedding party and then getting drunk after all the guests went home.

Wandering about, the three of us came upon the dining area set up at the periphery of the field. White sheets had been placed upon the rugs along the length and breadth of one side of the field. Servants were busily arranging bowls of oranges, apples, bananas, grapes, and dates. There were no knives or forks and no salt and pepper shakers. I recalled that the Saudis never add salt or pepper to their food after it is prepared, adding lime or lemon juice instead. They use salt and pepper sparingly in cooking, flavoring their food with tomatoes, raisins, orange rind, or carrots.

According to Monsoor, the main course—known as *kabsa*—was still being prepared. Monsoor described this as a portion of lamb on a bed of rice, surrounded by pieces of chicken, tomatoes, onions, and carrots, garnished with raisins and almonds, and bordered with hard-boiled eggs. It sounded delicious, and sharp hunger pangs reminded me of how late the Saudis usually eat their dinner.

Dinnertime finally arrived. The party suddenly moved to the food area as if by instinct. The Saudis quietly took their places, either squatting on their haunches or sitting cross-legged on the rugs with their legs tucked up under them. Much to my amazement I heard not a single cracking of a kneebone during this procedure. Some of them squatting comfortably nearby were in their seventies and eighties, but their limbs were much more elastic than mine.

Envying their limberness, I tried to emulate both procedures, much to the amusement of Sultan and Monsoor. Squatting was an absolute failure: I simply couldn't get down on my haunches and remain there. Sitting cross-legged proved equally uncomfortable. I couldn't get my legs under me at first, but when this was accomplished with the help of my friends on either side, both legs tingled and then went numb. I finally compromised by lying on my side and leaning on one elbow, Roman style. However, the Romans, as I recalled, were always surrounded by a bevy of beautiful women, comparable in no way to my present situation.

When everyone was assembled, a fleet of small Toyota trucks began to shuttle food back and forth from the main house, which was located some distance away. Servants brought huge platters of steaming hot *kabsa* and placed them on the ground before us. The guests began to eat from these platters with their hands. They ate sparingly in a slow, quiet, and deliberate manner, while conversing in undertones. They would reach for the food, always using their right hand, and tear off a piece of lamb or chicken. At times, they would squeeze a small ball of rice in the palm of a hand and eat it that way. Each tray was placed so that four people could eat comfortably from it, two on each side. The Saudis never chewed on the bones, but deftly picked them clean with their fingers. The lamb was tough but tasty, and the chicken perfect. The rice was a little sticky, probably from overcooking. Dessert consisted of fresh fruit and individual servings of a fruit and custard mold. The dates were especially sweet and succulent, and they were a perfect end to a very satisfying meal. I was grateful that nobody had tripped over my outstretched legs.

During the dinner, Mr. Daouk, clutching his prayer beads, roamed about, graciously greeting friends and making certain that there was enough food for everyone.

"How do you like it so far?" asked Sultan when we had finished eating.

"It's fascinating," I replied. "I've attended a lot of weddings in my life, but never one without any women. This is a new experience."

"It gets better," said Sultan with a smile.

In the distance I heard the beating of drums. It was coming from the other side of the field.

"Come with us," said Monsoor. "They are beginning the dance."

The three of us began to walk across the field. On the way, the boys stopped to greet friends and family members. Suddenly Mahmoud appeared and came over to shake my hand. He was smiling but he looked nervous.

"Are you enjoying the wedding?" he asked politely.

"It's unique," I replied. "Am I still invited to see the women's ceremony?"

"Sure," he said. "I will be leaving later in the evening. Sultan and Monsoor will tell you the plan."

Mahmoud was deluged by well-wishers, and Sultan, Monsoor, and I continued walking in the direction of the beating drums. There, under strings of bright lights, was a large area covered by impressive blue-and-gold rugs. We saw two lines of men facing each other about twenty feet apart.

One line of men carried round, bright-colored drums suspended by ropes around their necks. Facing the drummers was the second line of men, who were the chanters. Each chanter held a long stick in one hand, representing a spear, or carried a long, fierce-looking sword. In a minor key and in monotone, they recounted the glories of Bedouin life and of past battles. They chanted, to the beat of the drums, the many tales and parables handed down by word of mouth from generation to generation, the traditional way of recording history in an illiterate society. Some of these stories were a thousand years old, mostly unrecorded.

At first, the chanters remained in line facing the drummers. Then, one or two at a time, they began to dance as they sang. They really just pranced about as the spirit moved them, their long thobes fluttering in the breeze. Some carried what appeared to be feathery, multicolored pom-poms as they danced. Then some of the drummers joined in the dance, followed finally by the bridegroom and the wedding guests, who were cavorting around with no apparent pattern or style, and simply leaping up and down to express the Bedouin joy of life. Everyone was improvising. Anyone could do it. Of course, Sultan, Monsoor, and I joined the group, and touched by the excitement, danced about in frenzied abandon, although none of us knew what we were doing. There was no rhythm to the beat. It was not a war dance. It was what I would call "free expression," and it was a very primitive or a very modern dance, depending on how one views such things.

The dance had no beginning and no end. It seemed to go on interminably. People just dropped out from exhaustion. The excitement began to ebb. The chanters gave out one by one, and the drummers gradually lost their vigor. The dance did not end; it collapsed. Then it all dwindled into silence. The guests went back to their seats and began to converse as before. Somehow, I found this ending deflating, an anticlimax. My friends assured me, however, that the dancing would go on until dawn.

The silence was broken by a more familiar sound coming from the other side of the field. It was a mixture of rock and roll and belly-dance music. We went over to investigate. About one hundred men dressed in Western-style trousers, blue jeans, and colorful shirts had gathered. They were part of the work force imported from other countries by our host for his water-drilling operation. Most of them were from Lebanon; some were Palestinian.

They squatted on their haunches or sat cross-legged in a large circle on the huge oriental rugs. One man had a guitar. The others clapped to the rhythm of the guitar while two men performed a magnificent belly dance in the center of the circle. Everyone was caught up in the rhythm. As the clapping grew louder and louder, the dancing became more frenzied. The young men took turns at the belly dancing, each trying to surpass the other. It was quite a sight!

The Saudis looked on with curiosity and restraint. They did not participate in the hand clapping. This kind of dancing is considered licentious in Saudi Arabia and is forbidden. Within a few minutes the chanters and the drummers lined up again, and the Saudi dancing started anew, in competition with the Lebanese on the other side of the field.

After a while, I walked with Sultan and Monsoor toward the main house of the Daouk compound. It was a huge villa surrounded by lovely grounds, manicured lawns, and graceful palm trees laden with dates. The swimming pool was located in a separate enclosure. There were a number of smaller houses nearby for the servants.

"Let me show you where Sultana and Mahmoud are going to live," said Monsoor. He led me to a small cottage near the swimming pool. It was the "honeymoon cottage" Sultana had spoken of in the hospital.

"This is where they will spend their first night together," said Sultan. "They will come back here from the Intercontinental Hotel."

"We will bring you here after the wedding," added Monsoor, "so that you can take the first pictures of them at home, as Sultana promised."

"I have the camera in my pocket," I said, laughing. "Sultana didn't forget her promise. She is quite remarkable."

"Soon Mahmoud will be leaving for the Intercontinental to get Sultana," announced Monsoor. "He is very nervous about it—he doesn't like being around all those women by himself."

"Aren't the women mostly members of his family?"

"Sure," said Monsoor, "many of them are relatives. But still he will be one man among three hundred women."

"What should I do?" I asked. "How can I get to the Intercontinental?"

Monsoor and Sultan proceeded to unfold the plan. Around midnight, the family and friends would gather around Mahmoud, shake his hand and wish him well. This would be the indication that he was preparing to leave. At that point, Mahmoud and his father would drive to the Intercontinental Hotel in one car, and Sultan and the bride's father would go in another. Meanwhile, Monsoor and I would ride together in the Mercedes.

"We should leave before the others," warned Monsoor, "so that you can watch the women's party. My father has not been told about your little adventure, and he will be furious if he finds out. Also, it is very important that the women do not see you. If they catch you at the Intercontinental, looking in on the women's party, we will *all* be in trouble, including Sultana. Have you made all the arrangements?"

"Yes," I said. "I'll tell you about it later."

"Good," he replied. "Remember that what you are doing is strictly forbidden by our culture." It seemed as though the phrases "It is forbidden" and "It is the custom" were used constantly.

I assured him that both Sultana and her father had approved, and that Mahmoud knew all about it as well.

A short time later the men began to crowd around the groom and I knew that it was time to leave. For a brief, panic-stricken moment I could not find Monsoor.

"Where's Monsoor?" I asked Sultan.

"Right here."

I turned to find him hiding behind a friend, and grinning at my agitation. "Let's go," he said.

Quietly we slipped out the gate of the compound and drove off in the Mercedes. On the way to the hotel I outlined my plan for watching the women's party. An Egyptian patient of mine whom I had befriended happened to be the headwaiter at the Intercontinental. He had promised to show me a good hiding place, which would keep me concealed and yet offer me a perfect view of the proceedings.

"*Inshallah*," said Monsoor as we arrived at the Intercontinental. "Good luck, and *please* don't take any flash pictures from your hiding place!"

"I promise," I replied, feeling a little apprehensive about my undertaking. "Meet me in the lobby afterward!"

Inside the hotel I found Hussein, my headwaiter friend, waiting for me. He led me through the employees' entrance up a back stairway to a small balcony overlooking the ballroom.

"Here we are," he whispered. "If you stand behind these drapes, they won't be able to see you, but be very careful." Then, with a smile, he quietly disappeared down the stairs.

From behind the curtains, I looked down upon the scene below, which was strange, wondrous, and exotic. It conjured up a fantasy from the Arabian nights: hundreds of tall, elegant women, magnificently gowned in glowing silks and satins, brilliant with color. Since no men were present, the women were unveiled, and their combined beauty was breathtaking. Their graceful necks and slender wrists glittered with priceless jewels. Emeralds, rubies, and diamonds seemed to come alive with fire beneath the bright crystal chandeliers of the great ballroom.

Although my initial impression was that of grandeur, it soon became apparent that the atmosphere was relaxed and informal, much like the men's half of the wedding. Most of the women were sitting or standing in small groups, talking quietly. A few women were dancing, either alone or two women together. On a raised platform in the front of the room, a group of young women were seated in a semicircle, playing an assortment of instruments. Sultana was nowhere to be seen.

In the back of the room, looking like ghouls, sat a group of heavily-veiled onlookers dressed completely in black. These were the *mutfarra-jeen,* spectators who go to wedding parties without invitations. They are usually poor women who take vicarious pleasure in attending a grand celebration such as this. By Saudi Arabian custom, these women are allowed to attend a wedding providing they remain veiled. I wondered whether there was a man among them.

Several minutes later, Sultana appeared through a small side door. She was wearing a white Parisian gown embroidered with pearls and a white veil held in place by a diamond tiara. As she slowly walked toward the dais, escorted by her stepmother and several other women of both families, a drum began to beat. At the same time, the women accompanying the bride began a high-pitched, harsh, trilling sound, which was made by flicking the tongue rapidly back and forth over the roof of the mouth, to the accompaniment of shrill cries. Known as the *zeffa,* this ritual is a remnant of medieval pageantry designed to ward off evil spirits. It reminded me vaguely of a southern rebel yell.

As Sultana approached the dais in her lavish gown, glistening with pearls, I thought of the hours we had spent talking in the hospital, where she was not surrounded by all this glory. There she sat in a simple hospital robe, describing how sad it was that women lived in anticipation of these parties, where they could display their finery to one another and exchange gossip. Now, as she was escorted to one of the two thronelike chairs on the dais, she was committing herself to exactly this kind of life. From now on she would wait for events such as this, where women grasped at the few hours of conviviality allowed to them. This was her future. She had chosen to live as a Saudi Arabian princess. I wondered whether she had considered the price.

After a short time, Mahmoud and his father came into the ballroom and walked toward the dais with a slow, ceremonious tread. Then the groom mounted the dais and stood before his bride. Gently, he reached out and lifted her veil very slowly and deliberately. There was a poignant sensuality to the performance. In the old days, this might have been the moment when the groom saw his bride's face for the first time. Sultana looked at him impassively for a moment, then broke into a wide smile. The entire party laughed and applauded.

Following the traditional wedding ceremony, Mahmoud threw handfuls of small gold coins among the guests to demonstrate his joy. After a brief but mad scramble for the coins, the women approached the dais to congratulate the bridal couple. Suddenly, Monsoor and Sultan appeared in the room, and this caused the women to shriek a loud warning. They began to pelt them good-naturedly with gold coins and hard candies, which was to symbolize the throwing of stones to drive the men away and to protect their virtue. The boys drew back in feigned terror, and after scooping up the "stones" they ran from the ballroom.

Mahmoud and Sultana sat on the dais for several more minutes, and after receiving the felicitations of the guests, they rose to leave. Abandoning my secluded vantage point, I dashed down the back stairs to the lobby, where I found Monsoor and Sultan happily eating candy and counting their gold coins. After bidding goodby to Sultan, Monsoor and I drove back to the Daouk compound.

There we found the men's party continuing into the night, despite the fact that most of the guests had now left. The drummers and chanters were still at it, and a hardcore group of dancers seemed ready to stay until dawn. The belly dancing on the Lebanese side of the field was also going on with as much enthusiasm as ever.

After a while, Monsoor directed me to the "honeymoon cottage" that he had shown me earlier in the evening. There I was greeted by the servant who had stayed with Sultana in the hospital. She gave me a smile of recognition and showed me into the living room. Sultana and Mahmoud were sitting close together on a long couch, looking exhausted but happy. What astonished me was the manner in which Mahmoud had "taken possession" of his bride. He had placed his arm about Sultana's shoulder, as if to say, "She belongs to me now." Such a show of physical affection was strongly disapproved by Saudi culture, especially in front of other people. Clearly, they thought of me as a special friend.

Mahmoud asked if I would like something to drink. I hoped for champagne but was given a choice of fruit juice or coffee. Accepting the fruit juice, I listened as Sultana talked and laughed about the wedding party. Although she was clearly in an ebullient mood, there was a strangely stifled quality to her conversation, as if she felt restricted in the presence of her husband. It occurred to me that Mahmoud might never see the side of her that I had come to appreciate. The Sultana I knew, the budding young woman who had been so free and uninhibited, had now disappeared. I watched her with a feeling of sadness and joy.

"Did you bring your camera?" Sultana asked at length.

"It's right here in my pocket."

I took several pictures of the bridal couple, in which Mahmoud's arm was still firmly planted around Sultana's shoulder, as if to document his possession.

"I'll send you the prints," I promised as I prepared to leave.

The two of them stood up to say goodbye. Sultana thanked me for helping her to recover so quickly, and Mahmoud invited me to visit them when they returned from their honeymoon. I promised that I would but doubted that it was a promise I would keep. Something about the formality of this meeting made me realize that my close friendship with Sultana was already at an end.

I congratulated them and thanked them for inviting me to the wedding, and "for all the special privileges."

"Oh, enjoy your honeymoon," I said, turning to get a last look at Sultana.

She stood beside her husband now, with her arms at her sides and her hands clasped at her waist. Her smile was not of the kind in the hospital that had captivated and charmed me. It was fixed, contented, controlled. We caught each other's eye for a brief second, and then both looked away.

I left wondering if she would be able to fit her bright, active mind into the façade of ignorance and submission that was still a woman's only role in Saudi Arabia. I hoped that Sultana would somehow find meaning and freedom in her new and cloistered existence.

◊ *12* ◊

A HEAD ROLLS ON CHOP SQUARE

PERHAPS THE MOST SATISFYING facet of my job at the King Faisal Hospital was the chance I had to work with young Saudi Arabian medical students. At the time, the first class of doctors from the Riyadh Medical School were entering the internship period of the program, and this gave me a unique opportunity to influence the future development of the medical profession. The Saudi medical students were bright and eager to learn, and teaching them was an enormous challenge, for the students were not only learning medicine in a foreign language—namely English—but they lacked the basic knowledge that would be considered rudimentary in a technological society. For example, some of the students were so inexperienced that they had never seen a hypodermic needle until they went to medical school. Often, as I watched them struggle to make up centuries of experience, I remembered Bill Thompson's prediction that it would be years before the Saudis could be trained to be competent doctors. Somehow, this prediction became a personal challenge, and whenever I was frustrated at the slow pace of learning, I would think of Bill and then renew my determination to prove him wrong.

One of the students in that first class of doctors was a man by the name of Abdul Taleem. Abdul was a brilliant young man, who worked very hard and who spoke English well enough to make the learning experience a quick and painless process. Abdul often came to me when he had questions, and as the year progressed a bond of friendship began to grow between us. Often, we would sit in the cafeteria of the hospital talking over coffee, and our conversations would range from medicine to America and back again. When the school year ended, I quietly arranged for Abdul to receive an apprentice internship at the hospital—with pay—during his summer vacation.

As my friendship with Abdul developed, our conversations began to focus more and more on his experiences and perceptions of life in Saudi Arabia. One day, I mentioned that I was interested in purchasing a *khanjar,* one of the famous curved daggers that are distinctive of Arabia. At this news Abdul's eyes lit up, for he had grown up in Riyadh and knew every shop in the city.

"I know a perfect place to buy a *khanjar*," he assured me. "It is the antiques *suq* (marketplace) near Chop Square. There are many small shops there, and they have a large collection of swords and daggers. I will go with you this Friday and make sure that the shopkeepers do not try to cheat you on the price."

"Oh no, you don't have to do that," I said, as if to turn him down. In truth, I was delighted by his generous offer, but in keeping with Arab custom I was making a formal pretense of refusing his assistance. Both he and I knew that this was simply a matter of etiquette, and that I fully intended to have him accompany me.

"Of course I will come with you," said Abdul, smiling.

"No, no, I do not want to impose on you. I can do the bargaining myself."

"Like you did with the watch?" he asked, with a glint of humor.

I laughed. A month earlier, I had gone to the *suq* to buy a watch, and I had argued the trader down to a price I considered reasonable. When I later showed the watch to Abdul and told him the price, he was aghast at my naïveté. I knew that Abdul was a shrewd bargainer, and that he could probably talk a shopkeeper down to a price that was a fraction of what I would pay.

"All right," I said, giving in at last, "I would be honored to have you accompany me. But you must let me drive."

"Oh no," said Abdul, "you are a guest in my country. I must . . ."

We argued about this for a while longer, until I finally gave in. In America we could have made the decision in five seconds. With Abdul, the same decision took five minutes—but then it was also much more fun.

On Friday morning Abdul picked me up at my house for the shopping expedition. He was driving an old sports car, and I was initially apprehensive that he would be another of the suicidal Arabian drivers that I had come to fear. To my surprise, however, Abdul proved to be a model of driving decorum.

"You drive very well," I complimented him.

"Oh, this is nothing," he replied. "I am driving slow because I have heard you complain about the Saudi drivers. If you like, I will go normal speed."

"Normal speed?" I thought to myself. We were already going thirty-five in an urban area.

"Ah . . . no," I said. "Don't go normal speed. Drive slowly."

Since it was a Friday, the Moslem sabbath, the streets of Riyadh were comparatively quiet—which is to say merely overcrowded instead of jam-packed. Many of the shops in the market were closed today. Consequently, the traffic was light, and we could navigate the narrow sidewalks without being pushed into the street. When Abdul and I reached the shopping area, we found a space in an alley to park our car, which would have been impossible on a weekday. As we got out of the car, I noticed that Abdul did not lock the doors. When I reminded him of this, Abdul looked at me oddly; nobody in Saudi Arabia locked his car because cars were never stolen.

When shopping in Saudi Arabia, one must always plan the expedition around the prayer schedule, since everything stops during the five daily prayers. The prayer time changes from day to day depending on the time of sunrise and sunset. By consulting the *Arab News,* the English-language newspaper, I had learned that the prayer schedule for that day was 12:10 for the noon prayer, and 3:26 for the afternoon prayer. The Saudis are very precise about prayer time. (For some reason, the prayer information was always printed right next to the crossword puzzle.) Since the shops generally closed on Friday between the noon prayer and the afternoon prayer, we had to get our shopping done by noontime. It was now approximately 10 A.M., which gave us two hours.

With Abdul in the lead, we wandered through the maze of delightful little markets and shops that characterize the Saudi Arabian *suq.* As we approached the main shopping street, Sharah Wasir, I could smell the open sewers that ran the length of Sharah Batha a block away. Sharah Wasir had recently been renamed King Faisal Street, but the natives still used the old name, and a request for directions to King Faisal Street would probably have drawn blank stares. Walking down Sharah Wasir/King Faisal Street, I marveled at the small shops that sold everything from jewelry to incense to household goods. The shops, though quite shabby, often displayed the merchandise in a manner which was very impressive. This was typical of the Arab world, where advertising in newspapers is still a new and rarely-used technique, and where an impressive display of goods is considered the effective method of marketing.

The Japanese products were really bargains, particularly cameras, radios, calculators, hi-fi equipment, and watches. There was no sales tax on any of these luxuries.

As Abdul and I wandered among the shops, our conversation took an equally leisurely and meandering course. Inevitably, however, our conversation arrived at a discussion of the role that religion plays in Saudi Arabian life.

"These shops must all close at the noontime prayer," said Abdul. "If they don't the *matawa* (morals police) will come bang on their doors and make them close. Sometimes they may give a tardy shopkeeper a few whacks with their canes."

"What do you think of the *matawa?*" I asked, realizing that this was a highly sensitive question for a Westerner to ask an Arabian; Abdul, however, took it in stride.

"I think they are what you Americans call a 'pain in the ass,' " he said with a small smile. "They are orthodox Moslems who belong to the militant Wahabi sect, and they insist on following the old ways of a thousand years ago without exception. Sometimes, the things they fight for are good, but other times they stand in the way of progress."

"Would most people in Saudi Arabia agree with your assessment?"

Abdul pursed his lips. "Most of the young people would," he replied. "We understand the *matawa,* and we sympathize with them, but they are very aggressive about what they think is right. Last year, for example, two of them grabbed me on the street during Ramadan and cut my hair because they thought it was too long."

"You're kidding!" I exclaimed. "Did you do anything about it?"

He shrugged. "The *matawa* and the Wahabi are a force unto themselves. They are only ordinary people—citizens—but the royal family and police are very careful not to cross them. If I had complained of the attack, I knew nothing would be done. I didn't bother.

"You must understand Saudi Arabia," he continued, as if to answer my silence. "We are a very religious country. No other Islamic country is as strict about prayers as we are. The changes that the *matawa* see—long hair, blue jeans—are extremely threatening, and they react with ignorance and fear. I often disagree with them, but I also understand them. What they are is also a part of me.

"Wahabism has been successful so far but it won't last forever. There are too many foreigners and too many new ideas coming into the country to keep things as they are now."

As if to change the subject, Abdul suddenly pointed down the street. "That is the old Musmak fortress where King Ibn Saud won the battle to recapture Riyadh in 1902. There is a spearhead embedded in the gate that was supposedly thrown by King Ibn Saud himself. It has been left there all these years. This is called Thumayri Street, and it is named after one of Ibn Saud's men who was killed in the battle for the town."

The ancient fortress was built of mud bricks, and there were a few mudbrick houses in the surrounding area. On the other side of the street, some small shops displaying cameras, radios, and perfumes were open and doing a brisk business.

We finally arrived at Dira Square, the traditional center of Riyadh. The square was named Dira by the Bedouins, which means a grazing area. We all called it Chop Square because this was where the beheadings took place. Here, surrounding the large square, were several government buildings, including the Palace of Justice and the home office of the governor of Riyadh.

In addition to its official and rather grisly functions, Chop Square is also a center for most of the important *suqs* in the city of Riyadh. For example, the money changer *suq* is located right on Chop Square, and here the Saudi riyal can be exchanged for every currency in the world. Around the corner is the spice *suq*, where one can buy frankincense, aromatic herbs, and resins of every description. Nearby is a bazaar with a display of colorful silks from Damascus and the Orient.

To me, the most interesting of these market areas was the gold *suq*. Here, tiny shops line both sides of several long dirt paths, and each shop displays a dazzling assortment of gold jewelry that is hung from the ceiling and walls. Every available inch of space is devoted to gold in one form or another: mounds of rings, earrings, and small charms greet the eye, all made of 18-karat gold. The glitter and brilliance are nearly blinding. Never had I seen such an array. Women shrouded in black were picking over the mounds of gold, haggling with the shopkeepers over the price. Actually, each item was priced according to the weight, and in the end it was the scale that determined the price. The value of a gram of gold was set daily by the government. Still, the women bargained with the shopkeepers, if only out of a lifetime of habit. There was always the chance of a discount.

The most striking thing about the gold *suq* was the lack of security. All the gold sat in wide-open areas, without police or security guards to keep a watchful eye on the customers. The situation appeared to invite theft— and yet the shopkeepers felt perfectly safe. It was here in the gold *suq* that I truly understood what the Saudis meant when they said that they had no crime: it was a spiritual and emotional experience to feel such security and confidence among fellow human beings. My faith in mankind was being restored.

On the other side of the square, Abdul and I walked past the Great Mosque, a huge religious shrine of comparatively recent vintage, which was made of poured concrete and erected on the site of a smaller mud-brick mosque which had been there until 1850. Not far from the Great Mosque was the auction market, where slaves had been bought and sold until about fifteen years ago. This, I reflected, was the other side of the Saudi Arabian culture, for the same society that was so free of crime had, until recently, condoned the owning of human beings. I asked Abdul if he remembered slavery, and if his family had ever owned any slaves.

Slaves, Abdul told me, were treated differently from those in other countries. They were, for the most part, domestics and concubines. Many came from Syria, Iran, the Sudan, and Ethiopia.

Near the Great Mosque, we found the antiques *suq,* a large warehouse-type building containing countless shops that bought and sold antiques. Beneath the spacious roof, buyers and sellers bartered over the price in an Arabian tradition older than the most ancient object in the building. Following the maze of hard dirt paths, Abdul and I began to peruse the shops, looking for an appropriately old dagger.

Frequently, we would stop to talk with a shopkeeper, and we would rummage through dusty chests filled with daggers, old spears, rusted swords, and antique firearms. On the walls hung ancient ornate daggers in leather, silver, gold, or gem-studded scabbards, whose luster was long dimmed by age. Helter-skelter on the floor were large chests made of brass or teakwood and decorated with brass studs, often in floral designs covered by years of dust. Abdul said that most of the antiques came from Yemen, Syria, Egypt, Lebanon, and Persia. The camel-milk bowls, hollowed out of wood and tacked with decorative brass or silver studs, were from Saudi Arabia. Out of the semidarkness loomed ancient vessels of every size: brass and silver ewers, pitchers and coffeepots, all dull with the collected grime of time, having long outlived their days of glory.

After visiting perhaps a dozen shops, I found a curved dagger that I liked: it was approximately eight inches long, with a beautiful silver-and-gold-inlaid handle and a matching scabbard. The handle was decorated with silver threads shaped layer upon layer into geometric patterns, and filled with gold. The silver had tarnished from age, and the blade was dull, but the workmanship of the knife was superb.

Although I was delighted by the knife, Abdul had warned me not to express any interest. Rather, he told me that I should hand the knife to him, and signal my desire to purchase it by holding the tip of the blade. When I did this, Abdul eyed the knife quickly and then grimaced, as if I had handed him a truly unacceptable specimen. Holding the knife in a disparaging manner, Abdul began to discuss it with the shopowner.

The two of them were soon bargaining fast and furiously over the *khanjar.* Although the negotiations were in Arabic, I could follow the discussion by the gestures and the yelling. Abdul held up the dagger and pointed to the dull silver with his finger. The owner replied by emphasizing the gold filling and the fine workmanship. At one point, Abdul seized my arm and began to drag me from the shop. The owner seized my other arm and dragged me back. Finally, after much haggling, Abdul and the shopowner agreed on the price of 250 riyals, or about $85. To sweeten the deal, the antique dealer then served us some tea, congratulating us on an excellent selection.

"He was a tough one," said Abdul as we left the shop. "He wasn't fooled a bit—he knew that we wanted that knife and that we would pay his price."

"Well, even if we did not get the best deal, it's still a good buy," I said.

Abdul looked at me with a pained expression. To a Saudi, getting a good deal is often more important than getting the object that you are trying to buy. In a very important way, negotiations are a test of skill and ability: Abdul clearly felt that he had not done as well in this transaction as he should have.

As we walked back toward the Great Mosque the shops began to close their doors in preparation for the midday prayers. Saudis dressed in white thobes hurried past us toward the mosque, and the *matawa* banged on the shop doors with their clubs, announcing prayer time with the shout "*Salaat! Salaat!*" The streets around the Great Mosque were filled with cars, and drivers looked around frantically for places to park within walking distance of the mosque.

Abdul and I wandered through the crowd, taking in the sights and smells. In front of the moneychangers' *suq,* two falconers squatted with their hooded falcons, looking for customers. It seemed like an odd time for them to be selling falcons, but perhaps there was a Saudi nuance involved that was beyond me. When I pointed them out to Abdul, he laughed and told me a story about an American who had bought a falcon and taken it to his house in Riyadh. After a week or two, the American took the falcon out to the desert to see if it would catch a wild rabbit or bring down a stray bird. When he removed the hood, the falcon took off and was never seen again, presumably having been trained to return to the original owner.

"That bird didn't bring back a scrawny rabbit," joked Abdul. "He brought home 300 riyals!"

For the next hour, Abdul and I wandered through the deserted streets, talking as we toured the empty markets. Although everyone had gone to prayer at the Great Mosque, nobody bothered to lock up or otherwise protect his property. It amazed me that valuable merchandise could be left completely unattended in the open markets. Apparently, nobody would think of stealing, unless he was willing to have his hand chopped off in the bargain. It was like living in a fairytale, however, to find a land where people are basically honest.

The streets were quiet and everyone was praying. It reminded me of a Sunday morning in front of Trinity Church at home: peace and tranquility.

When prayer time was over, Abdul and I returned to Chop Square to watch the crowds leaving the mosque. Everyone was dressed in his Friday best, and the clean, bright clothing brought a festive air to the occasion. As we stood among the happy throng, the atmosphere in the square suddenly seemed to change. Soldiers began to appear, sealing off traffic and herding people into groups. There was a hum of excitement in the air.

"There's going to be a beheading," said Abdul in an excited whisper.

"Beheadings are always held on Friday, after the midday prayers," he explained, pushing forward in the crowd. "They announce it in the newspaper a day in advance to attract a bigger crowd. You're lucky, because most foreigners are not allowed to see a beheading."

"In that case, let's get out of here," I said, grateful for an excuse to leave the scene.

"Impossible," said Abdul. "We're jammed in here solid, and we'll just call attention to ourselves if we try to leave. Besides, our car is in the area which has been sealed off. Just stand still, and for God's sake don't take any pictures. It's absolutely forbidden."

Reluctantly, I began to realize that I was now about to watch a ceremonial execution. The thought was repugnant to me; Abdul, however, seemed to await the beheading with excitement and anticipation.

"How many executions have you seen?" I asked him with a shudder.

"In my life?"

"Yes."

Abdul shrugged. "Perhaps six or seven. I saw the first one when I was very young. It was a man who tried to rape a young girl. The last one was a month ago—they chopped a Yemeni for murdering his friend in a quarrel."

Listening to Abdul, I sensed an excitement in his voice that I found strange and upsetting. He discussed the matter as if an execution were some kind of spectator sport, like a soccer match. However, I realized that this was a reflection of Saudi culture, and I tried to observe it without being judgmental. After all, since I believed in capital punishment as a deterrent to crime, it was my duty to witness—at least once in my life— what I was advocating.

As we awaited the arrival of the condemned prisoner, I reflected on a tragic recent event that had led me to consider deeply my feelings about capital punishment and the role that it played in Saudi Arabia. Two months earlier, a woman at the hospital compound had been brutally attacked and raped in her own home by an unknown assailant dressed in Arab robes. The woman, whose husband was a member of the night staff at the hospital, was awakened from her sleep by an Arab man who held a knife to her throat and in broken English threatened to kill her unless she submitted. Thinking of her two young children in the adjoining room, the woman did not resist the attack. Afterward, the attacker left, but only after promising to return the following night.

After the attacker disappeared, the woman became hysterical and was taken to the hospital, where I was called upon to perform a physical examination. While the examination revealed that she had not suffered any permanent physical harm, the psychological trauma was clearly severe. My outrage at the cruelty of this act led me to a sense of grim satisfaction when the rapist was later captured while trying to attack another woman, this time a dietician in the hospital. The rapist proved to be an Egyptian who worked as an attendant in the surgical department, and who knew the comings and goings of the staff. In Saudi Arabia, the penalty for rape is swift and certain: death by beheading. Two weeks later he was executed in Chop Square.

Now, standing amongst the crowd in Chop Square, the image of the hysterical young wife in the emergency room of the hospital came to me again. However terrible is the reality of capital punishment! Although I was already certain that I would find it abhorrent, I was also conscious of the other side of justice, the obligation that society owes to the victims of crime. What was the appropriate price to exact upon an assailant for a cruel and vicious act? In America, I was convinced that the punishment was too lenient and the likelihood of retribution too uncertain to prevent violent crime. In Saudi Arabia, I was experiencing a society that applied harsh Koranic justice to social violators. The penalty for theft was amputation of the hand; the punishment for rape or murder was execution. The methods were exceedingly harsh, but none could dispute their effectiveness, or the striking contrast between Saudi Arabia and my "enlightened" but crime-ridden country.

I recalled a hospital dinner at which I had sat next to the Governor of Riyadh. We had talked about crime prevention and he had told me that Riyadh had the lowest crime rate in the world.

"Capital punishment," he had said in perfect English, "is a deterrent to crime—no question about that."

A murmur passed through the crowd as a police car appeared and slowly moved through the mob of people to the center of the square. When it reached its destination, it stopped, and the executioner emerged from the rear door. He was a huge and imposing man, well over six feet tall, and he was dressed in an immaculate white thobe with a black bandolier across his chest and a sash around his waist. The most striking thing about him, however, was his race: he was clearly a black man. His charcoal-black skin glistened in the midday sun.

"The executioners all come from one Ethiopian family," whispered Abdul, as if he anticipated my surprise. "They were slaves of the King many years ago. Now, of course, they are free."

Then an even greater murmur passed through the crowd.

"They're bringing the condemned man," said Abdul excitedly.

The crowd fell deathly silent as the condemned man was led from another police car toward the center of the square. The prisoner appeared to be a young man. He was dressed in a simple white robe and was wearing a black blindfold. His hands were tied behind his back. As he was led to where the executioner stood, a bare rectangular piece of cardboard was placed on the ground, and the condemned man was forced to kneel upon it. To my surprise there was no platform. I was startled by the bareness and simplicity of the procedure. In this last moment of his life, the prisoner seemed to despair, for he willingly knelt on the cardboard.

As the crowd watched and listened, a voice over the public-address system began the execution ceremony.

"There is no god but God, and Mohammed is the Messenger of God," intoned the voice from the Palace of Justice. It then went on to describe the murder committed by the condemned man, and the punishment required by Sharia law. Delivered in a monotone, the condemnation reverberated through the square like the voice of doom, and seemed to cast a cold chill in the midday heat.

The executioner slowly rolled up the sleeve of his robe, baring a large, muscular right arm. He then drew the sword in a graceful motion, letting the air ring with the clear, scraping sound of the blade leaving the scabbard. The sword was a curved, double-edged Arab blade, about three feet long, and it glistened brightly in the noonday sun. Holding perfectly still for an instant, the executioner nodded to his assistant, who stood beside the prisoner. At the signal, the assistant quickly lifted the sharp stick that he was holding and drove it into the side of the condemned man. As the prisoner's neck stiffened in reflex, the executioner was already in motion. He took several quick small steps—almost as in a ballet—and then with one long stride he raised the sword high and with a loud whoosh brought the sword down with all his strength, severing the head with one mighty stroke.

Bright red arterial blood spurted four feet into the air, and the head jumped forward into the crowd. The headless body convulsed and then toppled backward. For a moment there was a stunned silence, and then a single roar of approval rose from the crowd. Surprised, I turned to study the faces around me. There was no sense of pity or sorrow for the prisoner: he was a murderer, and he had received the proper administration of justice according to the Koranic law.

As I watched, the executioner's assistant picked up the severed head, examined it briefly, and then placed it on a nearby stretcher. After a couple of minutes, two men in uniform lifted the body from the pool of blood and placed it on the stretcher with the head. The body was then carried to a waiting ambulance, while the crowd quietly began to disperse.

As I stood in the rapidly emptying square, I tried to control my emotions, and to make some assessment of the compelling drama that I had just witnessed. It was really an abomination to destroy a human life. My initial reaction was one of revulsion: I had a physician's respect for the amazing and wondrous complexity of the human body, and to destroy it wantonly seemed like a sacrilege. I was reminded of the philosophy of Schweitzer and his "Reverence for Life." And yet this was the law of Saudi Arabia, a law that was more than a thousand years old. Against the sight of the headless body, I tried to balance the life he had destroyed and the grief he had caused.

While the square quickly settled into its normal pace, I stared at the pool of blood soaking the street. What a few precious minutes before had been part of a living, breathing human being was now soaking into the ground, already turning dark and sticky in the hot sun. The terrifying mortality of man weighed heavily on my mind.

Abdul seemed less affected by the spectacle—perhaps because it was so natural to him—but he was considerate enough to wait until I was ready to leave.

"It seems so strange to watch a human being destroyed," I said as we walked away, "and to be with people who want him to die, and let him die. I devote myself to saving life."

Abdul walked quietly beside me, through the bustling streets of the *suq*.

"It is normal for me," he said at last. "It is how we live in Saudi Arabia. They are old values, but we still follow them, still believe in them. We are changing slowly—now a thief sometimes gets forty lashes instead of losing a hand. In Saudi Arabia that is progress."

"Does the harshness of the punishment ever bother you?" I asked.

"Yes. But does it ever bother you when someone in your country commits a serious crime and goes unpunished?"

"Of course."

Abdul shrugged. "I believe in the punishment. It is how we live, and we accept it as just. Even the condemned man accepts that it is his punishment to die by the sword."

A melancholy descended over us, and as we walked through the marketplace on the way to our car, I looked at the stalls filled with valuable goods that had been left unattended an hour before. The streets were safe night and day, and the homes were safe. They did have a society in which there was very little crime—and what crime existed was usually attributable to outsiders. People could argue the merits of capital punishment and the value of life and draw different conclusions, but all will agree on one thing—the nature and dimension of the tragedy.

What happened today seemed so barbaric!

I'll never forget that young man's head flying through the air. I felt sorry for him. I also felt sorry for the raped women, and the murder victims . . . and for all humanity.

Whatever the morality, whatever the issue of right or wrong, there is, in the end, only the darkening spot of blood on the soil. In the end, there is only the stain of our own brief mortality.

EXPERIENCES OF A DOCTOR'S WIFE

ALTHOUGH I HAD TRAVELED seven thousand miles to Saudi Arabia and entered a culture entirely different from my American one, several major things did not change for me: I was still on the staff of a well-equipped hospital, where I spent most of my working hours; I still wore Western dress, the coats used by the hospital or suits or desert clothes for my day off; and I still had the freedom of movement I had known in America to visit any town or village in Saudi Arabia and feel safe and secure. However, for Ruth, my wife, coming to Saudi Arabia was like entering a different time frame.

Before leaving the United States we had spent an indoctrination period of several days in Nashville, Tennessee, where the company that provided management and personnel for the King Faisal Hospital had its headquarters. We attended informative lectures on the customs and habits of Saudi Arabians. A lecturer in psychology helped prepare us emotionally for problems we might encounter.

Ruth learned that women must conform in manner of dress. For example, in public she would be required at all times to be covered from neck to ankle, and to keep her arms concealed by long sleeves. It so happens that Ruth was accustomed to wearing hostess gowns at home in Boston. She found them comfortable in the evening, inexpensive, and not without glamour. Now she stocked up on several additional new lightweight, easily washable long dresses.

Few of the staff wives had foreseen the clothing problem and they tried to solve it with dresses poorly made by Riyadh dressmakers. These lacked style and wrinkled easily. Some women wore tailored thobes, which were long and straight, buttoning to a small rounded collar. After a time, however, this mode of dress was outlawed because it was actually a copy of the traditional dress for Saudi men and considered inappropriate for women.

Visas were essential for travel to Saudi Arabia and given with reluctance to women. Visitors were discouraged. Ruth was allowed to join me only because I had signed a definite contract with the King Faisal Hospital for an extended period of time. Even so, she waited what seemed an interminable time in London until her visa was finally granted. Only two flights a week went to Saudi Arabia, all heavily booked, and we despaired of her ever getting a reservation. But finally a telegram arrived stating that she was on her way.

Ruth later told me that the flight had been comfortable, but that most of the passengers were Arabs and seemed to resent the presence of an unescorted foreign woman. Sweet fruit drinks were served instead of alcoholic beverages and the only meal consisted of a bland dish of lamb and rice—the typical Saudi Arabian fare.

At one point in the trip, Ruth managed to change from her Western daytime dress into one of the long hostess gowns she had brought with her from Boston. I remember my first moment of surprise at seeing her step from the plane in a dress usually reserved for our late winter evenings by the fire.

After going through customs, we collected her luggage amid the din of the airport and the shouting of the porters of various sizes and ages arguing as to who would carry her bags. She was unused to all the confusion and pleased at last to settle into the quiet comfort of an American car. We drove to the Al Sharq Hotel, our quarters for the next six months.

When Ruth complained that the mattress was hard as a board, "an orthopedic specialist's dream," I told her about my connivance with the former occupant on her behalf. "If you were to see the room at the Al Yamama," I said, "you would take the next plane back to London. This is the Connaught Hotel by comparison."

I pointed out the several luxuries not available at the Al Yamama, such as the tiny refrigerator and a noisy, but most welcome, air conditioner. "When there is a power failure," I said, trying to be reassuring, "it is usually for only three or four hours." I learned later, however, that in some areas of the city the power failures lasted for days.

Ruth asked about the elderly men sitting outside the door. I told her that they did the cleaning and changed the linen. She soon learned that their concept of cleaning was to walk into a room with a can of Raid, swish it around the length of the room so thoroughly that the stench almost did us in rather than the cockroaches, and walk out. Sheets were changed several times a month, unless the attendants were tipped. That was the extent of the cleaning.

All general services in Saudi Arabia, such as waiting on tables, cleaning, or clerking, are performed by men, often Egyptian or Sudanese. When a Japanese restaurant opened nearby, we were pleased and surprised to find attractive Japanese girls serving as waitresses. However, the morals police soon intervened and the restaurant was quietly closed within a few days.

Cockroaches are not exactly my wife's favorite subject, but mention of them cannot be omitted. They were a constant source of torment during our entire stay in Saudi Arabia. Even when we finally had our own villa and kept it scrupulously clean, these creatures managed to invade each room. In spite of every precaution, they flourished and grew to a monstrous size. It was the only thing in that country which she dreaded.

Flies were plentiful and a constant nuisance. When Ruth told one of our sons how fast they were, he thought she exaggerated. However, it was almost impossible to kill a fly with a fly swatter. We depended entirely on sprays, and it always required a strong dose. Strangely enough, they could not tolerate the summer heat, and when it became very hot, the flies all disappeared.

One afternoon Ruth was invited to tea at the home of a patient of mine who was a general in the air force. The ladies were enjoying tea and pastries brought into a comfortable sitting room by a manservant. The general stood guard nearby with a fly swatter poised in his hand. One fly zoomed about constantly, apparently aiming at the pastries. The general used the fly swatter repeatedly but to no avail. The fly was still buzzing about happily two hours later when she left. Ruth told me that she hoped the general fared better with his anti-aircraft maneuvers.

When she visited them many months later, after she had learned a few Arabic phrases, they were immensely pleased. Ruth told them that she had recently finished the painting of my first patient, Prince Yusef, and that it was about to be framed. Nura, the general's wife, and her two daughters decided to accompany her to the framers. They were unusually attractive women, smartly dressed, in soft blouses and long graceful skirts. Just before they left the house, Ruth was astonished to see each of the women gather up a long sheer black veil. When thrown over their heads, the veils not only covered their faces, but reached nearly to the ankle, so that their clothing was almost completely concealed as well.

The driver took them to the shop where the painting was now hanging on a far wall with a border of green velvet and a carved wooden frame painted gold. Nura walked over to the painting to examine it. Only then, with her back to everyone else in the shop, did she carefully raise her veil for a moment to see the picture more clearly. The daughters did likewise. This was a family that had been exposed to Western culture. Their home was tastefully decorated, their clothes had been made in France, and their attitudes were Western. However, when they appeared in public, they conformed to Saudi customs without hesitation.

Friday was the one day of the week that we anticipated with particular pleasure, because it was a holiday and a nonworking day for most of us. We often made arrangements for drives into the country, and since the skies were nearly always cloudless, rain never interfered with our plans.

On one of our excursions, we had discovered a perfect spot for picnics. We now owned a comfortable green air-conditioned Pontiac, and on Friday mornings we would fill an insulated picnic hamper to take with us. Ruth prepared fried chicken and generous tunafish sandwiches on frankfurter rolls. Because we needed large amounts of liquid, we carried a container of water, a thermos of hot coffee, and another of iced tea. The hamper was placed in the trunk of the car and we were on our way. Ruth's usual costume was a long dress, a huge straw hat held in place with a colorful flowing scarf, and the most comfortable, sloppy-looking shoes she owned.

As we drove through the outskirts of Riyadh, we passed some unpleasant sights. There were junkyards of rotting automobile bodies, dozens of goats feasting on garbage, and shabby three-story apartment houses, whose balconies were almost hidden by an assortment of ragged laundry hung out to dry. Farther on, we came upon countless groups of sheds thrown together haphazardly with pieces of corrugated metal, wood, and cardboard offering little protection from the elements. Sometimes a tiny yard enclosed with metal sheeting extruded from a dilapidated dwelling where goats wandered about bleating like children.

Then the desert stretched ahead with almost no sign of human habitation. Occasionally we passed a small group of tents with an old truck parked nearby or a few camels grazing. The road continued on through endless miles of solitary desert, and we longed for the sight of a tree. Hawks circled high in the hot sky above us.

After passing long stretches of barren sand, we were suddenly overwhelmed by the sight of a magnificent ridge of mountains glistening in the sun, their tops as flat as though they had been sliced off with a knife. Parallel ridges in deep shadow ran down the sides like rivulets of water. Soon, past a bend in the road, the mountains rose above us on all sides. We parked our car in some shade and walked to an area where we could look deep down into a large valley which had been formed by the surrounding hills. This was one of our favorite places. Although we saw it on each successive trip, the spectacle of these majestic mountains rising from a land so flat and so monotonous filled us with as much excitement and awe the last time as the first.

The sun was high overhead and we began to feel pangs of hunger. It

Experiences of a Doctor's Wife ◊ *151*

was time, we decided, to drive to our favorite private picnic site. We turned off the main road and were soon surrounded by flat desert land again. We passed an occasional alfalfa field adjoining a small oasis or the remnants of a deserted mud-brick house standing next to an old well long in disuse. After driving by a number of small farms, we finally came to a familiar dirt road, which led to our secluded picnic area. The first time we had discovered this retreat we had driven with trepidation onto the private road, conscious of trespassing on the land of a stranger. It was a lovely secluded spot. We parked our car under the trees of a date grove and carried our provisions to a shaded area next to a clear, sparkling stream. (We later realized it was an irrigation ditch.) Soon a plump woman appeared with two small children. She had crossed the road from the farmhouse which stood on the other side of the highway. Much to my surprise she wore no veil. She beamed at us while her two children shyly peeked from behind her long cotton skirt. We sensed that she was pleased to have us use her land even though our communication consisted of only a few words of courtesy. We learned that her husband, a farmer, was busy at home. She made us feel quite welcome.

We spread a large blanket on the ground and placed our food, paper cups, and plates in the center while we stretched out on the border. Everything tasted delicious. It was a lovely, lazy part of the day and we enjoyed every moment. After lunch, we washed our hands in the stream and listened to the soothing sound of water pumps in the distance. Then we gathered our supplies together and placed everything in paper bags to be disposed of at home.

After tidying our picnic site, we walked along the footpath that ran the length of the farm until we reached the bulky metal pumps. The creaking monsters' constant action supplied the most precious commodity in the country, more precious than oil. The cool water jetted upward in a powerful stream that flowed to a maze of long ditches, the lifeblood of the farm.

Across the stream a huge deep-green field of alfalfa provided food for the animals, mostly donkeys, sheep, and goats. Farther on, there was a large field of lettuce, adding more color to our surroundings. I never realized until I came to Saudi Arabia how meaningful color can be in our lives. I found it difficult to adapt to the monotony of the desert brown and the absence of any other color. Even the houses were sand-colored for the most part. I was constantly attracted to the sight of anything green—even a weed.

One day after a rainstorm I glanced out of the hotel window and saw something green. I ran out and stared at it in rapture. It was a green weed! I realized that I had taken for granted our wealth of trees, endless fields of green, and miles of green farmland at home. In the surrounding drabness, green became the color we welcomed most, and this picnic site was an immense relief to eyes starved for the glories of the American landscape. Maybe the Saudis felt the same. Their national flag is green, the color of Islam.

From the first day on, either the husband or wife always came to greet us and made it clear that the area was reserved for our pleasure. One time when we arrived, we saw our host arguing with two men who had parked their car in our special place and were preparing to enjoy a picnic. After much gesticulating and shouting, he managed to make them leave, and we feared that our turn was next. But he smiled at us, sweeping his arm toward the vacated area. He simply wanted no one to invade our privacy. His wife several times sent her young son into the fields to cut huge bunches of lettuce as a gift for us to take home. We were much touched by their kindness.

In an effort to learn why the farmer's wife wore no veil I asked Abdul to join us on one of our picnics. He spoke to her at length and later told us that she wore no veil because she was not a Saudi. Both she and her husband were Egyptians. They were working the farm for an Egyptian cousin who had married a Saudi Arabian woman and later become a Saudi citizen. This qualified him to obtain money from the government to buy the farm.

Some weeks later, when we appeared for our weekly picnic and had begun to feel at ease with our new friends, I held a limited conversation with the farmer's wife, mostly in sign language. She was a heavy woman and walked with great difficulty. I explained that I was a doctor, *tabeeb*. With appropriate moaning, she pointed to her ankles, which obviously were swollen and were causing her constant pain. I tried to persuade her to come to the hospital, but she shook her head. She probably had never ventured far from her home. The faraway city of Riyadh was beyond her comprehension, a frightening unknown world.

Although I would have preferred to see her at the hospital, I realized that it was impossible. She would not have mentioned her problems to me if Ruth hadn't been present offering her encouragement. I promised to bring her some medication, and the following week gave her some pills, diuretics, to reduce the swelling of her ankles, with instructions in Arabic. When we appeared the next Friday, she smiled and thanked us, pointing to her ankles to indicate that they were much better. For our entire stay, this family remained for us an oasis of hospitality and their lovely farm one of our favorite places in Saudi Arabia.

Marketing in Riyadh proved a frustrating and time-consuming chore for the women. In the beginning, Ruth would laughingly tell me how awkward she felt dragging her long skirts through the dusty *suqs,* the native open markets, wondering if the hems would last for the length of our stay. But, after a while, her long dresses became a natural way of life, and when we caught a glimpse of visiting "foreigners" wandering about a hotel lobby, their short skirts struck us as almost bizarre and an affront to decency.

We often accompanied our wives on the shopping expeditions for food, primarily because a car was desirable. I usually supplied the car but contributed little else to this exercise, which was usually carried out in the evening.

There were few supermarkets in the city, and none to compare with the American concept. They were often poorly stocked, the selection was limited, and several were so filthy that, after several ventures, we avoided them when possible.

Spinney's supermarket was our favorite. It was run by Lebanese. Ruth always brought two aids from home. One was a shopping bag because none was provided by the store, and the second a plastic egg box, the sort in which eggs are usually packed in American stores. In Riyadh, eggs are sold loose, often broken. It amused the storekeepers to see us with our pink plastic egg box. Even so, the eggs had to be counted, for they weren't accustomed to selling them by the dozen.

The customers in food stores were mainly men. Upper-class Saudi women never appeared to market, a chore that was done by their male servants. In less-affluent families, the husband did all the marketing. As a result, courtesy was not only lacking but there were many signs of rudeness toward women, especially pushing and shoving.

Food in general was plentiful and not too expensive. There was a fair supply of frozen meat from Denmark, Australia, and New Zealand. Lamb and beef butchered locally was not aged and did not suit our Western taste. Canned goods, cereals, bread, and dairy products were shipped from the United States. Cookies, jams, and candies came from England and Germany. Fresh fish and shrimp were available at the fish *suqs.* Fresh fruits and vegetables from Lebanon were abundant and quite reasonable at the local open markets. Frozen vegetables were also available but they were expensive. Cheese came from Europe, butter from France, and milk in various forms from the United States and England.

At times, certain foods disappeared from the shelves for varying periods of time because of congestion in the port of Jidda, where there were limited docking facilities. Some ships waited as long as four months to find a berth before unloading. Perishables were simply thrown overboard. Ruth eventually learned to improvise with whatever finally made its way into the markets. In spite of the cost of shipping, which must have been considerable, the price of most items was little more than in America.

My favorite place to shop when Ruth was away was called Chicken Street. Here I could get chicken broiled on a revolving spit and ready to eat; nearby was an open market which carried fresh fruits and vegetables—a perfect setup for a bachelor dinner—not elegant but quite adequate.

Shopping was a favorite pastime for the foreign women. Although marketing for food was a chore, Ruth and her friends thoroughly enjoyed other shopping in Riyadh, finding it a completely new experience, often a challenge, and always an attraction. Hospital buses picked up the women at convenient locations near their homes and drove them into town, returning for them later in the day. The women always traveled in groups.

The real fascination lay in the bazaars. The one with the most appeal for Ruth was made up of a vast space crowded with mazes of alleyways, shops and stalls all under one roof. The open stalls were tiny, stood side by side, and were stacked high with their specialty products. For instance, there were dozens of shops that carried nothing but fabrics of every color, material, and pattern. Not only was the cloth displayed on shelves, but the floors were littered knee deep in the colorful lengths and bolts as the shopkeepers unwound length after length to find just the right one. Bargaining is the order of the day in every *suq* in Saudi Arabia, and soon Ruth learned to say with authority, "Too expensive" and "No, no, still too expensive." She said it was almost like taking part in a well-rehearsed play—the disdainful gestures of the shopkeepers, her own feigned indifference, while each recognized that they would eventually reach an agreeable price—but not too soon.

Ruth particularly enjoyed watching the buying and selling at the gold *suq*. Because gold was actually a bargain in Saudi Arabia, she bought several necklaces and two beautiful engraved gold bracelets. She told me later that she wished she had bought more. Time always passed quickly on these shopping excursions, and all too soon the women had to return to the buses for their journey home.

When Ruth had been in Saudi Arabia for several months and her days had settled into a comfortable routine, we realized that she was living a life very similar to that of a Saudi woman, almost a mirror image, except for the absence of the veil. We usually spent Friday together, and attended staff parties together, but for the most part we spent long hours leading separate lives. My work accounted for much of that time, but also included were the social invitations from Saudis that I felt I couldn't turn down—either out of courtesy or just plain curiosity—and to which I went alone or in the company of my fellow doctors. Ruth was very understanding of this situation and usually made plans to be with the other wives, just as Saudi women did. Eventually, we were invited together to some Saudi homes and went with pleasure, but this was the exception. Generally I went alone.

At times Ruth said the hotel seemed a little like a harem. It occurred to her that, far from being an immoral place full of jealousies and petty machinations, the harem probably had been a great source of companionship and comfort to the wives and concubines who comprised it. Just as is true today, the women were excluded from the company of all men who were not relatives, and rarely saw their husbands or had a meal with them. Therefore, the addition of another wife to a female household must have been a welcome event, someone with whom to gossip or exchange clothes and jewelry, or share the joy and burdens of motherhood. At any rate, Ruth delighted in the company of the other doctors' wives and in the activities they shared, and made many lasting friendships.

She has always led an active life and her life in Saudi Arabia was no exception. One morning a week she joined a group of eight women to study Arabic at the home of a Jordanian. They traveled by taxi in groups of two or more, the only safe way except for hospital buses. Usually they had an argument with the driver before they started. Because there were no meters, the price was determined at the outset.

Their Jordanian teacher lived with her family in a spacious home quite a distance away. She greeted them in Arabic and offered them tea, which they drank, and then they sat around a large dining-room table. Several of the women brought small tape recorders. Even though they took careful notes, pronunciation was so important that playback of the tape proved very useful.

Although Ruth did not continue beyond the first series of lessons and can speak few sentences properly, one of the expressions she found most useful was "slow!," a warning with which they all admonished cab drivers as they clung to the edges of their seats. Other obvious directions were "right," "left," "here," and "stay." Then there was "how much?," followed immediately with "too expensive," and "how are you?," "good morning," "thank you." This was not the extent of their vocabulary, but it was certainly more practical than "la plume de ma tante."

Each week a dozen doctors' wives met for lunch and bridge at the various homes. Some women were expert players and others were novices, but none had less experience than Ruth. She had never played previously. Consequently, before she would make a bid or play a card, she consulted half the players at the other tables. Most of them took all this good-naturedly, but some of the expert players withdrew discreetly to another room. The women were all friendly and congenial, according to Ruth, and felt that the main purpose of these luncheons was to socialize. The bridge playing, fortunately for her, was a secondary consideration. Some time later, however, the Recreation Center at the hospital instituted a series of bridge lessons to which Ruth subscribed, and within a year she became so proficient she was able to play the game successfully without outside consultation.

The Saudi Arabian government is apprehensive about the congregation of any large number of people. The right of assembly is a privilege which the Saudis do not yet enjoy. This restriction applies to the expatriate population as well. Consequently, when the wives representing every nationality living in Saudi Arabia decided to organize a series of monthly meetings, they met with considerable opposition because of their large numbers and particularly because they were women. Undaunted, however, the women decided to hold their meetings in the dining room of the Intercontinental Hotel to demonstrate that there was nothing secretive about their activities, and they adopted no official name.

Several hundred women met the first Monday of every month. They came originally from almost everywhere in the world: the United States, England, France, Germany, Korea, the Scandinavian countries, Japan, Italy, India, Lebanon, and Egypt, to mention a few. A different country was responsible for a program each month. Saudi women were welcome, but very few, if any, attended, according to Ruth. She considered these meetings to be really special and gave me a detailed account of them.

The doctors' wives arrived by hospital bus in the late morning and visited with each other over coffee before the program began. The programs varied enormously. There were fashion shows, using members as models. An English marine biologist and photographer involved in the exploration of underwater life in the Red Sea showed magnificent colored slides of coral, exotic fish, and other dazzling deep-sea creatures. Once they were entertained by a concert pianist from Germany. Another time they were given a cooking demonstration of the local food in India. Ruth's favorite program, she told me, was presented by a group from Japan, dressed in their lovely native costumes, who gave a demonstration of the tea ceremony and flower arranging. Ruth was charmed by these petite, graceful women in their colorful silk gowns, although they seemed out of place in Saudi Arabia.

When the program was finished, the women held a brief business meeting, presented various reports, and introduced new members. Then they all gathered for a leisurely lunch before dispersing to their various homes.

One of Ruth's most challenging experiences involved a tour of the Royal Guest Palace for some women who were coming with their husbands to Riyadh from various parts of the country to attend a medical conference. I was responsible for arranging the medical program and Ruth was in charge of the social activities. The Guest Palace had been the home of the late King Saud, whose reckless spending had forced him into exile. When he died, resentment was so strong that his former palace was left to disintegrate. Recently, it had been resurrected to be used as a Guest Palace for visiting heads of state. Algernon Asprey, the most exclusive interior decorator in England, was chosen for the task, which took three years to complete. Ruth had been told that the interior of the palace was spectacular but that women had never been permitted inside. However, she was determined to give the visiting wives the privilege of touring the palace and the grounds.

At first it seemed hopeless. Ruth was told that women would not be welcome and that the tour might be canceled at the last moment, either at the whim of the government or by the arrival of an important visitor such as Prince Philip of England, who had stayed at the Royal Guest Palace recently.

Ruth persisted, however, and permission was finally granted. She was then given a private tour of all but the living quarters on the second floor. The reception hall, she told me later, boasted the largest Persian rug in existence with the exception of one in the Palace of the late Shah of Iran. The air conditioner, she had been informed by her guide, was almost as powerful as the one in the Pentagon in Washington.

She went into raptures describing the great mansion. The ceiling of the main hall was at least three stories high, graced by a beautiful balcony and at least a dozen glowing crystal chandeliers. Each room had such massive proportions that no matter how elaborate the decorations they looked appropriate. Numerous salons led off the main hall, with miles of satin draperies at the tall majestic windows. Countless French silk-brocaded settees were scattered about, flanked by exquisite inlaid tables and beautiful antique chests carved from rare woods.

The dining room could seat hundreds of guests. Dozens of long tables were surrounded by carved high-backed chairs, and elegant, colorful bouquets of fresh flowers graced each table. Planeloads of flowers arrived each day to provide the magnificent floral arrangements found in every room.

The spacious offices that belonged to various heads of the Saudi government were decorated according to the taste of the occupants and ranged from ultra-modern to very traditional. "It was a dream world," Ruth concluded.

The afternoon following her private tour, the big event took place. Ruth had chosen four assistant hostesses and made green satin badges with attached name tags. The hostesses were the only local wives permitted to attend. The palace social secretary had limited the total number and Ruth felt that the out-of-town visitors should be given priority.

When the buses arrived, she stood at the entrance of the palace to greet the guests and then led them inside. They moved from room to room in silence, broken only by gasps of amazement at the lavish décor and at the priceless antiques selected by the London decorators. The tour took two hours to complete because of the immense size of the palace and the awe-inspiring surroundings. At the end, the women were ushered into a pale rose-colored French salon, where they were offered tea and delicate pastries. Then each guest, to her delight and surprise, was presented with a packet of charming souvenirs, consisting of beautifully packaged fragrances, soaps, notepads, and pens, each inscribed with the crest of Saudi Arabia. Printed in green were the words "Royal Guest Palace." The souvenirs had been made in France and, as usual, the French flair for drama and presentation was obvious.

When I asked Ruth one day which single event was most memorable during her stay in Saudi Arabia, she replied without hesitation. "The night at the Saudi Women's Club was one of the most extraordinary experiences of my life," she said with enthusiasm. "It was a night to remember!"

The Saudi Women's Club was the first of its kind in Saudi Arabia and was founded by the intrepid Queen Iffat. This courageous woman had overcome innumerable obstacles to bring it into existence. Clubs in general were illegal in Saudi Arabia, and a meeting of women was inconceivable. But Iffat's husband was King Faisal and her influence over him was considerable. Had he lived longer, Iffat might well have changed the course of women's lives in Saudi Arabia. She overcame the objections of the fundamentalists by dedicating the club to religion, charity, and health care, as well as educational, social, and cultural activities. The establishment of a club for women was a daring step forward, a complete break with tradition, and a totally innovative concept. The women loved it.

The clubhouse was comprised of two buildings on a large, walled-off tract of land. Members met in various rooms to carry on their charitable work, or gathered in a spacious auditorium for lectures, entertainment, or other programs. On one occasion, Ruth was personally invited to a lecture by one of the foreign speakers. She was Geneviève de Vilmorin, a charming young French woman from a distinguished family. As a correspondent and daughter of a diplomat, she had lived in many countries and had written books about the lives of a number of world leaders such as Chou En-lai.

On the particular afternoon that Ruth had been invited to attend, the subject of her talk was Farah Diba, now widow of the late Shah of Iran. Geneviève had known her well when she was a student of architecture in France. At that time, Farah Diba was plump, homely, and uninterested in men. However, she and the Shah fell in love and Farah returned to France many months before her wedding to be transformed. She lost weight, had her nose bobbed, and learned grooming and fashion. "The result was a romantically beautiful bride," said Geneviève.

Farah Diba was also a strong-willed woman and had begun measures to help liberate the women of Iran, until the Shah's ministers warned him of the possible dire consequences. She was immediately silenced and placed under surveillance by the police. Her freedom had ended.

"The women held their breath during that lecture," said Ruth. "The silence was ominous and the applause explosive."

That afternoon's lecture was one of several that proved illuminating and stimulating. They opened vistas into worlds some of the women never dreamed existed. The culmination was the social program held at night to celebrate the last meeting of the season. It was the first time that Western women had been invited to an evening event of the Saudi Women's Club. Several hundred attended.

The affair started dramatically when the guests, all women, were ushered through the entrance gates. Some of the Saudi women were dressed elegantly and others wore more simple, long gowns with long sleeves, as did Ruth.

The grounds had been completely covered with colorful oriental rugs. An enormous half tent had been erected at the far end. It had been woven of fine black wool by a group of Bedouin women, a task requiring a full year to complete. One could watch this painstaking process in a small area outside the tent, where some Bedouin women sat twisting the fine camel's wool onto spindles.

The airy tent formed a semicircle at the perimeter of which had been placed a succession of large cushions, mostly velvet, upon which about twelve Saudi women were seated. They were the hostesses. Some were dressed in native costumes, including bridal outfits from various regions of the country. The bridal gowns, rarely white, glowed with a spectrum of intense colors to complement the elaborate golden headdresses. Even their hands were covered with intricate gold weaving held in place by lacing over the fingers. The more wealthy Saudi hostesses were not in costume and wore magnificent Paris gowns, creations of the great couturiers. One was a lovely princess, who wore, at her throat, a delicate butterfly of diamonds, exquisitely hung on a fragile gold chain. Ruth said that the hostesses, as a group, were young and strikingly beautiful. They stood tall, slim, and graceful, with fine features and raven-black hair. What a pity, she thought, that they must always be veiled except with family, other women, and family servants.

Two docile-appearing camels stood outside the tent. Nearby sat a group of male servants fanning the flames of a wood fire with large bellows. Hanging over the fire were huge brass coffee pots whose steam smelled of cardamom and strong coffee. Black female servants, some of whom had been slaves, poured the spiced coffee into tiny, delicate china cups and passed silver trays of delicious stuffed dates while the costumes were casually paraded before the guests.

Nearly all of these Saudi women attempted to speak English, occasionally quite well, as they passed gracefully among their guests. Ruth and her English friend Joan Dann engaged them in simple conversations. After the fashion presentation, the president of the club, a poised young princess, greeted her audience with a speech, which she read with ease over a microphone. It was skillfully written and explained the purpose of the club.

When she had finished, the guests were shown into one of the two buildings, where round dining tables filled several rooms. In one large room, there were men standing behind enormous platters of steaming lamb and chicken, ready to carve and serve. Ten or twelve carvers were stationed every few yards at the serving tables, which were placed in a continuous line around three sides of the room.

The visitors noted with some amusement that the dining tables were later cleared by princesses and the more prominent hostesses in their exquisite gowns and glamorous coiffures. Ruth said she was certain that not one of them had ever so much as lifted a plate before. In their homes, they were surrounded by countless servants, so that any effort remotely domestic was clearly beneath them. Their endeavors to serve their guests at this lovely party probably were meant to convey friendship and respect.

After dinner, the women were ushered into a second building, where the auditorium was located. Joan and Ruth sat quite near the stage but were hardly prepared for the astonishing entertainment which followed.

A group of eight young Saudi women, seated in a semicircle on the floor at the rear of the stage, played an assortment of musical instruments from strings to primitive drums. Soon one of the musicians rose to sing. Her demeanor was joyful and the song, filled with enthusiasm, was accompanied by much rhythmic clapping. To Western ears, the dissonance was disconcerting.

During the next hour, young women in costume or in demure, long evening gowns appeared on stage to dance. Usually, two danced at the same time, circling each other with exotic movements, and occasionally showing an ankle! No pictures were allowed at any time. During one dance, the women loosened their long hair and swung their heads from side to side so that their hair flew back and forth in wild abandon, almost savage in feeling. The finale was belly dancing. They performed this dance with such elegance and grace that Ruth felt it should bear a more dignified name.

The party ended at midnight with the arrival of the buses and cars. Ruth and Joan said good-bye to their new Saudi friends, grateful at being given the opportunity to participate in the joy and warmth of the woman's world in Saudi Arabia. Outside the gates, Ruth noted a number of Rolls Royces with chauffeurs lined up in front of the tent. This was not a Cinderella fairy tale, she concluded. These coaches would not turn into pumpkins. Ruth's first comment when she arrived home was, "What a night!"

◊ *14* ◊

SOCIAL LIFE

IN APRIL I SAW the first rainfall in five months. It came down in torrents for a short time, flooding the dirt roads and dry riverbeds, and then disappeared into the thirsty soil. The average rainfall in this area is only two inches a year. The days were getting warmer, approaching 120 degrees in the shade. The sky was usually cloudless, and the air very dry. The blistered sidewalks and the cracks in the cement of new buildings in Riyadh attested to the ravages of heat and desiccation.

Soon after we arrived the critical shortage of living quarters for the doctors became a crucial issue at the hospital staff meetings. Finally it was decided to allocate the choicest housing by a point system: one point for each month of residency in Riyadh, and one-half point for each child under eighteen years. The largest villas were assigned to those who had been at the hospital longest and had the most young children. Since we had no small children, we didn't qualify for a villa until a year later.

Consequently, in the beginning many of us lived in sleazy hotels like the Al Sharq, where we had two rooms and a bath, or in apartments scattered throughout the city. One complex was called Zoo Road Apartments because of its proximity to the zoo, and another was named the Batha Apartments because it overlooked the open sewers, which ran the length of Shara Batha. It was located downwind from the sewers, and at times the smell was overpowering. The critical shortage in housing resulted in a runaway inflation. Rent for a three-bedroom house increased from $6,500 in 1979 to $25,000 two years later.

For six months Ruth and I had been living in the dismal Al Sharq Hotel a floor below Philip and Doris Westbrook. With the intense heat of summer just weeks away, we were anxious to move one rung higher on the housing ladder and were hoping that the Petromin Apartments would have an available place. This new complex was named after the Petromin Corporation, an oil conglomerate nearby. The Yemeni laborers had been working on the apartment building for two years, but were notoriously slow and unskilled compared to the German and Korean builders.

Finally, after six months we qualified for one of the Petromin Apartments. It had a fair-sized living room, two bedrooms, a kitchen, and bath.

Ruth was delighted with the closet space when we went for our first visit, but couldn't believe the mess in the bathtub. One of the Yemeni workmen had mixed paints there and it took us weeks to scrub it clean enough for bathing. We looked forward someday to moving into the more spacious hospital villas and then to the apogee of housing, the elegant Princess Sara Villas, which were still under construction. But one rung at a time.

Soon after we moved into the Petromin Apartments I had my first experience with a *shamal*. Ruth, after a short trip to London, was about to return and I was busy cleaning the apartment prior to her arrival. To make a particularly good impression, I vacuumed all the rugs and then proceeded to dust the furniture, but this seemed to be an exercise in frustration. The more I dusted, the more dust appeared. It became so thick I could write my name in it. Then I felt something stinging the back of my neck. I looked up and saw a fine stream of sand pouring out of a grate in the ceiling and covering everything in sight. I heard the wind howling and the sand beating upon the windows. The sun disappeared and everything outside was obscured by a heavy cloud of sand.

It was now pouring out of the grate in torrents. The Yemeni builders had installed contraptions called "desert coolers," which were supposed to bring in air from the outside. The coolers supplied no electrical refrigeration, but merely circulated the "cooled" desert air throughout the apartment. They remained invitingly open, giving the *shamal* free access to the apartment. Sand continued to blow in from everywhere, including the smallest openings in the window sills.

It took weeks to clean up. A thin layer of sand covered everything, and I even found some sand between the pages of books. When Ruth arrived the next day, she expressed disappointment. "You usually do better than this," she said. "There is sand in the cupboards, and I even found some in my tea."

She had never heard of a *shamal*.

I explained that a *shamal* can grow to great proportions, particularly in the Eastern Province, where unrelenting gales of sand swirl about for days, blasting the paint off buildings, knocking over trees, and forcing airplanes to fly at altitudes of 15,000 feet to escape the blinding sand and dust.

"I should have stayed in London," she said, "where I don't have to clean up after a heavy fog."

Power failures were common at the Petromin Apartments and always seemed to occur when the temperature rose to 130 degrees and there was no relief for days. At night, we gathered in the coolest available apartment, wearing bathing suits and carrying candles or hurricane lanterns. We talked of everything but the heat, and finally returned to our own apartments in a futile attempt to get some sleep.

But living in Petromin was an unforgettable experience. The apartment building was located then at the outskirts of Riyadh, and we were often kept awake at night by the howling of packs of wild *saluki* dogs that roamed that area. Arriving home in the evening was always an adventure. Because of the housing boom, the dirt roads leading to the apartment appeared and disappeared within hours as the bulldozers moved huge mounds of earth, often completely obstructing the entrance to the building.

There was little, if any, social life with the Saudis during our first six months in Riyadh, and the foreign colony kept largely to itself. The English had their own clique and welcomed every Englishman who arrived. Americans were less clannish but also tended to look after their own. The Egyptians and Lebanese kept entirely to themselves.

However, as time went on, personal friendships broke down national barriers. Dinner parties became more frequent as each group gradually accepted the other. Entertaining became more relaxed and more festive.

Dr. Compton, as Medical Director, had the largest villa, which was located in the city not far from the Intercontinental Hotel. He entertained more than a hundred people on Christmas Day at a buffet dinner at his home. A large Fourth of July party was held at one of the ten Campus Villas on the hospital grounds. These villas were walled off for privacy and had enclosed lawns and gardens maintained by the hospital staff. A large American flag hung in the garden above the buffet. There were about seventy-five people, including the English, a few Lebanese with their wives, and two Saudis who came alone.

Since Friday was the holiday, hospital parties generally were held the night before. They usually began at nine o'clock and ended at two in the morning. The only alcoholic beverage available was sadiki, "my friend," served in a fruit punch or with tonic water. We all missed our scotch, gin, and vodka. A buffet dinner followed at midnight, and later there was dancing to disco music.

On one occasion a tall, curvaceous secretary in a seductive white gown performed a belly dance. To our delight, two young Lebanese men, hospital technicians, joined in to demonstrate how it *really* should be done.

Since wine was not available we learned to make our own, and the bubbling sounds and smells of fermenting wine often greeted us upon entering an American or English home. One night at dinner I complimented my host on his wine. He replied, lifting his glass, "Ah yes, September was a good month." I invariably recall that remark whenever I'm selecting a vintage wine in some fancy French restaurant.

At times staff dinners were held in the hospital dining room, an attractively decorated room with superior food and European waiters, unusual for any hospital. On one occasion Queen Iffat, the wife of the recently assassinated King Faisal, arrived with two friends. She wore a simple black dress, no jewelry and no veil. Iffat was the Susan B. Anthony of Saudi Arabia. Against great opposition from the Wahabi fundamentalists, she succeeded in opening schools for young women and championed their education. She was the first to organize Saudi women's clubs, previously unheard of, to raise the standards of women in religion, culture, maternal care, and hygiene. This had been a landmark achievement made possible by her influence over her husband.

I had not seen Queen Iffat for about sixteen years, since her visit to Boston for a medical examination. I walked over to her table, where she sat talking with friends. She recognized me immediately and said, "It's been a long time, but neither of us has changed much."

I told her that I had brought her medical record with me from Boston "just in case." I could tell she was pleased.

I told her how much I admired the work she had done in Saudi Arabia, and how impressed I was with the hospital named for her late husband.

"You should see my son, Prince Saud, again," she said. "He works very hard." Prince Saud had been a boy when I had seen him in Boston, but now he was the Foreign Minister. He came to the hospital for an examination several months later. We talked about the recent oil embargo and the importance of Saudi Arabia to the Western world.

As time went on, we invited some Saudi men to our parties, and they invariably came alone. Although we had been advised not to inquire about a Saudi's wife or wives, I asked a close Saudi friend why they always left their wives at home.

"Several reasons," he said solemnly. "Not only is it against our tradition for a woman to appear among strangers unveiled, but she would be fearful that the other Saudis might see her and consider her an immoral woman or report the incident to her family. If she kept her veil on she would feel conspicuous and uncomfortable."

"What about the modern Saudi woman who has studied abroad?" I asked, thinking of Sultana.

"A more emancipated Saudi woman will attend a party with her husband," he said, "providing it is a small group and she knows all the women. The host usually makes the arrangements to preclude the presence of a stranger, and tells his guests the names of those he is planning to invite.

"You must remember, a man might be educated, but his wife could be illiterate and would feel out of place," he concluded. He did not mention his own wife nor did I press him to talk more personally.

In accepting an invitation to a Saudi home, I always waited for my host to invite my wife. If he didn't I would be expected to go alone. Ruth was understanding in this temporary acquiescence to Saudi traditions.

On our first Christmas, a prince, a former patient, came to the Al Sharq Hotel carrying wine, scotch, and vodka camouflaged in a shopping bag filled with old newspapers. Without a word he deposited the bag on a table and departed. It is illegal to import, possess, or drink alcohol. Consequently, many Saudis overcompensate by drinking heavily while they are abroad. When they drink at home it is called *munkar*, moral turpitude. The Committee for the Encouragement of Virtue and the Elimination of Vice tries to control the alcohol problem, but never invades the privacy of a home.

The Saudi royals were usually freer in displaying their liquor than they were in displaying their wives. The one exception was a dinner Ruth and I attended at the home of a sheikh who was a patient of mine, as was his wife. His daughter was married to a prince whom I had treated in the clinic. So for all practical purposes I was considered a member of their extended family.

Many of the wealthy Saudis are careful not to display their wealth. The sheik's opulent villa was concealed by a plain six-foot concrete wall. We drove through the gates into a lovely walled courtyard, a miniature oasis of palm trees and soft grass. At the entrance to their villa, the sheikh, his wife, and daughter waited to welcome us. The women appeared unveiled and beautifully dressed in long gowns. The prince, too, greeted us warmly.

We entered the villa and were shown some of the main rooms of the house. There were large Chinese rugs on the floors, and the walls were covered with textured carpeting. Continuous seating was arranged around three sides of each room, with comfortable armchairs and countless velvet cushions. The reception hall was handsomely decorated, with French-style furniture and velvet-covered chairs made in Lebanon. Large mirrors, rarely seen in Saudi Arabia, with elaborate gold frames dramatized the effect.

When we returned to the sitting room a manservant wheeled in a silver trolley. It was stocked with a choice selection of liquors of every description.

Fortified with drink, we went into the dining room, where I was shown to the head of the vast table. We sat on high-backed blue velvet chairs. In the center of the table was an immense silver platter which held a whole roasted lamb on a bed of steaming white rice. On one side was a large serving dish filled with layers of succulent fish. Another platter held a spicy mixture of mincemeat encased in rolls of tender grape leaves. The sheikh's wife served the dessert, which consisted of a refreshing combination of fruit and custard, tastefully molded.

After dinner we returned to the living room, where a servant, bearing a golden tray, served us small cups of strong coffee.

Then the sheikh brought in his collection of prayer beads, which were made of semiprecious stones of all colors strung on gold chains. About fifty of them were arranged in velvet drawers and no two were alike, either in size or color. The sheikh asked me to select one for myself. After great deliberation I chose a set of carved coral beads, which I have to this day. Then they showed us some photographs of a house they were in the process of buying in London—a huge old mansion probably enormously expensive. Before we left, our hostess gave Ruth a beautiful turquoise-and-pearl ring. She said shyly that she was studying English and Ruth promised to learn Arabic. They became good friends.

A number of Saudis who had studied abroad returned to Saudi Arabia with American or European wives. Sadly, many of those marriages ended in divorce, often because the Saudi abroad and the Saudi at home are two different people. The Saudi identifies with his family and community far more intensely than his counterpart in the West, and although he may stray from the traditional way of life when he is outside the country, eventually he returns home. There the foreign wife finds that she has married a stranger, and a schizophrenic one at that by American or European standards. The government had recently forbidden Saudis to marry non-Moslem women.

In all instances of mixed marriages in which the wife was American or European, Ruth would be included when they entertained. An example of such a marriage was that of His Excellency Dr. Bandar Akkad, a cabinet minister with a Ph.D. from Stanford, considered to be one of the most important officials in Saudi Arabia outside the royal family. Dr. Akkad thought of himself as a "technocrat" rather than an aristocrat. He was multilingual, a poet and a philsopher as well as a brilliant executive. I met Bandar when he was a patient at the clinic and we became good friends. His wife was English but had lived in Saudi Arabia since childhood. Her father had been a construction engineer during King Faisal's reign. Bandar had met his future wife when they were both studying abroad. She became a Moslem when they returned to Riyadh, is his only wife, and bore him two sons. Ruth and I were very fond of her.

Although Bandar came from a very wealthy family, his home was unpretentious. I was impressed with his collection of English and American classics. His library would do credit to a professor of literature in the U.S. He was very proud of his books and obviously enjoyed discussing them with his guests.

An Egyptian woman later served an excellent dinner. There were no alcoholic beverages. During dessert he told us about his youth, and that as a young boy he had had great difficulty with his eyes.

"There were no doctors whatever in my town when I was young," he said, "and I would have gone blind if my parents hadn't sent me to England for medical care. You know, we are criticized for developing our country too rapidly. We are often disorganized and wasteful because we're in such a hurry. But we have to make up for years of lost time. There are still many blind people in my town today who are without adequate medical care. We have a long way to go."

As I look back, that dinner party, which included the wives, exemplified the social behavior of the modern liberal "Westernized" Saudi, whom the religious fundamentalists oppose. We later invited Bandar and his wife to our Petromin apartment for dinner. I had told him which Saudis would be there, so that he would be comfortable in bringing his wife. When he arrived he removed his long brown *bisht* or robe, edged with gold, which he wore over this thobe, and said, putting us all at ease, "Where shall I put my tent?"

We also had invited a Saudi doctor and his wife who had studied in California for eight years, a Lebanese businessman and his wife, and an American couple. All I had available for cocktails was sadiki and some homemade wine, which everyone pretended to enjoy. Dinner consisted of shrimp cocktails, steak flown in from Australia, vegetables, salad, and ice cream.

Conversation turned to Iran, where Ruth and I had visited recently. We had noticed that Americans were very unpopular in Iran, and had felt the animosity even though the Shah was supposedly our friend. "I tried to buy Iranian caviar," I said, "but they refused to sell it to me. However, we were able to buy some beautiful rugs in Isfahan."

"The Americans," Bandar said prophetically, "are making a mistake by backing the Shah of Iran. They are mistaking a mirage for an oasis in Iran, and an oasis for a mirage in Saudi Arabia. In this country we are American-oriented. We admire and respect the U.S. and send our children there to be educated. Crown Prince Fahd has sent four of his sons to the University of California. But still we feel considerable bias against us in the U.S." I expressed my regrets that this was so and embraced him warmly when he left. The next day one of his assistants brought me two pounds of Iranian caviar packed in ice.

Bandar and I had many other conversations. Once I asked him if he thought the new generation of urbanized foreign-educated young Saudis would maintain their strong family loyalties.

"I'm not sure," he replied, "but I think they will. A Saudi is known by the family to which he belongs. However great his talents and dedication, a man without a family to back him does not count for much in his community. The proof is that after we travel far and wide we all eventually return home. I was away for more than eight years studying at various universities, but I returned to my country and my family.

"Family members protect each other's interests. A brother continues to concern himself with his sister's affairs even after she has married, and the closeness of brothers and cousins is proverbial. Young people are also expected to care for their elders and to respect them, an obligation which is often idealized as a pleasant and honorable duty." I myself felt privileged that he would speak so openly with me.

When I asked him about the hostility of the fundamentalists toward the foreign community, he acknowledged a deepening schism between them and the modern Saudis as well.

I told him that most of the homes to which I had been invited belonged to Saudis who had studied abroad but that some of the desert Bedouins had been most friendly.

"That's because you are a doctor," he said. "You probably helped them."

"Even though I'm an infidel?"

"You are a benign and friendly infidel," he said, laughing. "Maybe they will convert you to Islam."

When Bandar mentioned conversion to Islam I remembered a conversation I had had with Bandar's wife in the clinic a month previously. She told me that she felt insecure in her marriage because she was a foreigner. Although she had embraced Islam and had produced two sons, she realized that her husband was free to have three more wives if he wished.

"He is too intelligent and too loyal to do that," I assured her, and this assurance proved to be justified.

We had a totally unexpected social visit with an Arab one sunny morning when Ruth and I were walking down a street near the University of Riyadh. A stranger in Saudi dress approached us and started talking in English. When we told him we were Americans he insisted that we come to his home nearby for coffee. On the way he said that he had studied engineering at Cal Tech and was very partial to Americans. He obviously loved being able to converse once again in the language of his formal education. He served us coffee, which he had prepared in another room. We heard him speak to his wife but we did not meet her. He said he hoped to visit California again someday.

I didn't know it at the time, but soon I would be invited into the home of a Saudi who had never seen a foreigner before in his lifetime. It would take place in the far-off Asir Province near the Red Sea.

A month later I was on my way to Khamis Mushayt, a small town located in the Asir, a mountainous region along the southern Red Sea coast, near the Yemen border. It was about five hundred miles southwest of Riyadh, adjacent to the vast desert called the Empty Quarter. I flew there at the invitation of Dr. Stewart Randall, an American doctor, who was working in a military hospital in this isolated area. Because there was no telephone service between Khamis Mushayt and Riyadh, Stewart had contacted me by radio several weeks before about an American nurse who was suffering from severe abdominal pain. He wanted to have her flown to our hospital in Riyadh for diagnosis and treatment. We made the necessary arrangements for her hospital stay and our tests subsequently indicated that she had a blockage of one of the small blood vessels to the intestine. We were able to treat her successfully and she returned to Khamis Mushayt. Now I was on my way to visit their hospital and to examine my patient. I was pleased to be able to explore this picturesque part of the country.

Moussa, from the transportation department of the hospital, had arranged for a first-class ticket for me, which he had confirmed by letter. Ten minutes after I had checked in at the ticket counter, I was paged and the agent, a Saudi, told me I must yield my first-class ticket for a second-class one. Suspecting my place was being taken by a royal I refused and showed him Moussa's letter of confirmation.

When the plane's departure was announced, I boarded and proceeded to the first-class section, which had four empty seats. Soon the Saudi agent came aboard, accompanied by a short Bedouin guard in a khaki uniform carrying a gun and looking very uncomfortable. I felt sure that the gun was not loaded. The guard appeared more apprehensive than I was as he shifted his weight from one leg to the other. The agent insisted that I go second class. I refused and told him to get another guard and to carry me off, because I would not budge.

"Two guards will be necessary," I said, "because I weigh eighty kilos and this guard is pretty small and thin." As we were talking a royal entered the plane with a wife and two children. He sized up the situation immediately and put his children in second class.

The agent suddenly changed his tone. "Sorry about that," he said as he turned and left. The Bedouin guard followed with a look of relief. By a strange coincidence, when I later deplaned at the airport near Khamis Mushayt the music from the plane's loudspeaker greeted me with George M. Cohan's "I'm a Yankee Doodle Dandy"!

In the hour-and-a-half flight we passed over part of the huge and forbidding Empty Quarter, the largest sand desert in the world. This sea of deep shifting sands, the size of Texas, extends from the Yemen highlands on the southwest border of Saudi Arabia to the foothills of Oman nine hundred miles to the east. It also stretches for five hundred miles from Yemen in the south to the Arabian or Persian Gulf in the northeast. The "desert within a desert" of 250,000 square miles is so enormous and desolate that it remained unexplored for more than a thousand years until Bertram Thomas, and later Harry St. John Philby, both Englishmen, crossed it on camels. Thomas was the first to cross the Rub Al Khali in 1930, and Philby followed two years later. In a letter to the marshal of the British Royal Air Force in 1926, T. E. Lawrence suggested that the RAF fly over it to "mark an era of exploration." "Nothing but an airship can do it," he wrote, "and I want it to be one of ours that gets the plum."

My first view of the Empty Quarter fulfilled all my expectations of what a great desert should look like. The sand dunes appeared as enormous billows or huge ocean swells of fine sand, a mile across, sometimes rising from the level plains to a peak of two thousand feet. The prevailing north winds transformed the windward side of the dunes into steep, curved slopes, too vertical for a camel to climb. Other dunes took the shape of domes and crescents, or formed long spectacular deep red or rust-colored parallel escarpments called *urug* (veins) by the Bedouins. In some areas the dunes appeared cream-colored, white, or red in every imaginable shade. Several peaks shone with green-tinted gold. In the flat areas the sand appeared rippled or whorled like immense fingerprints of some celestial giant, or the ridged bottom of an ocean. Yet the only vestiges of organic life were limestone oyster fossils from some ancient sea millions of years ago.

As we made our approach to Khamis Mushayt we passed over a large canyon whose steep walls consisted of parallel layers of rock similar to those in our Grand Canyon in Arizona. The fine sand covering the bottom of the canyon and the cliffs glistened white like snow. Just before we circled to land I could see the rugged mountains of the Asir, ten thousand feet high, which border the Red Sea along the southwest coast of Saudi Arabia and form a watershed for the entire Arabian peninsular plateau. In this southern area, the coastal plain called the Tihama appears. It rises gradually from the sea to the mountains. With twenty-five inches of annual rainfall, there is enough water to permit cultivation of the land without irrigation.

The well-watered slopes of the Tihama plain are the most productive region of Saudi Arabia. The slopes and the mountains behind them are extensively terraced to make the best use of the land. Coffee, grain, fruits, and vegetables are cultivated at five hundred feet above sea level on the terraced slopes of the western side of the mountains facing the Red Sea. The eastern slope is gentle and melds into a plateau region which drops gradually into the Rub Al Khali, the Empty Quarter. A number of lava beds and huge craters on the surface of the eastern plateau give evidence of fairly recent volcanic activity. This is certainly a land of contrasts—topographically as well as socially: the Red Sea and a fertile plateau on one side of the mountains, with lava beds and a frightful desert on the other.

Stewart Randall met me at the small airport at Abha and drove me to his home near the nondescript military hospital in Khamis Mushayt where he worked. The houses all looked alike, built of cement and stucco and lined up like pill boxes. They were comfortable inside except for the lack of air conditioning.

Stewart and his wife originally came from Jersey City. They had been in Jakarta in Indonesia for two years and in Khamis Mushayt for two years and were leaving for Jidda in a few months. They both loved to travel.

My patient, Edwina Parnell, had recovered completely. She invited us to dinner in her apartment and announced she was celebrating my visit by taking several days' leave from the hospital to show me around. There were of course no restaurants and all entertaining was done at home. The next day, after a visit to the hospital, where I briefly examined Edwina, the Randalls, Edwina, and I set out for a picnic in a Swedish van driven by a friend of Edwina's named Hisham.

As we drove west out of town I noticed beds of black rocks of all sizes and shapes piled on top of each other, similar to the volcanic rocks I had once seen in Iceland. Soon we found a spot for our picnic covered with lush vegetation and overlooking a huge canyon with the Asir Mountains beyond. Mary Randall served an excellent basket lunch of fried chicken, potato salad, and coffee. After lunch, while exploring, we came upon a large dilapidated relic of what once had been a grandiose palace, now in ruins. Stewart told us that the palace had been used as a holiday hideaway by King Saud, his wives, and concubines, but had been deserted since King Saud left the country in 1964.

"Did you know," Randall asked, pointing into the distance, "that Yemen is only a few miles away? We are practically on the border." He said that many Yemeni are riddled with parasites. In some areas the boys are thought to menstruate because so many have blood in their urine caused by bilharzia, a parasite which attacks the urinary tract, or the intestinal tract and the liver. The disease spreads by the passage of contaminated human waste into shallow, slow-moving water channels where snails breed. The parasite is transformed into the infective form within the snail and later returns to the water, where it penetrates the skin of humans working or bathing in the infested area. Finally the parasitic worm invades the blood vessels and organs of the human hosts.

There are more than a half-million Yemeni working in Saudi Arabia, according to Randall, many in poor health with a life expectancy of about forty years. Because they are not permitted to bring their wives into Saudi Arabia, they are subjected to long periods of sexual abstinence. Consequently, homosexuality is common among them, and a number have been executed for rape.

"Not long ago, three Yemeni were beheaded in Riyadh for rape on a single day," he added.

"Let me tell you," I said, "about some experiences I have had with the President of Yemen and the former Prime Minister." They frequently came to Saudi Arabia to consult with the King and Crown Prince Fahd. Lieutenant Colonel Ibrahim Al-Hamdi at that time was President of North Yemen, which has very strong ties with the West and with Saudi Arabia, while South Yemen has a Marxist government and its army is Soviet-trained. Actually North Yemen was bankrupt and practically defenseless against the Soviet-backed South Yemen. The Saudis were so concerned that they purchased $400 million worth of military equipment from the United States and had it shipped to North Yemen, accompanied by one hundred American military advisors.

While these transactions were going on, I received a call from the palace asking me to see Judge Abdullah Al-Hagri, the former Prime Minister of North Yemen who was serving as an advisor to Al-Hamdi. He was a short, stocky man about sixty years of age, wearing a white thobe and a large white turban to give him additional height. Around his waist he carried a colorful belt with a large vicious-looking curved dagger. He told me he was in the process of writing a constitution for the Republic of Yemen.

"It won't be as liberal or academic as your Constitution in the United States," he said, "but I'll do my best under the existing conditions in our country."

I examined him on a number of occasions, testing him for bilharzia infection. I also examined his wife and a twelve-year-old son—one of eleven children. The day before he left Saudi Arabia he brought me five pounds of coffee grown in his native land and gave me a formal invitation to visit his capital. He embraced me warmly when we parted.

Six months later Al-Hagri and his wife were gunned down in his car in front of the Royal Lancaster Hotel in London on a Sunday morning. According to the authorities, his killing was politically motivated and carried out by professionals. The London press emphasized the Libyan connection, since Al-Hagri had opposed the Libyan-sponsored plans to create a single Yemen republic, which would constitute a takeover by the Soviet-dominated South Yemen.

Several months later I examined President Ibrahim Al-Hamdi. The Saudi press had been reporting President Hamdi's talks with Crown Prince Fahd, hailing Saudi-Yemen friendship. The Chief of Security personally escorted the President to my office, having indicated beforehand that all possible precautions were being taken for his safety. He was a medium-sized man, about thirty-eight years old, and much to my surprise clean-shaven and wearing a dark blue suit, blue tie, and white shirt. And he carried a briefcase like a Manhattan banker. He appeared to be the strong, silent type who keeps his emotions within himself. He was suffering from high blood pressure, which was readily understandable. When I examined his retinal blood vessels with an ophthalmoscope he demonstrated absolute control of eye movement.

"You're a very disciplined person, Mr. President," I said to him.

"I should be," he replied. "I'm a lieutenant colonel in the army."

After appropriate tests and x-rays I prescribed medication, although it alone could not solve his problem. I saw him only on two occasions, always under heavy guard. Eighteen months later, President Al-Hamdi was killed by the explosion of a booby-trapped briefcase, similar to the one he carried with him when he was in my office.

We continued our explorations the next day, driving about ten miles west of Khamis Mushayt to some terraced farms on the slopes of the Asir Mountains. They were irrigated by channels of water descending from terrace to terrace where men, women, and children were working in the fields side by side. The women were in the majority, unveiled in the privacy of their family. All wore the broad-brimmed hats characteristic of this area.

The houses of mud construction were grouped together in family units of five to ten and were three or four stories high. Wooden shingles were embedded into the mud at six- to eight-inch intervals, overlapping each other and protruding from the sides of the house, giving it a rippled appearance. The wooden shakes slanted downward to protect the mud from the weather. The most picturesque part of the scene was the brilliant colors of the houses: pastel shades of green, brown, red, yellow, orange, and blue. The crenelated roof lines shone a brilliant white, and the small square windows were outlined with red, pink, or yellow. It reminded me of a child's first painting of houses in watercolor.

As we walked about admiring the village, a man about forty years old approached us. He was dressed in the traditional thobe and sandals but he wore a large straw hat instead of the red-checkered ghutra and agal. An intricately worked leather belt circled his waist and supported a carved silver dagger. Edwina's friend Hisham acted as our interpreter and told him we were admiring the houses and that we were Americans. The man said he was a farmer and that he had never been outside the Asir or seen foreigners before. He name was Rashad. We all shook hands, nodding our heads and smiling. Hisham told us that Rashad wanted us to visit his home. We were delighted and followed him to a pink-and-green house with white trimming. He took off his sandals and placed them on a stack of similar sandals outside his colorfully decorated door. We followed suit as I recalled some of the pertinent instructions in the *Sand Script*, the hospital bulletin, titled "Visiting an Arabic Home."

Your host may embrace you or shake hands with both men and women. Do not ask about his wife and daughters, or where they are. If you must, ask about his "family." Saudi women stay in the background. However, if your host introduces you to the female members of his household, he may be following Western customs, to put you at your ease. His wife may show great affection for your wife and children. However, should she not stay, do not ask if she is coming back. Never tell your host that the adult female members of the household are pretty or beautiful as this may cause offense.

When you enter the house or living-room your host may remove his shoes.

If so, do the same.... Let the host lead the way to the living-room. Do not follow close behind; there may be ladies who do not wish to be seen. If you are a lady join any ladies who may be present; they may be sitting apart from the men, and it is customary that you sit with them, unless this is otherwise indicated. When sitting, men should cross their legs, and women sit to one side with legs tucked under, never showing the soles of the feet to anyone's face.

The living room was a large rectangular room with colorful Turkish rugs covering the floor. There were no chairs, but a number of large tufted pillows were arranged along the walls. The ceiling was made of wood, with suspended wooden beams about one-half inch thick, which were painted in many pastel colors. The walls, too, were painted with two-foot-wide stripes of pink, blue, green, and yellow to match the ceiling beams. Rashad said they had electricity, but it was *mafi* (out of order). There were two small square windows, edged with white, close to the ceiling on the outer wall.

Three women wearing black veils and black *abeyyas* entered the room. They were barefoot. Rashad introduced them and to my surprise we all shook hands. Hisham said they were two of Rashad's wives and one of his sisters. They left as quietly and as quickly as they had come, and we never saw the women again. In accordance with the *Sand Script's* admonitions we did not inquire further about them.

The men sat on one side of the room and Mary and Edwina sat on the other, with their legs tucked under them as prescribed by custom. I remembered that at the parties given by the Egyptians or Lebanese the women sat in a row on one side of the room and the men sat on the other. Mixing eventually took place when dinner was served.

Rashad served us the usual coffee with the help of one of his sons. Thick chunks of cardamom floated in it because he didn't have enough time to filter it properly. In the royal households one servant is assigned to making, filtering, and serving coffee, and that's all he does. It apparently takes time and skill, and Rashad had prepared the coffee at a moment's notice. I accepted a second cup to be polite. Three cups is the limit according to Saudi etiquette. The guest signals that he has had enough by shaking the empty cup with rapid little movements of the wrist.

Rashad told us he was a tenant wheat farmer and that wheat was one of the major crops in the Asir area. He also planted barley and corn on occasion. He said they had ample rain in the summer months, June to September, and were seven thousand feet above sea level.

Stewart asked Rashad if he grew *qat*, a green succulent plant cultivated in the Asir at altitudes over four thousand feet. Its leaves have a narcotic effect. Rashad said that the government controlled the production of *qat* and he did not have a permit to grow it.

After Rashad's son served tea, we congratulated our host on his home and thanked him for his hospitality. I think he would have liked to ask us many questions but was too shy to do so. We all shook hands with him and his son, put on our shoes waiting for us outside the doorway, and departed.

On Thursday, shopping day, people came to Khamis Mushayt from long distances to buy fruits, vegetables, nuts, and spices at the outdoor *suqs*. Some traveled seventy-five miles or more to take part in the festive mood of the marketplace, with its array of straw hats, pottery, goatskin water bags, and beautifully carved silver knives and bracelets. We created a sensation because most of the people had never seen foreigners in Western dress before. They gathered about us in small circles wherever we went, staring at the clean-shaven light-haired men in trousers and shirts, and the unveiled, white-skinned women. Some of the men carried guns; others wore elaborately tooled belts with carved silver daggers. When I decided to buy a dagger, the men gathered about, anxious to help me select the best one. All this was carried out in pantomime, since by now I had lost Hisham and Stewart in the crowd.

The men were in a holiday humor. When I finally made a choice, they helped me put the belt on and fix the silver dagger in place. Then they applauded. Now I was one of them. It was all done in fun, in the spirit of the carnival.

In the afternoon we went to see the Queen of Sheba Mountain, where it is said the Queen of Sheba camped on her way from Africa to Israel to marry King Solomon. On the way home I saw a young shepherd wearing the conventional thobe and a straw hat. In addition he carried an open umbrella to protect himself from the sun.

"Now I've seen everything," I said. "Maybe he learned that from Haile Selassie, who often carried an umbrella, and Ethiopia is really nearby."

"Only four or five hundred miles," Hisham said.

The most charming area of the Asir was the mountainous region to the south, known as Sooda, which I saw on my last day in Khamis Mushayt. Here there were many farms with terraced fields, and the women do absolutely *all* the work. The men sit around and enjoy a life of leisure. No one questions this. I contemplated taking up permanent residence here, but I didn't think Ruth would approve of anything beyond a one-day visit.

◇ *15* ◇

BLOOD MONEY

WHEN I ARRIVED at my office one morning, I found an unusual document on my desk. It was typed in Arabic and looked like an official proclamation. I called my secretary over the intercom.

"My Arabic is a bit rusty this morning," I said. "Do you have a translation of this?"

"I'll be right in," she replied. Her voice wasn't as cheerful as usual.

Manda came into the office. She looked worried. "I wanted to break the news to you gradually," she said as she handed me a paper. "This translation was stapled to the Arabic cablegram on your desk."

It began, "In the name of Allah, the most compassionate, the most merciful," and went on to say that one of our patients had died in the hospital recently and that her husband accused four doctors of "causing her death." He claimed that "the doctors should pay him blood money."

The cable directed them to appear for trial in the Department of Forensic Medicine in the Ministry of Health. Two doctors whom they named were ordered to appear on a Sunday night at 7:30 P.M. and two on a Monday night. It was signed by the Director of Forensic Medicine.

I explained to Manda that the term "forensic medicine" meant legal medicine. The physicians named in the suit for blood money were Dr. George Rogers, a specialist in internal medicine, and three other doctors: the physician in the clinic, the reception physician, and the physician on call.

Manda placed a cigarette in her cigarette holder, lit it, and leaned back in her chair. She was very loyal to our department and appeared upset by the cable.

"What is this business about blood money?" she asked. "I never heard of it before."

I explained that, when a person is killed by accident or by intent, his next of kin has the legal right to demand blood money, which is a set payment to compensate for the death. According to the old Sharia law, the family of the victim can bring charges against the accused for the right "to retaliate in kind" by killing him. However, this form of retaliation is now discouraged by Islamic law and the acceptance of blood money by the family of the deceased is considered preferable. For example, when someone is killed in an automobile accident, a very common occurrence in Saudi Arabia, the person responsible pays blood money to the victim's family and often goes to prison as well.

In the old days, when the tribes were fighting and killing each other, a neutral tribe would intervene and make peace by having the tribe who lost fewer men in battle pay blood money to the other side for their surplus of dead bodies. This prevented further feuding as a means of retaliation.

Blood money for an ordinary life had been about 1,200 riyals ($400, U.S.) in 1936, but the value of a life, in view of inflation and the increased cost of living, had now risen to 40,000 riyals ($13,500, U.S.). In some Moslem countries, the amount paid increases with the social status of the deceased, but not in Saudi Arabia.

"You're not involved in this trial," said Manda, exhaling a cloud of smoke. "Why did they send a copy of the cable to you?"

"Because the patient was in the care of the Department of Medicine when she died and I'm the chairman of the department," I said. "We'll have to make a thorough investigation of the matter to determine negligence or malpractice. Dr. Compton probably sent this to prepare me for the bad news. We will be hearing from him soon, you can count on it."

Two hours later Hugh Compton called. "Did you receive a copy of that cable from the Ministry of Health?" he asked, but before I could answer he continued. "The reputation of the hospital is at stake. The blood money itself is not the issue. The hospital carries insurance to cover it.

"The question is whether this was a preventable death. I want to make certain we did everything possible for this woman," he said. "At least fourteen people participated in her care during the eight hours she was in the hospital. I intend to get written testimony from everyone involved: the doctors, nurses, the resuscitation team, and so forth.

"I want you to appoint a peer review committee to determine if there was negligence on the part of anyone in the management of this patient," he concluded. "We have less than a week to get this done. Then, we'll have a meeting and put it all together."

I appointed a committee consisting of four specialists to consider whether there was negligence or malpractice on the part of the physicians, the nursing staff, or members of the other hospital departments. Our main concern, however, was possible negligence on the part of the physicians in charge of her care who were named as defendants in the cable.

The committee learned that the patient, Tadra Zaki Shibat Hashin, a forty-five-year-old woman, came to the hospital reception desk with her husband requesting admission to the clinic at about 3 P.M. She had a letter from her doctor stating that she had pneumonia in the lower lobe of her left lung. Dr. Zabbar, the reception physician, referred her to the primary-care doctor in the Family Health Center to determine whether she should be admitted to the hospital. This was in accordance with an established policy to screen all patients before admitting them because the hospital was usually filled to capacity and·the referring physician's letters were sometimes misleading.

Dr. Tabil saw the patient at 3:30 P.M. in the Health Center. She complained of a sore throat and cough, complicated later by shortness of breath and chest pain. She did not cough blood, she said, but her coughing had become worse despite the medicine. Dr. Tabil examined her and noted a blue discoloration of her skin, indicating an oxygen deficiency. She was enormously obese, weighing 194 pounds and measuring less than five feet in height. His findings on physical examination indicated pneumonia, but he was puzzled by her subnormal temperature, her very low blood pressure, and very rapid heart rate.

Dr. Tabil ordered the appropriate x-rays and blood tests, and then called Dr. Rogers, the specialist. They reviewed the x-rays, which revealed extensive pneumonia involving both lungs. The electrocardiogram was normal except for the rapid rate.

Although the patient said she preferred to go home, Dr. Rogers insisted on admitting her to the hospital immediately. He ordered oxygen-inhalation therapy, an oral antibiotic every six hours, and a number of blood tests. She arrived on Ward B-3 at 4:30 P.M. and died shortly after midnight about eight hours later.

With the benefit of hindsight, the peer committee felt that Dr. Rogers did not appreciate at the time the gravity of the patient's condition and did not institute adequate and appropriate treatment. The low blood pressure, the low temperature, rapid pulse, and shortness of breath suggested that she had an overwhelming bloodstream infection secondary to her extensive pneumonia and that she was in septic shock prior to her hospitalization.

The committee was of the opinion that Dr. Rogers had not been negligent but that there had been a serious error in judgment on his part. Whether massive doses of antibiotics intravenously and more supportive therapy would have saved her life was conjectural, particularly in view of her morbid obesity and the extent of her infection.

A few other points came to light during our investigations. Dr. Rogers had instructed the Egyptian nurse assigned to the patient to call Dr. Saban, the medical physician-on-call, if the patient's condition should deteriorate, and then, if necessary, to report back to him. However, because of language difficulties, the special nurse apparently did not understand and never called Dr. Saban, who had been available in the hospital all night, and who, actually, had visited Ward B-3 on his rounds. Later, when the patient's blood pressure fell precipitously, the head nurse herself called Dr. Saban. He started an intravenous infusion shortly before midnight, but within a half hour the patient became unconscious. Emergency resuscitative measures by the anesthesiologist team were to no avail.

The patient's husband had been called several hours earlier and notified of his wife's critical condition. When he arrived in the hospital and was informed of her death, he became extremely irate, accused the staff of negligence, and threatened litigation for blood money.

Dr. Rogers, who was at home, had heard nothing further from the special nurse or from Dr. Saban and assumed that all was going well with his patient. A language difficulty on the part of the special Egyptian nurse had been a contributing factor, the committee decided after they took her testimony.

The final opinion was that this patient's illness in all its fulminant gravity had not been recognized immediately and that she was not given appropriate treatment. This was attributed to a tragic sequence of misjudgments and mischances which could not fairly be ascribed to any one individual's negligence.

The Arab doctor who wrote the report concluded: "It is also the considered opinion of the committee that the final outcome of this patient was probably predetermined regardless of the treatment administered."

I must admit that I too had a gut feeling that this patient would not have survived in any event, but I had not thought of it in the Moslem sense—that the final outcome "was predetermined."

I had considerable respect for the manner in which the American corporation which managed the hospital carried out its mission of health care. All of my professional life had been spent in hospitals associated with medical schools, including the University of Chicago and Harvard, but none of them, in my opinion, had the managerial talent to compete with that of the King Faisal Hospital. Our doctors at the university hospitals were more academic, more research-oriented, and more world-renowned, but the administrators at the King Faisal Hospital demonstrated considerably more expertise, particularly in the face of supply shortages, problems in communication, and complex cultural and religious differences. I was, above all, impressed by their dedication to achieving the highest possible level of health care in the face of almost insurmountable obstacles.

A few days before the trial, Hugh Compton called a special meeting of the Medical Advisory Board. He presented the report of the Peer Review Committee and the detailed testimony of everyone involved in the treatment of the deceased. Hugh emphasized the confidentiality of these reports and of all business transacted at this session. After some discussion, the board accepted the conclusions of the Peer Review Committee that there had been no negligence but that the patient had not received adequate and appropriate treatment because of misjudgment on the part of Dr. Rogers.

Then Dr. Compton called on Galal Abu Nassera, the legal advisor to the hospital. Galal was a brilliant young man, an Egyptian who was a full-time employee. He told us that malpractice or negligence resulting in the death or disability of a patient was considered a civil liability. According to high royal decree, the compensation, called blood money, was fixed at 40,000 riyals (about $13,500) in case of death. Lesser amounts were paid in the event of disability or the loss of an extremity.

"Negligence or malpractice on the part of the physician is always considered an unintentional error ascribed to lack of precaution, neglect, or misjudgment," he said. "If the physician treats a patient by methods not generally accepted by the profession or if he fails to perform certain duties essential to uphold the quality of his profession and its Islamic nature, he is also liable.

"If guilt is decreed, the sentences imposed for civil liability may be the payment of blood money; a reprimand or censure; expulsion from the country; or all three.

"The physician is criminally liable," he added, "if he performs an unauthorized abortion; prescribes narcotics without a medical reason; fails to notify the police in cases of bullet wounds, suicide, rape, or narcotic abuse; or forges birth or death certificates. If an abortion is necessary to save the patient's life, two physicians, one of which must be a specialist, should agree as to the urgency of the abortion.

"Criminal liability is punishable by imprisonment, the payment of blood money or fines, and expulsion from the country in the case of foreigners. Bail is accepted in some cases but the guarantor may go to jail if the defendant jumps bail."

A few minutes of silence followed Galal's dissertation. Some of our American doctors had come to Saudi Arabia to avoid paying exorbitant premiums for malpractice insurance. In California, many physicians were forced to pay from $75,000 to $100,00 a year! The memory of these enormous insurance premiums still rankled in everyone's mind. The next question naturally was "Who pays the blood money?"

Galal said the hospital carried insurance to cover the professional liability of its physicians. The hospital would pay "any compensation or civil obligation and shall pay the sum determined by the court, promptly, without waiting for the insurance company to settle the amount."

There was an audible sigh of relief. The hospital apparently was confident of its ability to select a superior cadre of physicians which would not get involved in these suits.

Since expelling foreigners from the country was a common procedure in Saudi Arabia, Galal said that it was in the hospital's interest that the physician not leave the country prior to testifying before a body of competent investigative authorities.

"Leaving the country, however, should not be interpreted as a confession of guilt," he added.

Dr. Compton pointed out that in any case of unexplained death the family should be urged to have an autopsy performed. If they refused, the legal advisor should be notified and requested to take appropriate action.

After the meeting was adjourned, I called George Rogers and asked him to come to the office. George was a friend of mine and I felt obliged to prepare him for the worst. He came from Leeds originally, was a competent physician, and had worked in hospitals in Nigeria, Uganda, and Iran before coming to Riyadh. He was about fifty years old, tall, lanky, and balding, with hazel eyes and gray hair.

I told him that there was a possibility he would be dismissed from the hospital and forced to leave the country within a week after the trial.

"That wouldn't give you much time," I said. "You might think about selling your car and shipping your valuables home.

"But there is some good news, too," I added. "The hospital will pay the blood money, if you are found guilty." I told him about Galal's presentation at the Medical Advisory Board Meeting. "I thought they would take it out of my salary," said George. He looked relieved.

"As I think back on it," said George, "the patient led me astray when she said she wanted to go home. I had no idea at the time that she had such a serious infection."

Maybe she wanted to go home to die, I thought. That seems to be the tradition here.

"Then, because of language barriers, the nurse did not notify me in time to allow me to re-evaluate the patient's treatment," he said. He also told me that he was preoccupied that night preparing a lecture for a hospital meeting the next day.

"Galal, Hugh Compton and I will probably accompany you to the trial, for moral support," I said. "Galal knows a great deal about the law. You might want to talk with him before the trial. I've made an appointment for you to see him tomorrow."

He thanked me and left. I felt unhappy about his situation and sorry for him. There was no question in my mind, however, that he had made a mistake in evaluating his patient's condition and in treating her so haphazardly. To err may be human, I thought, but to forgive would not be divine—not according to the Koran.

The Saudis basically are gentle, sensitive, law-abiding people. Swearing at a Saudi is a criminal offense and punishable by a fine. A hearty slap on the back may be construed as assault and battery. Striking a Saudi, even in self-defense, is illegal and may lead to a jail sentence, fines, or deportation. The use of abusive language in public may be punished by imprisonment. In the event of an auto accident, both drivers are jailed pending an investigation. Anyone found drunk in public is jailed and deported, if he is a foreigner. Moslems caught drinking alcohol are lashed.

In Riyadh, however, there were very few civil police to enforce the law. Only an occasional Saudi in military uniform might be seen directing traffic. But the *matawa,* the morals police, were everywhere and not only enforced the law to the letter but at times exceeded their jurisdiction.

The next day George and I went to Galal's office. He told us that George would be tried under the Sharia law, the Islamic legal code, whose judgments are both secular and spiritual. It condemns thievery, protects private property, lays down inheritance procedures, and generally defines the rights and obligations of its citizenry.

Interpretation of the law is carried out by the Ulema, a body of religious scholars who are the highest authority on legal matters. The Grand Mufti is the Chief Judge, the leader of the Ulema, and a descendant of the founder of the fundamentalist Wahabi movement. This ultra-conservative body is chary of innovations in interpreting the Koran, particularly regarding ethics, morality, and religious matters.

Galal said that the court would be presided over by a *qadi,* an Islamic judge appointed by the Grand Mufti. The *qadis* are religious scholars of Islamic law who have graduated from a Sharia college and from the Supreme Judicial Institute in Riyadh.

"How is the jury selected?" asked George.

"There is no trial by jury under Islamic law," said Galal. "The *qadi* is both judge and jury. His function is to establish the facts. The defense and prosecution are not adversaries. They are there to help the *qadi*. The accused can have a lawyer if he wishes, but it is the *qadi* who takes the initiative in clarifying the defendant's case. It is he who asks the questions and cross-examines the witnesses."

"In a way, the *qadi* is both the judge and the lawyer," I said.

"We're searching for the truth," said Galal, "not some lawyer's embellishment of the truth. In the West the juries are often swayed by the oratory of the lawyers, and verdicts are based on emotions rather than upon facts."

"Do Sharia courts handle all litigation?" I asked.

"No," said Galal, "there are special courts in several fields. For example, there is a court for the settlement of commercial disputes, which handles business matters. But business law must conform to Sharia law, and if there is a conflict, the Sharia law takes precedence. Labor disputes are handled by the Ministry of Labor, where there are special labor courts for industrial disputes. The Ministry of Health has jurisdiction over grievances involving legal medicine such as ours."

"What about trials for murder?" I asked.

"Under Islamic law," said Galal, "homicide is not considered a crime against society, in which the state moves against the criminal. It is rather a crime against the family of the victim. The Sharia law recognizes the right of the victim's family to press charges against the accused.

"The defendant must be found guilty of a premeditated act in order to be convicted of murder," he continued. "At least three *qadis* hear the case together. If convicted, the murderer must pay blood money, and serve a prison sentence, or he might be beheaded, if the relatives of the victim demand it. This prevents long-running feuds between families.

"Beheadings are not infrequent," he concluded. "There are beheadings the first Friday of each month in Riyadh, Jidda, and elsewhere. Many of those beheaded are foreigners from Yemen and other countries. Some are beheaded for rape and others for murder."

"You have been very helpful," I remarked as we prepared to leave. "Let's meet Monday night and go to the Ministry of Health together."

"Good idea," said Galal. "I am going with Zabbar and Saban on Sunday night, but that hearing will only be the preliminary to the main event on Monday. After all, Dr. Zabbar, the physician at the reception desk, and the physician on call, Dr. Saban, have little, if any, direct responsibility."

George nodded silently as we left.

We met at the front desk on Monday night at seven. I volunteered to drive. Galal sat up front with me, and Hugh Compton, George Rogers, and Tabil, the primary-care physician, sat in back. Everyone was in a lugubrious mood except for Galal, who couldn't stop talking.

He told us that the trial hadn't started the night before until nine o'clock. "Haste comes from the devil," he said. "We are never on time." It was an aphorism I had heard before. "Besides the qadi or judge," Galal continued, "there was a panel of three doctors from the Riyadh Medical School and the Deputy Minister of Forensic Medicine. The qadi first questioned the complainant, the husband of the deceased, and then Zabbar and Saban. He concentrated on Saban, the physician on call, to determine why he had not tended to the patient earlier. Saban explained the language difficulty with the Egyptian nurse and that he had been available all evening but had not been called. Then the doctors asked him a few questions regarding the emergency call system at the hospital. Since Zabbar and Saban were Moslems under oath, the hearing went smoothly. They adjourned at eleven o' clock."

We arrived at the Ministry of Health in twenty minutes. It was located on Airport Road across the street from the Al Sharq Hotel. Galal directed us to a room on the fourth floor in the Department of Forensic Medicine. It was a dimly-lit medium-sized room. The white walls of plaster were beginning to peel. In fact, there were cracks in the walls and signs of deterioration everywhere although the building was relatively new. I remembered that the Saudis do not believe in maintenance. They prefer to rebuild.

The room was spartan in appearance. The white walls were bare except for an Arabic inscription on the wall. Beneath the inscription stood a desk-like table laden with books and papers. This was apparently the qadi's table. About six feet away, on the same level, was a rectangular table placed perpendicular to that of the qadi. This table was surrounded by straight-backed chairs arranged to face the qadi. There were a few wooden benches and chairs scattered in back for the spectators. The room was otherwise bare and austere.

It was seven-thirty, the designated time for the trial. Nobody else had arrived.

"The trial won't start for another hour, until after the evening prayers," said Galal, as we sat down on the hard benches.

I asked Galal about the Arabic inscription on the wall. He said that it read, "Justice should be applied equally among all people."

"That's a democratic principle," I said. "I hope it means that justice *is* applied equally to all people."

"It is," Galal reassured me. "Some of the Sharia laws are similar to yours in the West and some quite different. Under Islamic law, a person is innocent until found guilty. However, the right of habeas corpus is not recognized. In cases involving death or serious injuries, the accused is usually jailed for considerable periods, often until the day of trial. In minor offenses, the police will accept a bond."

Turning to George, he said sympathetically, "In an argument between an infidel and a Moslem, the testimony of the Moslem is given greater credence because he testifies under oath upon the Koran. There are no Christian Bibles in Moslem courts. The oath is taken very seriously. If a Moslem refuses to take an oath on the Koran, he jeopardizes his case. However, confessions are accepted to establish guilt.

"Two witnesses are necessary to prove a point except in cases of adultery, which require four eyewitnesses," he added.

"What rights do women have in your courts?" I asked.

Galal looked embarrassed. "I wish you hadn't asked me that," he said. "As a witness a woman counts as half a man."

"And she gets half as much inheritance as her brothers, according to your laws," I added. "I thought the inscription on the wall says that 'justice should be applied equally among *all* people.' That must mean that you still don't consider women as people."

Hugh Compton rose to the occasion. "The Sharia laws go back over a thousand years," he said. "How can such an antiquated legal system adjust to present-day situations?"

Galal went on the defensive. "Your constitutional laws in the U.S. are over two hundred years old and you are constantly revising them or interpreting them in the light of the twentieth century," he said. "Our Sharia laws are equally flexible and have been subject to reinterpretation according to the need. We have made many adjustments to cope with the industrialization of our country and foreign influences.

"The Sharia law has been modified to accept advances in technology, such as the airplane, telephone, photography, and television, which are not specifically prohibited in our source books and are therefore not against the wishes of God. The protection of traditional values is more important to us than the perpetuation of specific prohibitions. Our government has stood firmly in favor of modernization as long as Islam is not undermined, but we will not compromise our morals and our ethics."

Galal told us that commercial and civil codes had begun to supplement and to replace the Sharia. Royal decrees, the Grievance Board, and other secular administrative courts were taking over jurisdiction in the business fields.

"However, in any conflict between religious and secular or political considerations of the law, those of religion still take precedence," he emphasized. "The Sharia, for example, forbids the charging of interest on loans as usury but the banks may instead impose a 'service charge,' which is not specifically prohibited by the Koran. However, if the loan is in default, the bank can only demand repayment of the principal in a Sharia court, but not the interest or 'service charge.'

"We are making compromises," he said, "and in all matters that do not affect the basic faith or devotional rituals the Sharia is a flexible legal system. In fact, a number of Moslem nations are moving away from decadent Western-type legal systems and adopting the Sharia. Pakistan, Oman, North Yemen, Libya, Sudan, Kuwait, and Nigeria, for example, are changing their statutes to conform to the Sharia."

"Some of the penalties specified by Sharia law are medieval and barbaric," said Hugh, "although they are apparently proving to deter crime. We have read a good deal in the American newspapers about the beheading of rapists and murderers, the stoning to death of adulterers, amputation of a hand for theft, and public lashings for lesser crimes."

"Actually, few hands are amputated in Saudi Arabia except in cases of repeated thievery," said Galal. "Poverty can be used as an excuse to mitigate the penalty. If the thief repents, the *qadi* may reduce the sentence to imprisonment. Highway robbery is a very serious offense, however, and is punished by having alternate hands and feet cut off. In the past if there was bodily harm to the victim, the criminal was liable to execution by crucifixion. In Saudi Arabia, this was extremely rare.

"If caught drinking alcohol or using drugs, Moslems are whipped in public and imprisoned," he added. "Foreigners are imprisoned and then evicted from the country. Two Englishmen caught selling liquor recently were publicly flogged and jailed. The aim of the whipping is to humiliate the criminal in public. Trafficking in drugs is a serious crime punishable by flogging, imprisonment, and occasionally by death."

Galal emphasized again that many of the beheadings, amputations of hands, and public whippings in Saudi Arabia involved foreigners from Moslem countries. "These countries have recently repudiated Western values and are establishing Islamic law," he said. "There is a definite revival of the Sharia throughout the Moslem world. This growing clamor for a return to Islamic law involves Egypt as well, and Sadat is polarizing the religious forces when he warns them that 'religion and politics cannot mix.'

"Sadat is making a fatal mistake," he concluded. "Islamic law will prevail."

During our conversation, George kept looking at his watch. It was now eight-thirty and nobody else had yet arrived. "They should be here soon," said Galal. "I'm sure we'll start before nine."

Twenty minutes later, the judge came into the court attended by another man carrying some books and by a young man whom Galal identified as the court secretary. The *qadi* was dressed completely in white and wore a white robe trimmed with gold thread, denoting his high office. He had a gray beard and a kind, gentle face.

The *qadi* sat down at the table and began to read some of the papers the young secretary had set before him, presumably yesterday's testimony. In a few minutes the others straggled into the room and took their seats at the rectangular table facing the judge. George and Tabil joined them. Galal identified the complainant, a short, heavy-set man with a black beard and wearing a dark thobe, who was sitting next to Dr. Tabil. No particular seating arrangement was necessary because there were no lawyers or prosecuting attorneys. I remembered that Galal had told us that the defendants and the complainant were not adversaries under Sharia law. They were just there to state the facts and to tell the truth. Consequently, George, Tabil, and the complainant sat on one side of the table and the panel of three doctors who had come in together sat on the other. Finally, the Deputy Minister of Forensic Medicine arrived and took his place at the head of the rectangular table.

The *qadi* stood up and called the court to order: "In the name of Allah, the Most Compassionate, the Most Merciful." He then asked the complainant to swear upon the Koran to tell the truth. Tabil, a Lebanese, was similarly sworn in, with his hand on the Koran. The young clerk standing next to the *qadi* asked Rogers to raise his hand and swear to tell the truth, but there was no Bible to swear upon.

The *qadi* asked the complainant why these doctors should pay him blood money for the death of his wife. The complainant stated with emotion that his wife was able to walk into the hospital and that within eight hours she was dead. He said that Dr. Rogers attended her only once during that period and that no other doctors saw her until Dr. Saban was called shortly before her death. The *qadi* asked the clerk to read in English the testimony that Dr. Saban had given to the court last night. He told George through the interpreter that they were all here merely to get at the truth and asked him whether he wished to confirm or to deny the testimony of the complainant or of Dr. Saban. George replied that he had nothing to say at this point.

The next two hours were spent questioning Rogers and Tabil as to the

extent of the deceased woman's pneumonia and the treatment administered by Dr. Rogers. The *qadi* asked all the questions, with the clerk
serving as the interpreter. Although the court secretary was busily recording the proceedings, both the *qadi* and the Deputy Minister took notes
during the entire hearing. After the extent of the patient's disease had
been established, the next questions centered on her treatment and why
Dr. Rogers had attended her only once. The three doctors took turns
asking very pertinent questions as to the adequacy of Dr. Rogers's treatment and why he or his associates had failed to re-evaluate her condition
during the brief period of her hospitalization. Dr. Rogers's reply was that
he had not appreciated the crucial nature of her illness, and, not hearing
from the nurse, thought her condition was satisfactory.

"Was this an error in judgment?" asked one of the doctors in English.
"Yes," replied Dr. Rogers quietly. Finally, the *qadi* asked Dr. Rogers if he
had anything further to say. When he answered in the negative, the *qadi*
looked him squarely in the eyes and asked, "Do you think she might have
died, according to God's will, regardless of the treatment?"

"Yes," replied Dr. Rogers. "In view of her enormous obesity, the extensive involvement of her lungs, and the fulminant nature of her disease, she
might have died in any event."

The *qadi* listened intently to the reply. Then he stood up and said,
"*Maktub* [It is written]. *La ilah illa'llah* [There is no god but God]."

The court was adjourned.

It was midnight. We drove back in relative silence, each enveloped in
his own thoughts. I asked George whether he thought the trial was fair.
He said he thought it was fair considering the language barriers, but that
the doctors had asked him some tough questions.

Hugh Compton said that, in his experience and in the view of the entire
expatriate community in Saudi Arabia, the *qadis* had a reputation for incor-
ruptibility and justice. "There is considerable faith even on the part of the
foreigners in the essential fairness of the Sharia procedures," he said.

"When will we know the outcome?" asked George.

Galal said that the handling of these cases was fairly prompt. "We
should have the verdict within two weeks," he said.

After determining guilt or innocence and the right to compensation, the
qadi attempts to arrive at a fair assessment of reparations acceptable to
both parties or to pass sentence. He has available case books of legal prece-
dents which spell out the facts of the case, the legal principles involved,
and the decisions of the Sharia courts.

The *qadi* would also take into account the judgment rendered by the panel of physicians who had questioned Dr. Rogers. Finally, he would discuss his verdict with the Deputy Minister who had attended the trial and with the Director of Forensic Medicine before passing sentence.

In more serious cases, the *qadi* suggests punishment but does not pass sentence independently. All papers pertaining to the case are sent to the district emir or governor of the town or province involved, who is often a prince. With the consent and advice of the local Ulema, the emir then pronounces sentence.

"Is there a right of appeal?" asked George.

"Appeals courts automatically review all Sharia cases involving serious punishment," replied Galal. "Further appeals may be made to the Supreme Council of Justice, the highest judicial court in the kingdom."

Two weeks later Hugh Compton called George Rogers and me to his office. "I have bad news," he said to George. "We have just received a cable from the Director of Forensic Medicine and the Minister of Health, stating that Dr. George Rogers has been found guilty in the case of Tadra Zaki Shibat Hashin. They demand the payment of 40,000 riyals in blood money and the expulsion of Dr. Rogers from Saudi Arabia within fourteen days. The cable was sent to the Director of the King Faisal Hospital this morning.

"I'm sorry about this," said Hugh. "The hospital will pay the blood money and we'll get you the exit visa and help you in any way that we can."

George merely said, "I expected this. I have already sold my car and sent some things back to England."

I couldn't help thinking that the handling of this case had been expeditious compared to a parallel situation in the United States. The trial here took place within two months of the patient's death, and a verdict was reached and judgment passed within an additional two weeks. At home it would have taken two years at least, and the judgment might amount to anywhere from $100,000 to millions of dollars, if the physician was found liable. Meanwhile, he would be paying $50,000 to $100,000 a year in malpractice insurance!

As we left Hugh's office, George told me that this was the first time he had ever been subjected to a lawsuit. "There's always a first time," I said, hoping mine would never come.

While we were awaiting the verdict an article had appeared in the *Arab News* in Riyadh, stating that "the hand of a convicted culprit was chopped off here Friday, for committing theft." A note was issued by the Governor of Riyadh, saying that Ahmad Al-Tizani stole a car engine, and "upon his confession the Supreme Court passed the judgment to cut off his right hand from the palm joint—which was done after the Friday prayer at the Justice Square in Riyadh."

Shortly thereafter I found another article in the same newspaper under the headline "Two Criminals Are Beheaded in Riyadh." The two men were identified by name. The statement issued by the Riyadh Governor's office said that "they had kidnaped and raped a boy and had confessed to their crime after being arrested by security men. . . . The Higher Judicial Council directed that the two men deserved death for the rape alone and also deserved death for kidnaping and frightening the boy and his whole village. . . . The government approved the court's sentence and it was carried out in public after the Friday prayers in keeping with Saudi tradition."

Both articles stated that the culprits had confessed their crimes.

The hospital had two more encounters with the Sharia law. One involved a suit against an American doctor who was finally acquitted in a trial for blood money. The *qadi*, however, passed sentence upon the doctor in the form of a "Letter of Reprimand and Censure."

The other related to a young, attractive American secretary, who had circulated letters criticizing certain hospital regulations, a common practice among malcontents. Unfortunately, however, she was found guilty of possessing hashish and was jailed. She remained in prison for four months and was never brought to trial.

"They never tried me for anything," she said, "and I never was convicted." Since there is no habeas corpus in Saudi Arabia, she remained in jail until she was eventually freed through the intercession of her congressman. She was then evicted from the country. The young woman admitted, however, that she was not mistreated at any time. They fed her well, supplied her with reading material, and she had access to a radio.

"But four months in prison is a long time," she said.

16

DESERT ADVENTURE:
"DR. GRAY, I PRESUME"

> The Beduin of the desert, born and grown up in it, had embraced with all his soul this nakedness too harsh for volunteers, for the reason ... that there he found himself indubitably free. He lost material ties, comforts, all superfluities and other complications to achieve a personal liberty which haunted starvation and death.... In his life he had air and winds, sun and light, open spaces and a great emptiness. There was no human effort, no fecundity in Nature: just the heaven above and the unspotted earth beneath. There unconsciously he came near God.
>
> T. E. LAWRENCE, *Seven Pillars of Wisdom*

"THANK GOD IT'S THURSDAY" echoed around the hospital halls at the end of every Thursday in imitation of the "TGIF" of the States, which welcomes in the weekend. But in Saudi Arabia, Friday is the only holiday of a six-day work week, and it comes none too soon and ends all too quickly. It took me a while to adjust to working Saturday and Sunday, and I frequently lost track of time. Although the pressures here did not equal those in the United States, we all felt that it was a long week and took advantage of the twenty-four-hour respite as best we could.

The Saudis spend Friday, their Holy Day, the same way we spend Sunday in the Christian world. The men, dressed in their "Sunday best"—white thobes and white ghutras—attend services in the mosques in the morning and spend the rest of the day with their families and friends at home. The women generally pray at home. In the afternoon some of the men take their wives and children out for drives or find secluded spots in oases for picnics. On these trips the women remain veiled and usually sit in the back of the car so that nobody on the outside can see them.

The American and English community spent Friday either recuperating from a party the night before or taking short trips into the desert, which has a timeless quality that seems to transcend the differences in our cultures.

One Friday, Philip Westbrook and I were in an exploring mood. Our wives were on a holiday in England, so we decided to rough it in Philip's Landcruiser, which was sturdy and well-equipped for desert travel. Abdul Taleem, the medical student, joined us, along with a Bedouin security guard from the hospital, named Nizar, with whom I had become friends. We had plenty of water and a picnic packed for us by Nizar. We started out on the Mecca Road, Philip and I in the front, with Philip driving at his usual breakneck speed, and Abdul and Nizar behind. Philip wore gloves to protect his hands from being burned by the steering wheel, which seemed to absorb the sun.

"This highway runs from Riyadh southwest to Mecca," Abdul told us, leaning forward, "and then to Jidda on the Red Sea, in all about six hundred miles."

"Lots of traffic here during the *hajj*," added Nizar. He went on to explain that the *hajj* is a five-day pilgrimage performed at least once in a lifetime by all Moslems and is one of the five pillars of Islam. "Every year, two million Moslems come to Saudi Arabia from every corner of the earth for the annual pilgrimage to the holy cities of Mecca and Medina. They come by bus, automobile, airplane, camel, or on foot. The airports are jammed, and this road to Mecca," he gestured to the empty road stretching out in front of the Landcruiser, "is crowded with pilgrims and with cars and trucks piled high, with luggage tied to the roofs."

The *hajj*, Abdul told us, is observed from December 11 to December 15. The official government holiday is from December 8 through December 19. But the *hajj* is more than a pilgrimage in this country. It is a historical pageant, a mass vacation, a political symbol, a state of mind. The *hajj* is televised and draws as much attention in Saudi Arabia as the World Series or the Democratic National Convention in the States. To a Saudi, the pilgrimage symbolizes the world of Islam and Saudi Arabia's place in it.

The Saudis are aware that their forefathers were the first Moslems and that Mecca and the holy cities of Saudi Arabia are the holy cities of Islam today as they were in the seventh century. Consequently they regard themselves as guardians of tradition and protectors of the faith and its holiest shrines. What matters to them most is their faith, the world of Islam, and their special place in it. The hotels go unattended, the dining rooms close, the mail is not delivered. Everything seems to stop, everything, that is, except the oil.

"The pilgrims are dressed all in white," said Abdul. "A man wears an *ihram,* which consists of two large white seamless towels, one of which is worn around the waist and the other over one shoulder. A woman wears a new white dress, white stockings, and white shoes. She covers her head with two headcloths—a small rectangular one, in which all of her hair is tied, for not one single hair should be seen; and a larger cloth which is wrapped around her head and face. The only parts of a woman which may show are her hands and feet.

"The government attempts to help the pilgrims in every way possible," he added. "On the Dhahran Road outside of Riyadh, they built a *hajj* camp, a tent city to house some of the pilgrims, who may pause there for a few days during their long and arduous journey to Mecca. In order to raise funds for the trip, many carry with them rugs woven by hand in Iran, Afghanistan, and other countries, which they attempt to sell along the way."

Several months later, during *hajj,* I recalled Abdul's fascinating account, so Ruth and I decided to drive out to the *hajj* camp. We arrived in early afternoon. The grounds were a mass of color, with Oriental rugs spread out over more than an acre. Some were ruby red, others sapphire blue, glowing like jewels on the sand. Silhouetted against the horizon in the background were rows upon rows of tents. Sitting cross-legged in front of their wares were Afghans, Pakistanis, Iranians, Mongolians, and others in flowing robes and turbans, waiting to sell their carpets, saddle bags, handicrafts, prayer beads, and jewelry.

After the usual bargaining exercise, we finally bought a rug. It depicted a stream of camels marching in orderly rows on a desert background. There were also elephants, ducks, and tigers in the dignified procession across the storybook carpet. We left the scene at dusk. The day had grown cold and the sky was darkening with clouds. As we drove back to the teeming city, we were met by a wondrous sight. High in the distance appeared the huge dome of a mosque. It looked like a mirage, startling us with its unusual color, a misty pink against the soft gray of the sky.

Shortly after *hajj* I was having dinner at the Intercontinental Hotel and noticed that the eyes of the headwaiter were red. When I asked him about it, he said, "I have just come back from the *hajj* and I wept most of the time. I couldn't stop crying. It was the only way I could wash away my sins, but now I feel pure and clean. It was a wonderful experience." He felt, he told me, that he was in a state of grace and purity. There is a deep conviction that once the pilgrimage is completed the *hajji,* or pilgrim, is completely purified of all his sins and is like a newborn again, free of all spiritual defects. If a Moslem dies during the pilgrimage, he is promised a place in Heaven.

But today, as we continued our explorations along the Mecca road, we saw almost no other cars. After driving southwest of Riyadh for five miles on the asphalt road, we passed an old settlement of about fifteen mud-brick houses. Most stood two stories high with spacious walled-off roofs, where the families often had their evening meals. High triangular or round holes served as windows for ventilation. A few minutes past the settlement we came upon a cluster of four identical villas perched side by side on a hill to our right. They glistened white in the sun, each with identical pillars, a red roof, and a manicured garden.

"Those are the villas of a rich merchant and his four wives," Abdul said. "When people see those villas they know they are on the Mecca Road. It's a landmark that has been here for many years."

We then crossed a bridge spanning a dry riverbed and continued southwest along its tributary. Abdul explained that there were no permanent rivers. Ancient riverbeds, called *wadis,* flooded occasionally after a heavy rain and ran for only a short time. The water seeped through the porous surface and was trapped above the impervious rock layers underground. Consequently, there were reservoirs of good water under much of the Arabian Peninsula, particularly in eastern Saudi Arabia, where artesian wells and springs were common.

About ten miles from the outskirts of Riyadh we came upon the Tuwayq Mountains. The escarpments appeared as a line of steep cliffs about a thousand feet high rising precipitously from the desert floor and running roughly north-south from Riyadh for about four hundred miles. It was a magnificent sight.

"The Tuwayq escarpments are capped by limestone deposited by ancient seas which once covered this area. There are shell fossils here 150 million years old. I'll find one for you," Abdul said.

"How do you know all this?" I asked, turning to look at him in amazement.

"I studied geology at the university in Riyadh," he said, pleased. "Let me finish my lecture. The bedrock formation of the escarpment slopes downward as it goes east, causing the rainwater to run off and to form wadis leading to Riyadh. This same bedrock extends to the Eastern Province and to the Arabian Gulf, becoming thicker and deeper as it approaches the Gulf. The lower layers, thousands of feet underground, contain the trapped oil."

Nizar took over. He told us about a deep natural cavern just south of Riyadh with an underground river at its bottom.

"The river undermined the limestone escarpment many centuries ago until it caved in," he said. "Now it is fed by rainwater running off the foothills of the Tuwayq escarpment in front of us." This natural waterhole was called Ayn Heet by the Bedouins, and I learned later that, in a way, it contributed to the discovery of oil by the American geologists.

Because we had no set schedule or itinerary, the escarpment seemed like a good place to begin our explorations. Philip turned off the road, found a track, and drove into the desert in the direction of the escarpment looming high above the desert floor. After a while we parked the Land-cruiser by the side of the track, and carrying canteens filled with water, we began to walk to the foot of the cliffs a mile away in search of fossils.

As soon as we left the car, each of us moving silently forward in the 130-degree heat, I was struck by the awesome cathedral-like silence of the desert. An absolute stillness enveloped us. As we proceeded further into the desert a feeling of incredible isolation and timelessness swept over me, as though I were reaching back into eternity. The primal allure was the empti-ness and the solitude—something uniquely magnificent about the desert which was conducive to soul-searching meditation.

We trudged along on the hard sand for about an hour in silence, Nizar and Abdul leading the way, Philip and I slowly falling behind. The skies were cloudless and the sun blazing and relentless. I had been accustomed to the humid summers of Boston, but here the heat was dry like an oven. The sweat evaporated as soon as it left our pores and the heat seemed to come from within. Our desert boots made the only sound, leather scuffing on a carpet of sand. In the distance the horizon shimmered and every depression in the landscape seemed to flicker like a small body of water.

"Mirage," said Nizar.

Suddenly I had a feeling of impending disaster. I had to get away from the sun or I would die. I stopped to search in all directions for some shel-ter, but no shade was in sight and I could barely see Philip's truck. In desperation I called to Nizar, who turned in alarm. "Can you find a spot of shade somewhere?" I pleaded. "This sun is getting to me. I'm not sure I can continue."

Nizar hurriedly retraced his steps toward me, concern on his face. He shaded his eyes with his ghutra and looked about. He wore no sunglasses in spite of the brilliant light. "We're in luck," he said, pointing with his stick. "I think there are some stones about a half mile ahead which might give us a little shade. Our car is too far away."

I looked in the direction he pointed and saw nothing except more desert, with or without my sunglasses.

"Let's go on before I pass out," I said, catching up to him and Abdul. "I can't even see your stones." Philip too was breathing hard beside me, nodding in agreement.

"You need some Bedouin blood, Dr. Gray," Nizar remarked with a grin.

Sure enough, following him, we came upon a small irregular pile of stones about two feet high. "It's not much," he said, "probably a grave marking, but it will give you some shade."

Mercifully there was just enough shade to shield two heads from the sun. I could tell that Philip was as grateful as I for the respite. We both sprawled out on the hot sand with our heads against the rock pile, our legs still in the intense sun. Slowly the sand cooled beneath our bodies, and my panic abated. We all drank some water from our canteens as memories of Western movies and the cliché of the empty canteen came back to me. Water had never tasted like this.

Then Nizar and Abdul said they would go on ahead to look for fossils, promising to return within a half hour.

"What if the shade disappears?" I asked, trying to guess the angle of the sun's rays.

Nizar squinted up at the sky and reassured me. "It will still be here when we return."

We watched them walk off, pointing and talking as if they were on a New York City street. After they were gone Philip confessed that he too had been about to panic. "Thank God you said something. That sun is really treacherous today." He wiped his forehead with his sleeve. "I've taken trips into the desert before without mishap, but the heat wasn't like this. You'll learn after you've been here for a while that people don't tan in this part of the world. They just burn, probably because of the intensity of the sun, coupled with the dryness of the air." I determined to use plenty of PABA sunscreen.

While we waited for our friends to return, an elderly Bedouin with a small herd of camels passed about three hundred feet away. He paused to see if we were alive and well. Then, reassured when he saw us sit up and wave, he continued on his way.

Abdul and Nizar soon returned, holding out some shell fossils for us. They were gray and feathered with the skeletons of ancient organisms.

"I'll take one back to MIT for Carbon 14 dating to check on your 150 million figure," I said, teasing Abdul. I thanked him and put the fossil in my pocket.

"Give or take a few million years," he said.

Desert Adventure: "Dr. Gray, I Presume" ◊ *199*

Refreshed by our rest, we returned to our Landcruiser and sat in its ample shade while we had our lunch of fruit and cheese. A lone Arab rode by sitting astride a donkey, his feet almost touching the ground. Abdul said he was probably returning to a nearby encampment.

Next Abdul suggested that we visit an area called the "Pink Sands" and then continue on the Mecca Road. At the Pink Sands the desert stretched before us like waves in the ocean or like low, undulating dunes—the classic sand desert of Western imagination pictured in the movies: Peter O'Toole riding over the desert as Lawrence of Arabia. The sand was as fine and soft as powder.

Abdul told us that the desert is never as uniform as the word implies. The sand may appear gray-brown in color, granular and flat like that surrounding the escarpment, or it may be soft and pink, forming ripples and flat dunes as it appeared here. I recalled that in the Empty Quarter, the dunes may be as high as six hundred feet, and the sand mountains, often one thousand feet high, are separated by valleys many miles wide.

Returning to the Mecca Road, we saw a small open Toyota pickup truck parked on the side of the road. In the back of the truck two camels sat on their haunches, looking very haughty as they gazed out beneath their long eyelashes onto the desert. Their Bedouin chauffeur was nowhere about. I shall never forget that sight. The camels had come a long way in the twentieth century!

A few minutes later we slowed down near a group of mud-brick houses and tents. Fifteen or twenty children, their thobes fluttering in the breeze, ran to greet us. They motioned for us to turn off and come into their village, laughing and chattering as they jumped about our car in excitement. Several held their arms out as if to block our way as they pleaded with us to stop and visit with them.

"They think we are all foreigners because of our clothes," Abdul said. Both he and Nizar were wearing blue jeans, tan cotton shirts, and desert boots.

The girls disappeared immediately, but the boys gathered about us as we left the car and directed us to a large tent. On the way we passed a truck. Curious, we approached the back to look inside. The boys immediately formed a line of defense in front of the curtained entrance, crying out, "*La la* [No no]." As Nizar and Abdul watched in amusement, the boys made it clear that it was forbidden for me to look in, but not before I caught a glimpse of veiled women in black, sitting in the back of the truck shelling peas and cutting up onions and tomatoes.

In the tent the elder of the family sat cross-legged on an old faded rug, smoking a water pipe. A young man about twenty-two joined him. Before we could utter a word, he said to the old man, "Tabeeb, Mustashfa Malek Faisal [A doctor from the King Faisal Hospital]."

I was astounded. Here we were in the middle of the desert in a tiny Bedouin encampment with no identification whatever, yet someone had recognized me.

Just then a middle-aged man with a graying beard, resplendent in his white thobe and ghutra, appeared in the entrance of the tent and moved to shake my hand. I immediately recognized him as a patient at the clinic whom I had been treating for high blood pressure. He had just arrived from the mosque and had told the young man, his son, who we were. My patient's name was Hussein Lateef.

After I had introduced my friends we all sat down on some large cushions. As usual, I had difficulty pulling my legs under me on the carpet. Hussein told Abdul and Nizar that he was pleased they were there to interpret because he spoke no English. Some of the older boys of the family served us coffee and later sweet tea. Then they brought us plates of dates, covered with flies but delicious nevertheless. I had become accustomed to waving my hand over food before taking a bite. Hussein invited us to stay for dinner, but we declined.

"We have just had our lunch," I explained through Nizar, "and we would like to get back to Riyadh before dark."

"You and your friends, then, must have a meal with us next Friday," he said, his eyes searching my face for assent.

I thanked him and said we would be pleased to come. After urging us to eat more of the dates, Hussein rose and beckoned us to join him. We left the tent and proceeded to an alfalfa field of about two acres, surrounded by date palms, and irrigated by a network of narrow channels. A Bedouin in bare feet was digging a new sluice. He changed the direction of the water by merely piling dirt in one of the channels to form a new "gate" or valve. Hussein explained that the alfalfa was grown perennially, and was used as feed for the animals.

He next directed us to a large artesian well, which his father had dug years ago. A gasoline pump circulated the water. There were several such wells in this oasis, Hussein told us proudly, but none larger than this. Nearby, mud-brick houses two stories high, with sheds attached for the livestock, had been built many years ago. They adjoined each other so the outer walls could be used for defense against raiding nomads. I also realized at that moment that, not so many years ago, we would have been killed as intruders, rather than welcomed as friends.

Desert Adventure: "Dr. Gray, I Presume" ◊ *201*

The villagers were mostly members of Hussein's family, seminomadic herders who spent the dry season in this oasis and then moved out onto the plateu with their flocks in late winter and spring in search of grazing areas.

We watched a young Bedouin herd pathetic-looking humped cattle into one of the sheds, scattering the chickens before them. In the distance several camels wandered about. Nearby small herds of sheep and goats grazed on the scrub grass. Hussein told us that sheep provided most of the meat in Saudi Arabia as well as milk, cheese, and laban, a yogurt product.

"These sheep grow hair rather than wool," he said, running his hand over the matted coat of one. "And we weave their hair to make blankets and clothing."

"What about the goats?" I asked.

"We drink their milk and make tents and rugs from their hair. The tent we were in was made of goat hair."

As we completed our tour we came upon two donkeys tethered to a post out in the open, under a merciless sun in a sandy area where they could not graze. When I asked Hussein about this he said the donkeys would refuse to work in the sun once they were kept under cover for any length of time. I admitted to him that the animals did look comfortable and apparently had adjusted to the intense heat.

"Just like us," he replied, his hand sweeping in the direction of the staring children.

It was now five o'clock and time to start back to Riyadh. As we returned to the jeep, Hussein excused himself and hurried off in the direction of the herds. He returned in a few minutes carrying a young squirming lamb across his shoulders, two feet in each hand. It was a parting gift, he told Abdul, as he tried to stuff it into the back of the Landcruiser. Philip said, "No, no" to anyone who would listen, as the lamb kept finding its feet, attempting to jump free of the car. I thanked Hussein profusely but explained that we had no facilities in Riyadh to butcher the lamb or to cook it. He agreed to take back the animal providing we join him the following Friday for dinner with his family. "We'll be here," Philip assured him. We shook hands with all the men and expressed our gratitude for their hospitality.

As we drove off we could hear the rhythmic thump thump of the water pumps, the heartbeat of the desert.

On the way back to Riyadh we drove slowly, as though hypnotized by the beauty around us. The desert glistened blood-red and gold in the setting sun. In the distance the escarpments shone with a purplish hue, casting undulating shadows upon the desert below in an infinite variety of colors: orange, brick-red, burnt-brown, pink, and gray.

Now and then we stopped to drink in the view or to allow goatherds and shepherds to cross the highway with their herds as they returned home at day's end.

The following Friday, as planned, Philip picked me up at my Petromin apartment in his Landcruiser, and then we collected Abdul and Nizar. I had just spent a sleepless night without electricity and of course without air conditioning. At that moment I would have given anything for a day at the seashore rather than a day in the hot desert, but there was no water within hundreds of miles. At least I was getting away from my stifling apartment.

Philip, full of vim and vigor, drove at his usual mad pace until we reached the desert, where once again he slowed down to absorb the beauty around us.

"The desert looks different every time you see it," Nizar said. "It depends on the light and time of day."

With his unerring sense of direction, Philip found the village without difficulty. The children greeted us by darting around our car and calling to one another, and my patient, Hussein, embraced us as old friends, his hands on our shoulders pulling us close. "Welcome," he said in Arabic, "I'm glad to see you." Nizar and Abdul took turns translating as Hussein introduced us to the men in his village. Most of them were members of his family, and as is the custom among seminomadic Bedouins, they moved as a unit. About twenty men were gathered around a line of bedraggled trucks. No women were in sight, but remembering last week's experience, I suspected that the women were concealed in the back of the trucks. How could they stand the heat, closed in like that?

Hussein told us that he had planned a picnic dinner in the desert a few miles away. We joined the caravan of trucks, camels, and donkeys and proceeded ten miles into the desert to a tiny oasis of palm trees and faded green scrub grass. The trucks were then arranged in a circle to shield us from the sun. Threadbare rugs were placed in the center of the circle. The camels and donkeys, which the children had ridden, roamed about nearby.

Preparations for dinner began immediately. Two men picked up a lamb, slit its throat, and hung its head down from the back of the truck. They cut the skin at the base of the hind legs, peeled it downward over the head, and then threw it out into the desert to attract the flies away from the carcass. Working quickly with very sharp knives they eviscerated the animal and proceeded to butcher it, expertly cutting it up and jointing it for cooking. Some of the others built fires away from our circle and then placed parts of the lamb on spits for roasting over the open fires. The older boys started smaller fires to boil water for tea and to cook some of the lamb in a large black pot which sat on three stones.

Meanwhile, the younger boys brought us fruit, nuts, and dates as we sat cross-legged on the carpets. I assumed my usual position in such situations by lying on my side and leaning on the elbow as I had learned to do at Sultana's wedding dinner. Abdul and Nizar smiled at my ineptitude.

"The English are much more flexible than the Americans, as you can see," remarked Philip.

"And the Arabs are the most flexible of all," said Abdul, watching a very old man tuck his legs under him with ease.

Soon the boys brought us cardamom coffee and later sweet mint tea. They made the coffee by roasting the beans and pounding them into a powder, which was then added to boiling water. A few crushed cardamom seeds were added to the brew, which was then poured into a smaller pot. A piece of palm fiber stuffed into the spout served as a strainer. Hot cardamom coffee was always served black and unsweetened in handleless cups, even when the temperature in the desert reached 140 degrees.

The dates were particularly delicious. I reminded Nizar of the day we first met. I had recently arrived and was curious about the date palm trees in front of the hospital, near the gatehouse where Nizar was on guard duty. After answering several of my questions—when were the dates harvested, how often, and so forth, Nizar took off his shoes, picked up a paper bag, and ran up the tree on all fours. Ten minutes later he came down with a bagful of dates. They were sweet and succulent. I hoarded them in the refrigerator for a week. From that moment on Nizar and I had become friends.

Hussein asked if we would like to try some camel milk but suggested that we drink only a little because it was very rich and might upset us. We walked over to the camels and Hussein milked one of them in long white streams into a basin. The milk was warm, frothy, and very creamy. The high fat content probably contributed to the peculiar taste. A little went a long way.

Upon our return, the men were carrying large platters of chopped tomatoes, carrots, and onions from the back of the trucks to add to the lamb simmering over the fire. Apparently the women were preparing the food in the trucks, out of sight, as they had last Friday.

The hours passed quickly. As we talked and walked about the oasis,

Philip and I noticed that we were on display. The Bedouins were watching us with as much interest as we were watching them. "Many of them have never seen a foreigner before," Abdul said, amused. "They are curious— you probably look more unusual to them than they do to you."

The red-checkered ghutras of the men, their gray thobes, and the colored rugs stood out in contrast to the monochromatic desert sand around us. Even the trucks blended into the distant landscape.

Finally, we made ourselves comfortable in a large circle on the rugs. The men removed their sandals and sat cross-legged with their feet tucked under them.

As Hussein removed his sandals, I noted the branding marks on his heels. He told me that branding his heels had cured his headaches.

"It must have taken your mind off your headache," I said. "The Chinese stick needles in far-off places on the body, too, and sometimes it works. It's called acupuncture."

Several men joined in the conversation. Nizar and Abdul continued to serve as interpreters. Each time Philip or I said anything they all leaned forward for the translation. They told us the most popular treatment was branding. Branding on the abdomen cured diarrhea, on the chest it cured pain and coughs, on the back it cured backache, and so forth. They branded their infants for colic and their sick camels as well.

"You complained of headaches when you first came to see me," I reminded Hussein. "Branding your heels did not cure your high blood pressure, which caused your headaches in the first place."

Hussein admitted that he felt better since he had been taking the medicine.

"High blood pressure, by the way, is rare in Saudi Arabia, maybe because of the low salt diet and the loss of salt in perspiration," I said.

"They are also under less stress than we are," Philip added.

Hussein's tribesmen loudly came to Hussein's defense, testifying to the wonderful cures wrought by branding men and animals. I told them that many patients in the clinic were covered with these branding marks.

"The next best treatment is to drink camel's urine, particularly for gastrointestinal problems, abdominal pain, and constipation," Hussein said solemnly, as if sharing his most precious secret with us. "It is also very effective as an eyewash and for healing wounds."

I leaned toward Philip and said quietly, "They may have something there. The urea in urine has some disinfecting properties, but camel urine is probably no more effective than human urine as far as I know."

Philip looked unconvinced as the others joined in again, gesturing and telling stories of how camel's urine had healed their sores, each one trying to outdo the other.

Then Nizar told us that the Bedouins believe that certain smells, particularly pleasant scents, have a harmful effect on wound healing. When I asked Hussein about this he nodded, saying, "The smell of a woman is very dangerous."

"No wonder," I said, "that camel's urine is so beneficial."

They all laughed politely. Hussein added that camel's urine was also an excellent health tonic and hair wash, and killed head vermin instantly. One of his family hastened to confirm this, pointing to his head and nodding vigorously.

I asked them about circumcision, having found that some clinic patients had been circumcised with unfortunate results. Hussein told us that circumcision is performed when a boy is between three and a half and seven years old. The day is observed as a family holiday, with a festive meal to celebrate the boy's becoming a "proper Moslem."

"It usually takes place in June when a dry northwest wind is blowing and the wound is more likely to heal quickly," Hussein said. In some areas the festivities continue for a week in the boy's home. In the evening the women and girls may dance about with each other. The men, of course, go elsewhere to celebrate. On the eighth day the family gathers and an operator who has experience with this procedure cuts off the child's foreskin with a razor or sharp knife. The wound heals in a week to ten days, although it occasionally turns septic because of flies and poor hygiene.

"How do you treat the infection?" I asked, dismayed by this barbarism in the guise of medicine.

"A mixture of salt, ashes, and camel dung," Hussein said. "But the wealthier Saudis in the towns now take their boys to a doctor for the circumcision." I could tell that his tribesmen didn't approve of this.

Abdul said that some tribes used to circumcise the girls to prevent sexual stimulation and excitement. The women who performed the operation passed a needle and thread through the clitoris, which was pulled outward to its full length by the thread and then amputated close to the body.

"Where do you learn these things?" I asked Abdul.

"The gynecologist in the Riyadh Medical School told us about it," he said.

I told Hussein I was surprised that so many Bedouins came to our hospital for medical care. "Do you think a doctor can save a man's life if he is very ill?" I asked.

"Never," replied Hussein vehemently. "Only Allah can save a man's life. When a man's time comes, he must die, 'as it is written.'"

Philip asked if any other men of the tribe had ever gone to the hospital. As soon as Nizar had translated the question they began shaking their heads vigorously. None of them had ever seen a doctor before except for Hussein, who was apparently considered a nonconformist by the other tribesmen.

Abdul said that the Koran admonishes the faithful to stay in good health and that physicians are acceptable from the Islamic point of view. "Until very recently, there just weren't any doctors in Saudi Arabia except for the few imported from Egypt and Iran, and they weren't very competent. That's why I'm studying medicine," he said.

"But all the Saudis we have treated have been very cooperative and grateful," I said, "even though they think of the doctors as infidels." Philip nodded in agreement.

"There are some Bedouins like these who won't go to a Western doctor under any conditions," Abdul said, shrugging his shoulders. "Hussein is an exception."

"The women come in for treatment providing their husbands accompany them and give their consent," Philip said.

"There is nothing in the Koran which forbids the Moslem seeking medical care," Abdul said. "But the outcome according to Islam is predetermined by Allah. The physician's role is secondary."

"*Maktub*—it is written," echoed Nizar, not needing to translate.

"The Western doctors don't object to some help from above, but we don't depend on it," Philip said.

"That's the difference between us," Nizar said. "We live and die according to God's will."

Although it would be improper for me to speak to my host, Hussein, about his women I couldn't refrain from asking Abdul, "How do the women manage? They are treated terribly and seem to be at the bottom of the pecking order."

"They have more influence than you realize," Abdul replied in English to cover up my indiscretion. "First of all, the Arab women are very prolific. An Arab woman is not happy unless she is pregnant. Consequently the birth rate is very high. A Bedouin woman may have fifteen children, four or five of whom will survive. Since she must produce sons to avoid divorce, she may be continuously pregnant throughout the first fifteen years of her marriage. The women in her tribal family help with delivery. There is no midwife as such. Infant mortality has been estimated as high as 70 percent in some areas, and the death rate of women in childbirth is correspondingly high.

"Poor hygiene and quack cures, a thousand years old, are responsible," he said. "But public-health programs for maternity and child care have been organized by the Ministry of Health, and the Saudi Red Crescent Society, like your Red Cross, provides first-aid services and mobile hospitals. Education of the women is the solution. Only the modern westernized women practice birth control, and that also depends on educating the women."

While we were conversing in English the tribesmen were chatting among themselves or tending to the lamb still roasting before the fires. In a few minutes the older boys appeared with huge platters piled high with lamb on a bed of rice surrounded with chopped tomatoes, cucumbers, onions, and pieces of lemon. There was a strong aroma of turmeric and cinnamon.

The Bedouins mashed the rice and lamb together and put it in their mouths with the fingers of their right hand. "Only the right hand is used to handle food," Abdul told us. Philip and I followed their lead. The food was tasty although the lamb was tough. And I found it disconcerting to see the children watching us hungrily as we ate. Hussein chose tasty pieces of meat and placed them on our plates with his fingers, urging us to eat more. When we had our fill, the children eagerly took the trays and picked them clean. I made a point of watching them return the trays and leavings to the women in the trucks. Only the women's hands could be seen as they reached out for the trays. I wish I could have thanked them for their part in our feast but it was impossible.

After dinner the Bedouins formed a line and began to dance and sing. Some carried long sticks and a few beat on scraggly drums. The performance reminded me of the chanters and drummers at Sultana's wedding, less professional though no less genuine. Much to the amusement of everyone, particularly the children, we joined in the dance, swaying with the line of men as the drums beat louder and louder.

At three-thirty in the afternoon one of the older men gave the call to prayer:

> *God is most great.*
> *I testify that there is no god but God.*
> *I testify that Mohammed is the Prophet of God.*
> *Come to prayer!*
> *Come to salvation!*
> *Prayer is better than sleep.*
> *God is most great.*
> *There is no god but God.*

Each line but the last was repeated twice. Then the men brought out their goatskins containing water to make their ablutions. First they washed their faces, hands, and feet, then sucked water into their nostrils, put wet fingers in their ears, and passed wet hands over the tops of their heads. The washing procedure was performed exactly in that order each time. If no water was available they would go through these washing motions with sand.

The old man who had greeted us in the tent the Friday before led the prayer. The others lined up behind him in two horizontal rows and faced east toward Mecca. They first stood upright, bending forward with their hands on their knees, then knelt on the rugs and bowed down until their foreheads touched the ground. They performed these ritual movements several times while reciting the formal prayer (Sura I of the Koran):

> In the name of God, the Compassionate, the Merci-
> ful.
> Praise be to God, Lord of the worlds!
> The Compassionate, the Merciful!
> King on the day of reckoning!
> Thee only do we worship and to Thee do we cry for
> help.
> Guide us on the straight path,
> The path of those to whom Thou has been gracious;
> With whom Thou are not angry, and who go not
> astray.

They repeated this verse as they prostrated themselves again and again. Since the Saudis pray five times daily, it's no wonder they are so limber, I thought, looking at their leader, who must have been in his eighties. The prayer ritual is superb exercise.

The older boys joined the men in prayer. Nizar prayed too, but I could see that Abdul's heart was not in it, although he joined the others on a small rug. I caught his eye for a moment, and there was a flicker of an understanding smile—he belonged to the modern generation of Saudis. Nevertheless, he too in his way believed in the One Great Almighty God, indivisible, all-seeing and ever-present, although he didn't pray regularly.

After prayers we had some dates and other fruit to top off the meal. The time had come for us to depart. We shook hands with everyone, including the boys, who shyly came forward to stare at our pale skins and hairless faces. I reminded Hussein to keep his appointment at the clinic to check on his blood pressure. He asked us when we could come again. I told him that our wives would be returning to Riyadh soon and perhaps we might bring them next time. His enthusiasm waned perceptibly, as I knew it would. Bedouins are traditionalists, and I couldn't expect him to break a thousand-year-old tradition in a matter of days.

On the way home we talked about the Bedouins and their impact on Saudi Arabia. "The Bedouins, the desert people, were the original Arabs and they remain the most 'Arab' of all," Abdul told us. "The majority are Sunni Moslems, who observe the strictly orthodox, puritanical traditions."

"But why is Saudi Arabia so different from other Moslem countries?" I asked.

"Remember," Nizar said, "Saudi Arabia is the birthplace of the religion. Here is where it all began, with Mohammed in Mecca and Medina. The men we were with today are direct descendants of the Bedouins who conquered what is now known as the Arab world in the seventh century. They have kept the Arab character unchanged and undiluted for more than a thousand years by intermarrying with their cousins."

"Wahabism has been the dominant creed in this country since the eighteenth century," Abdul said, "and its puritanical interpretation of Islam has already caused some trouble. In the late 1920s the followers of King Abdul-Aziz revolted because he was adopting too many Western innovations, such as telephones, radios, and airplanes. King Ibn Saud crushed the revolt. Later he reassured the Wahabi, who had condemned the telephone as the devil's invention, by reading the Koran to them over the telephone."

Philip and I were amused by the King's ingenuity. Then Abdul continued, "Now, fifty years later, at the other extreme are the Saudis who have studied abroad or traveled widely in the West. This new generation of young people want to adopt Western technology and to modernize our country. Education has to be the catalyst."

As we drove on through the desert, each lapsing into the silence of his own thoughts, I couldn't help but appreciate how fortunate I was to be a doctor. Here in the middle of the desert we had chanced upon a Bedouin village and found a warm and hospitable friend. We came from different worlds, but the bond between a doctor and his patient is universal and recognizes no boundary of language or culture.

I went back over the day spent with Hussein and his tribe. The Bedouins, as children of the desert, were clinging to a primitive simplicity and purity. Their temperance and abstinence, their contented poverty and contempt for luxury were, until very recently, the dominant mode of life in Saudi Arabia. They still adhered fanatically to the doctrine of Wahabism, which preaches a revival of Islamic simplicity and an extremist fidelity to the rigors of the Koran: "Woe to them who . . . gathered gold and count it up, who supposeth their riches will render them immortal. Nay truly will they be flung to hellfire." (*The Koran,* Sura CIV)

These fundamentalists believed literally in hellfire and were ready to fight and die for their religion. It was this fanaticism which might eventually erupt into a confrontation with the forces of modernization and "westernization." That they were on a collision course I had no doubt. And indeed within a year some of these religious extremists would seize the Great Mosque in Mecca because they felt the regime was selling out to the corrupt values of the West.

I said goodbye to Abdul, Nizar, and Philip, and watched them drive off through the dark streets of Riyadh. After a day in the desert I could understand why some Arabs still preferred to wander the sands as nomadic herders rather than live in the cities. But I was back in the city now and wondering whether there would be electricity and air conditioning in my apartment that night.

17

ARAMCO—WHERE IT ALL BEGAN

IN RECENT YEARS the new developments in medicine have been meteoric. The hospital administration recognized the necessity of keeping abreast of these advances and encouraged its physicians to attend two major medical conferences a year anywhere in the world. Some traveled as far as Japan or Australia, but I limited myself to meetings in the United States and Europe.

Because some of the medical problems we faced were unique to Saudi Arabia and the Middle East, we decided to organize a series of annual conferences for doctors throughout this area. The First Arabian Peninsula Medical Conference was to be held in Dhahran in the Eastern Province, where the Aramco (Arabian-American Oil Company) headquarters were located. Aramco was chosen as the first site for the meeting because it had the best facilities and had contributed more to the health of the Saudi Arabian people in the forty-five years of its existence than had been accomplished in the previous thousand years.

Aramco sent one of its "Flying Camels," a twin-engine prop jet, to fly us from Riyadh to Dhahran on the shore of the Arabian Gulf, also known as the Persian Gulf, about 250 miles away. There were twenty-five of us aboard the plane, including a few wives. Unfortunately, Ruth and Ron Lambries's wife, Pam, were in London at the time. A young Aramco employee, a Saudi named Naman, greeted us in perfect English and gave us a running commentary on the oil fields as we flew over them. On the way, we passed over the Ghawar oil field, the largest in the world, with a productive capacity of five million barrels of oil a day. Naman told us that it was 150 miles long and 25 miles wide at its broadest point. This one field holds more oil than can be found in the United States including Alaska.

"We produce and export more oil than any other country," he said proudly. "We have more than one-third of the world's reserves."

When asked about the flares of burning gas below, Naman told us that they could be seen a hundred miles away and that a very costly project was under way to recover the gas, which would add about 10 percent to the earnings on every barrel of oil.

In the next hour we bombarded Naman with questions about Aramco and its history. He was both obliging and knowledgeable. It was a story, he said, of the American pioneering spirit, technical ingenuity, and tenacity.

In 1932, when King Abdul-Aziz Ibn Saud finally unified the country into the Kingdom of Saudi Arabia, the government was practically destitute. The only outside income came from pilgrimages to Mecca, which yielded less than $2 million a year. Faced with increasing financial problems, King Ibn Saud, in 1933, granted a sixty-year concession for the exploration of oil to the Standard Oil Company of California (Socal). Although he distrusted foreigners, he had learned that the Americans had recently discovered oil in the neighboring sheikdom of Bahrain in the Arabian Gulf. The oil concession to Socal covered all of eastern Saudi Arabia, including the territorial waters of the Arabian Gulf. In 1923, ten years earlier, King Ibn Saud had given a similar concession to a British company to explore for oil in the Eastern Province, but they never exercised the rights, and the agreement was canceled four years later.

"The British don't like to think about this now," Naman said.

In the fall of 1933, an American vanguard of eight geologists and surveyors entered Saudi Arabia. They sailed across from the nearby island of Bahrain in native boats called dhows to explore a dome-shaped hill on the border of the Arabian Gulf, which they had spotted on clear days from Bahrain. It was named Jebel Dhahran. They thought there might be oil beneath it.

King Ibn Saud provided a guide and an escort of twelve soldiers to protect each pair of explorers and to keep them, in turn, away from the Saudis. He still hoped to avoid exposing his people to foreign influence. The Americans lived mostly on imported canned food, and traveled by trucks and by camels, avoiding the towns and villages, where Wahabism flourished and infidels were resented.

Because few maps of the country existed and those that did were faulty, the Americans brought in small planes and explored the region by aerial photography. At first the Wahabis violently opposed this procedure, which they interpreted as the making of false images forbidden by the Koran. King Ibn Saud finally intervened on the Americans' behalf.

Soon drilling equipment was landed from barges on the shallow sandy shore near Jebel Dhahran, and in the summer of 1935 the first well was begun. The temperature in the shade climbed to 130 degrees and the nearest drinking water was eleven miles away. After drilling in vain for ten months to a depth of 3,200 feet, they abandoned the well. During the following two years, six more wells were drilled at Jebel Dhahran without success. By the end of the fourth year, in 1937, about fifty Americans were living in camps of huts at Jebel Dhahran, expecting orders to pack up and go home at any moment. But fate and American tenacity decreed otherwise.

Although King Ibn Saud was vaguely interested in what the Americans were doing, his most pressing concern at the time was water rather than oil. The Americans already had drilled many artesian wells for him, a small operation compared to drilling for oil. Therefore, when he invited some of them to come to Riyadh to drill for more water, the Americans willingly obliged.

Two of the geologists, on their day off, went to visit the waterhole called Ayn Heet, which Nizar had told us about on our desert adventure. It was located near Riyadh and was a good place for a cool swim. Ayn Heet was a deep cavern formed by the collapse of the roof of a water-worn cave some hundreds of feet underground. At the bottom, about 150 feet down, was a deep, dark pool of water. Almost everyone from our hospital visited Ayn Heet at one time or another. To reach the pool, we had to clamber down a steep, zigzag path, which had been used for centuries by travelers who came to fill their water skins. It was at this waterhole that Ibn Saud and his forty men watered their camels before going on to recapture Riyadh on that historic night in 1902.

Thus the two geologists went to visit Ayn Heet as tourists more interested in it from the historical point of view than the scientific. But many monumental discoveries have been made purely by accident. "Chance favors the prepared mind" is a well-known aphorism; Horace Walpole called it "serendipity." The number of such discoveries in medicine are legion. The first use of ether as an anesthetic is an example. The discovery of the greatest oil field in history is another.

As the geologists approached the bottom of the path leading to the pool, they chanced upon a cap-rock formation at the water's edge which was similar to that known to exist in Bahrain. They had been searching in vain for this type of impervious rock formation for four years. Now their discovery in Riyadh of the same type of cap rock found in Bahrain meant that oil must be trapped somewhere between these two points. Armed with this information, they decided to deepen the seventh of the abortive wells in Jebel Dhahran. In March 1938, after four and a half unproductive, thwarted years, they struck oil at 4,727 feet, nearly a mile below the surface of the hill.

"They discovered an ocean of oil," said Naman, proudly.

Meanwhile, Standard Oil of California had sold half its concession interest to the Texas Oil Company (Texaco) in 1936. The new merger was named the Arabian-American Oil Company—Aramco—in 1944. Four years later, two more oil companies joined Aramco, which now consists of Standard Oil of California, Texaco, Exxon, and Mobil.

Aramco's discovery of the vast deposits of oil, its advanced technological skills, and the mutual benefits derived from both helped establish a cordial relationship between Saudi Arabia and the United States. Formal diplomatic relations with the American government began during World War II. King Ibn Saud was the only independent Mid-Eastern ruler friendly to the Allies. However, the wartime restraints on the Aramco operations and the reduced pilgrimage traffic to Mecca had brought the country close to bankruptcy. Financial support was granted to Saudi Arabia in the form of loans made through Aramco, the United States, and England. Bankruptcy was prevented, and by 1943 the Saudis were receiving loans under the United States Lend-Lease program.

As the war progressed, Saudi Arabia was drawn closer to the Allies. In February 1945, King Abdul-Aziz and President Roosevelt met briefly on the U.S. cruiser *Quincy* in Great Bitter Lake, Egypt. One month later, Saudi Arabia declared war on the Axis powers. In 1950 an agreement between Saudi Arabia and Aramco specified a fifty-fifty sharing of oil profits, the first of its kind in the Middle East.

"So you see," concluded Naman, "Aramco was instrumental in establishing a liaison between the United States and Saudi Arabia which goes back thirty years."

When we were about twenty-five miles west of the Gulf, Naman pointed out Abqaiq and Qatif, the originating points for the Trans-Arabian pipeline, which carries oil a thousand miles north to the Mediterranean. Then the Arabian Gulf came into view. Suddenly, almost like a mirage, the Aramco headquarters at Dhahran appeared, sprouting up out of the great desert beneath us. Soon, a few miles east of Dhahran, we could see the modern commercial city of Al-Khobar. Finally, Naman pointed to the huge port city of Dammam, the capital of the Eastern Province, just north of Dhahran.

The airport at Dhahran is relatively small but impressive. A series of graceful Arabian arches, such as seen in classic Islamic architecture, dominated the approach as we landed. The airport had been designed by a Japanese-American architect, Naman told us. The airfield itself, he said, had been constructed by American engineers in 1946 as a U.S. Strategic Air Command base. It had been a vital stop between Egypt and India on the Allies' supply route to Japan during the war. Before leaving, Naman showed us the Aramco hangar nearby, which housed a fleet of nine Flying

Camels, including two large executive jets, which flew from Dhahran to New York.

Our Aramco hosts greeted us warmly at the airport. Since there were no hotels in the vicinity, they had arranged for us to stay in their homes during the two-day meeting. Ron Lambrie and I had already made plans to stay at the home of a friend, Dr. Mel Gilbert, whom we had met previously in Riyadh. As Mel drove us from the airport to the Aramco compound, he told us they expected forty visitors "from the outside." Some doctors would be coming from Jidda, eight hundred miles away, and others from nearby Kuwait and Bahrain.

The compound, where thousands of employees and their families lived, was completely enclosed by high, endless wire fencing. Security guards at the main gate waved in recognition as we entered what looked like a suburban California town. It included a very sandy golf course, a driving range, tennis courts, hobby shop, swimming pool, library, dining hall, commissary, and a combined barber shop and beauty parlor.

"Tomorrow I'll show you our hospital and clinic," Mel promised. We stopped briefly at the Aramco headquarters, a low, U-shaped building with hundreds of small offices. "This is where the action is," said Mel, smiling. We then quickly drove past the service area, which contained a power station, laundry, garages, and a central air-conditioning plant.

But the homes impressed me most. What had originally been a camp of huts in Dhahran was now an attractive suburban city. Every nail, board, and pipe came from halfway around the world. This was "Little America" transplanted to Saudi Arabia and obviously thriving. We drove along well-paved, immaculate, curving roads lined with neat rows of modern, ranch-style houses. Some were painted a mellow orange; others were brown or green with broad windows edged with white. Long verandas nestled in the shade of palm trees. The homes all had carefully sprinkled, smooth lawns surrounded by jasmine hedges or clumps of oleander heavy with bright pink blossoms. Boys and girls in shorts were walking about in groups, riding their bicycles, or roller-skating. The sight made me homesick.

Mel's house was on a quiet corner and was somewhat larger than the others. He had been with Aramco for many years and was the Assistant Medical Director. His home was spacious and tastefully furnished, containing many mementos from the various parts of the world in which he had worked. His wife, Mary, was in the garden, tending to her flowers. She was an attractive woman originally from New England. Mel was a Canadian. They had two children who were attending college in the United States.

"I'm glad you're back," she said to her husband after welcoming us. "I need the car to do some shopping."

Ron and I expressed surprise.

"Oh, women are allowed to drive within the compound," she explained. "It is part of the original agreement with King Abdul-Aziz. We also can buy bacon, ham, and other pork products at the commissary. I know you'll want some with your eggs for breakfast tomorrow."

Mel explained that in a sense the Aramco compound was extraterritorial U.S. "The women are not allowed to drive cars outside the compound," he said. "In the old days, we could get wine, beer, and liquor, too, but the government put an end to that twenty-five years ago."

Ron and I said we would like to accompany Mary shopping. When we arrived at the commissary, we were overjoyed to see the various cuts of fresh meat neatly arranged under the glass counters. The display of bacon, ham, and sausage looked unreal, almost like a mirage. For more than a year, the only meat we chanced upon in the Riyadh "supermarkets" were packages of frozen beef from Australia, Denmark, or New Zealand, piled up in a large freezer. Here, meat, fresh fruit, and vegetables arrived by the Aramco planes weekly.

"People always want desperately what they can't have," I said, half aloud. "Actually, at home we don't eat pork more than two or three times a month. Now, I can't wait until breakfast tomorrow."

"If you carry some of these packages," Mary said as we left, "maybe I can be persuaded to serve some cocktail sausages with our drinks tonight."

At six o'clock, we had sadiki cocktails and hors d'oeuvres, including shrimp and plenty of sausages, with a tangy sauce which Mary kept replenishing. Mel had invited a number of Aramco friends, mostly administrators and doctors. The men wore colorful shirts open at the neck and the women wore casual cocktail dresses. Everyone was in a festive mood. I could sense the intimacy and communion among them. Many had spent the best part of their lives together here, some for twenty years or longer. A mix of fierce loyalty to Aramco, selfless dedication, and pride in their achievement bound them together in enduring friendship.

These men, I would learn, not only discovered the oil in Saudi Arabia but brought about an economic, social, and humanist revolution without inciting a political one. From the start, Aramco's pioneering specialists (engineers, sociologists, and health scientists) became involved in a situation that had no precedent. They developed principles and policies designed to cope with problems which bore no direct relationship to the oil industry.

I had expected to find a clique of tycoons wallowing in oil money. Instead, I discovered a family of dedicated professionals imbued with ideals worthy of the Salvation Army—pioneers in the basic needs of human beings and in their fulfillment.

Such a person was Tom Frazier, a slight man in his fifties with a deep tan, a small mustache, and blue eyes. He was about to retire after thirty years with the company.

"I've always lived on Aramco property," he said, "both before and after I was married and raised a family. But life in the early days was quite different than it is now. It was a pioneering undertaking. We were a small group of Americans sitting in a small community out in the desert. World War II had not been over very long. Materials to do the work were not readily available. Food had to be imported from the United States and, of course, fresh fruits and vegetables were hard to come by. The air conditioning was not reliable, and you can imagine what summers in Dhahran were like. Riyadh is bad enough but Dhahran gets insufferably hot. So these kinds of hardships, if you want to call them hardships, brought us together. There was a much more cohesive spirit, a oneness, in those times. When you did anything socially, you did it with everybody in the community."

When he arrived in 1947, about four hundred Americans were living in Saudi Arabia, he told me, but very few wives. The turnover rate was phenomenal because of loneliness and the non-availability of family housing. "We were losing about 30 percent of the American work force every year. Chartered airplanes came in with a full load of men and promptly left with a full load. Now we have about two thousand Americans living here with their families, and very few want to leave."

I asked Tom about the Saudi work force.

"That was one of our most challenging problems," he said. "The Arabs are nomadic by nature and the idea of coming to work every morning at seven o'clock and working five and a half or six days a week came as a severe shock. The concept of staying on and working month after month until vacation time seemed utterly absurd to them. At the end of one week, as soon as they were given a bag of silver riyals in payment, they would just disappear."

"How did you get them to do any manual labor?" I asked, reaching for another sausage.

"Well, the Arabs who worked for us," said Tom, "particularly the Bedouins, had very strict rules about things they would or would not do. Anything involving dirt, such as sweeping the floor, or anything that they looked upon as menial they were disinclined to do. The Bedouins were very proud. They lived in the desert, tended their flocks, rode their camels, and bartered. If we asked them to dig a ditch in which there was to be a sewer line, they absolutely refused.

"Most of our workmen were the Shiites," he continued. "As you know, they are a minority group in Saudi Arabia. There are only a few hundred thousand in this country, townspeople, farmers, and artisans who settled near here in Qatif and Hofuf. The Shiites were more adaptable to the needs of our industry and did the manual work for us which the Bedouins rejected.

"It took thirty years," he concluded, "but we now have almost 25,000 Saudi Arabians working for us. For the most part it is a very stable and dependable work force."

"You know," one of the doctors standing next to me said, "this aversion to working with the hands has spread to some of the Egyptian and Lebanese physicians. They sit and talk to the patients about their symptoms for hours but are reluctant to use their hands to perform a physical examination. It is weird."

Tom nodded as he refilled his scotch and soda, and continued: "The most valuable insight into the Arab mind and culture came from a Professor Bader from the American University of Beirut. It was 1948 and I was living at a very barren outpost built on a sand dune in Abqaiq. We were doing all our drilling and exploration from this point. 'You're a young man,' Professor Bader said, 'and you will be facing situations with the Saudis that will defy your ability to understand them because their traditions, culture, and value structure are fundamentally different from those of the Western world.'

" 'You Westerners,' he said, 'have a historic advantage over the Arabs. You have taken the concept of reason from the Greeks; the teachings that man can be the master of his own destiny from the Romans; and your religion from Judaism and Christianity. Then you synthesized all three: reason, man's ability to determine his own destiny, and religion into one mix. It's not a perfect mix,' he added, 'but you brought them together rather well.'

" 'After the death of the Prophet Mohammed,' Professor Bader continued, " 'the Arab people withdrew almost completely from Western civilization. While the Western world was going through the Renaissance and its humanistic revival, the Arab world remained isolated, embracing Islam alone. They rejected Aristotelian logic and reason. They did not accept the concept that man can control his own destiny. They based their whole system of life, including their jurisprudence, on the teachings of the Prophet.'

Aramco—Where It All Began ◊ *219*

" 'The Arab thinks with his heart rather than with his mind,' the professor concluded. 'The gesture of putting his hand over his heart when he talks to you is meaningful. He is emotional and theological rather than analytical.'

"Everything this Arab scholar told me proved to be true," Tom said. "An Arab can do a damn good job of running the refinery or managing a plant, but when you ask him to do a staff job involving planning, research, or reasoning, he can't do it. He hasn't the ability to work out, say, a new policy for compensation of employees, or to make a study involving industrial relations. He can't be analytical."

"He could run a hospital but couldn't develop a policy for its management. Is that it?" I asked.

"Exactly," said Tom. "Another problem we had was to get the Saudis to cooperate with other Saudis who were not in their tribe or immediate family. Western society often takes cooperation for granted. As far as I know there is no word in the Arabic language for cooperating. Here again, we go back to religion. Every Arab maintains a very close personal relationship with Allah. He doesn't go to that deity through a pastor or a priest or a leader of the flock. No, he goes straight to the deity. There is no intermediary."

Mel was standing by listening to our conversation. "That's absolutely true," he said. "A Saudi woman would bring her five children to the clinic when she came for medical attention. My God, we would have twenty-five of these women around there, each with five children. It was chaotic! And our staff would say, 'Now, look, madam, why don't you leave your children with your next-door neighbor, and then when she comes to the clinic, you can look after her children?' Never, never! Oh, no! Now, if it was her sister or cousin, then that would be fine."

"In keeping with this concept, originally there was no such thing in Saudi Arabia as a corporation outside the family," added Tom. "The idea of an Arab giving you money to manage for him in a business undertaking was inconceivable. Family is the cohesive unit here, and, of course, it is a patriarchal system where one man sits at the top and calls all the shots for the family. And they are absolutely committed to the one-man rule. But the idea of working together is completely foreign to them. Of course, this is reflected throughout the Arab world. You see the Syrians are always quarreling or fighting with the Lebanese; the Iranians with the Iraqi; the Saudis with the Libyans, and so on. Although there is an Arab League, the Arab nations never pull together in a cohesive manner. Neither do the oil-producing countries in OPEC.

"One of our main problems," he said, "was to get the Saudis to come out of the desert and to identify with us as employees. A Saudi's identity and loyalty were always with his tribe.

"For us, the beginning years were a crucial period. We had an industry to run and we needed people on hand to run the refinery, the drilling rigs, the separator plants, the power plants—and we needed people upon whom we could depend.

"Well," he said, putting down his glass, "those were challenging times, exciting times for the few of us stranded in a strange and hostile desert world."

"It seems impossible," I said. "What was the solution?"

Mel interrupted us to say it was time to leave. "We're going to a reception and dinner in honor of our guests at Don Mason's house. I hope you're all hungry by now."

"Actually, I'm not very hungry," I said. "I've eaten every sausage in sight."

Then I turned to Tom. "I hope we can get together tomorrow," I said. "I'm just beginning to realize that, if it weren't for Aramco, Saudi Arabia might still be a backward, destitute desert country today. I don't think people at home realize this." We arranged to meet for lunch the next day.

On the way to the reception, Mel and Mary told us a little about Don Mason. He was a physician at Aramco who had lived here for more than twenty years. He and his wife, Betty, were excellent tennis players.

Their home was truly impressive, surrounded by tall trees and beautiful gardens. On one side was a large illuminated swimming pool bordered by flowers. The interior of the house exuded international luxury. Rugs from Iran covered the floors and handwoven silk carpets hung from the walls. There were exquisite oriental screens from Japan and a breathtaking display of old English china and antique silver.

Sudanese and Pakistani servants passed among the guests with drinks and trays of hors d'oeuvres. Two buffets were laden with food, one in the dining room and the other in the candlelit garden. Don, our host, was a tall, slender man in his fifties, athletic in appearance, very quiet and relaxed. He introduced us to some of the doctors and other people from Aramco. I told him how impressed I was by his work.

"It's been an uphill battle," he said, "but we've made some progress. We still have a long way to go." We then discussed several patients he had sent me with difficult diagnostic problems. We had talked on the phone about some and corresponded about others.

Ron and I wandered about in that sea of strange faces. Everyone wore a badge listing the individual's name and point of origin. The guests were mostly doctors and technicians from hospitals all over the Arabian Peninsula.

I finally met Betty Mason. She was an attractive woman and looked every bit the tennis player she was. She and Don had four children now living in the United States. After spending so many years in Saudi Arabia, she told me, she was more than ready to go home.

"But you have a beautiful home and servants, and those will be difficult to duplicate in the United States," I said.

"There's nothing to do here but play bridge and tennis," she replied. "It's a stultifying environment: the same small group of people here year after year; the heat and the humidity; the flies and the sandstorms; and the endless talk about oil and hospitals. It's enough to drive a person to drink. I don't know why I'm telling you all this," she added, "but sometimes I think I'll go stark, raving mad unless I can go home."

I told her that I understood perfectly and that my wife was in London at this very moment for probably the same reasons. "Let me get you some dinner," I said.

"That sounds like a good idea," she replied. "Thank you." I asked one of the Sudanese to bring us some food from the buffet. Then we sat down at a table near the pool.

"This life is hard on women, particularly after our children have left," she said, "and now Don wants to stay on another five years!"

"Why don't you go home more often?" I asked.

"I just came back," she said. "It's the returning which is so difficult. I really love Don but sometimes I wonder . . ."

Some Aramco friends came over to say goodbye.

"I'll ask Ruth to call you," I said, as we finished our dinner. "There is a patient in the hospital who is the Lieutenant Governor of the Eastern Province. He invited us to be his guests next month and I couldn't refuse. Ruth is coming with me and I'm sure she'll want to meet you."

"That would be wonderful," Betty said with enthusiasm. "And thank you for the shoulder," she added as we parted.

On the way home, I told Mary about our conversation.

"I feel exactly the same way at times," she said. "It's difficult but I try to make the best of it."

"Thank God for that," said Mel fervently.

Bright and early the next morning we had a good breakfast of sausages and eggs that Mary had promised and then set out for our medical meeting. It was held in a large conference room in the library building, which could accommodate 250 people. The first day of the meeting would be devoted to a discussion of the major health problems in Saudi Arabia and Aramco's effort to combat them. On the second day, the physicians of the King Faisal Hospital would discuss recent advances in the diagnosis and treatment of some of these conditions. Slide and moving-picture projectors were made ready for each lecturer and microphones were stationed in the aisles to accommodate speakers from the audience. The conference room was filled to capacity.

In an introductory speech, the first speaker pointed out that, when Aramco arrived, no statistics or data existed on which to base estimates of the incidence of disease in Saudi Arabia. Most illness and death went unreported because there were no physicians to report them. Aramco was the first to set up a system for collecting vital statistics.

I knew this was the richest oil company on earth but I never had realized the scope of its involvement in public health. We learned that Aramco was the principal non-government provider of medical care in Saudi Arabia, and had two hospitals and a number of clinics dispersed throughout the Eastern Province. All company employees and their families were eligible for free care. Over a half million clinic visits were made annually and 90,000 patient days of hospital care were provided. Other clinic facilities nearing completion would accommodate an additional 700 outpatients daily.

Dr. Mason showed us a projected design of the new addition to the Dhahran Health Center, which when completed would add 150 beds to the center's 110-bed capacity and would include a new dental clinic and provide more sophisticated diagnostic and treatment capabilities.

"We are responsible for the health of about 25,000 employees and 75,000 dependents," he said, "of whom approximately 80 percent are Saudi Arabians."

Subsequent speakers pointed out that malaria, tuberculosis, and parasitic diseases had presented the most serious problems in the early days. It had soon become apparent that work in the Eastern Province would be impossible unless malaria was eradicated. Aramco in conjunction with WHO (World Health Organization) set about with mobile units to destroy the mosquito larvae and to eliminate the breeding areas. Subsequently, the incidence of malaria in the Eastern Province fell sharply, and malaria is now practically nonexistent.

Tuberculosis had been widespread, particularly in the towns and cities, a chest specialist reported, and progress had been slow. In 1955, however, when specific drugs became available, Aramco arranged for a team of experts to bring in special equipment from the United States to take chest x-rays of twenty thousand Saudi employees and their families. With the new treatment tuberculosis was practically eradicated from the Eastern Province, although tuberculosis-prevention centers are still maintained.

An eye surgeon told of the early days when more than 70 percent of the population suffered from some form of trachoma. Since the disease can be cured, if treated early, Aramco established a trachoma center at Dhahran which proved very effective.

A parasitologist gave a presentation on dysentery and other parasitic diseases which had affected almost 50 percent of the population when he first came to Saudi Arabia. The company set up a center to combat these infestations, as did the Saudi Arabian government, which, with Aramco's help, instituted control stations all over the country. Aramco's pioneering efforts in public health were also directed toward promoting sanitation, improving sewerage facilities, and supplying better water to the towns and villages.

Mel closed the meeting with a description of their teaching and training programs. In 1957, television had been introduced into the Eastern Province, offering educational programs devoted to languages, health, sanitation, and home economics. Closed-circuit television was now used extensively.

At the coffee break, I told Don Mason that I had never considered oil moguls as medical missionaries. "I'm really impressed. You have accomplished almost the impossible in a relatively short time."

"It's been more than twenty years," Don said. "I've spent practically all of my professional life here and am thinking about going home. As you know, Betty is very anxious to leave. She told me she talked to you about it last night."

I told him that I could understand her viewpoint. "Maybe you can arrange to continue your work here on a part-time basis or as a consultant," I said.

He then told me that he was interested in doing some research on cancer in Saudi Arabia and wondered whether the Harvard School of Public Health would be willing to collaborate on such a program.

I told him that, since the School of Public Health had already established such a precedent with their successful research on trachoma, they might be interested in his cancer research as well. "The government here will probably be willing to finance your research," I said, "and you could continue to work here part time."

Don thanked me for the encouragement and said he would keep in touch.

Tom arrived at precisely one o'clock to drive me to his home for lunch. He seemed as pleased to talk about the epoch-making days at Aramco as I was to listen.

"Where did I leave off last night?" he asked as we approached his car.

"You were telling me how you were able to motivate the Saudis to abandon their nomadic tribal life," I said. "It seems impossible to me."

"Well, it wasn't easy," Tom said, "and it took time. The first thing we had to do was to define our objective—our philosophical approach."

"What was that?" I asked.

"We decided that the crux of our policy in Saudi Arabia was to make the welfare of the Saudis our primary goal rather than to make as much money as possible," he said. "We knew we were going to make an awful lot of money in any event, but we didn't want to kill the goose that laid the golden egg.

"Our objective was to do as much as possible to benefit the host country so that the Saudis would want us to stay. We didn't want to be imperialists. We were already witnessing the dissolution of the British Empire. And then there were the French, Dutch, and Belgians who were being unceremoniously thrown out of the countries they had dominated. So we decided to conduct ourselves in such a manner that we would be acceptable and desirable guests to the Saudis without exerting any political force whatever."

I told him that I had never realized until today how much Aramco had done for the health and well-being of the Saudi Arabian people. "Some of the things you did were almost miraculous," I said, "like getting chest x-rays of twenty thousand Saudis in the middle of the desert twenty years ago when tuberculosis was so prevalent."

Tom told me that in the early days, when an employee was found to have active tuberculosis, he was discharged, given termination and disability pay, and sent home to die. Since he was contagious, he would be ostracized by his whole community. Consequently, some Saudis when found to be tubercular refused to leave. The only way to get them off the job was to call in the soldiers, who would drag them off screaming as though they were about to be executed.

"It was pathetic," he said. "I'll never forget it."

"Getting back to last night's discussion," I said, "how did you go about converting nomadic illiterate Bedouins into a stable, effective work force? Most of them, you said, would work for a week, pick up their bag of riyals and head for the desert and their families."

Tom described a series of benefits and rewards in keeping with Aramco's policy of contributing to the welfare of the workers. They established the "semi-annual continuous service award," which was a bonus for those who stayed for six months or longer. Then they started a thrift plan in which the employee could put away 10 percent of his income and the company would match it.

"The concept of saving for the future was not in the Saudi Arabian ethos," said Tom. "'Allah will take care of me and my family so why worry about saving money or insuring against catastrophe? That's ridiculous!' It took a while but eventually all the employees participated in the program.

"Accident prevention was another challenging problem," he said. "The Arab people, believing their destiny is in the hands of Allah, ridiculed accident-prevention measures such as wearing a helmet or dressing in trousers rather than thobes, which would get caught in the machines. Their philosophy was 'If you're going to get killed, you are going to get killed. It's all up to Allah. Why cut my shoulder-length hair?' People were getting killed and maimed and the accident rate was catastrophic.

"Finally, we decided to give a gift such as a watch or a transistor radio to those who were accident-free for a certain period of time, and in a year and a half the industrial accident rate fell precipitously. It worked like a charm.

"Several people in the administration felt," he continued, "that the greatest contribution we could make in generating goodwill would be to provide some kind of housing for the people, who lived in tents or shacks made out of scraps. They developed a housing loan plan by which the company loaned the employee 80 percent of the cost of his house interest-free, and then gave him the remaining 20 percent outright as a gift. Saudi contractors, in addition, were given interest-free loans for construction of these projects along with expert technical advice.

"Well, you can imagine what happened in the board rooms in New York when this came out," Tom said, laughing. "They raised hell but we persisted. In the past twenty-five years, Aramco granted $95 million in loans and more than 8,600 employees have become homeowners. I'm proud of that." He hesitated, then shook his head. "But to this day I don't know that the Saudis are happier than they were when we first came here, largely because they are going through this terrible trauma of change.

"The standard of living in the Eastern Province, of course, is much higher than anywhere else in Saudi Arabia," he added.

"And they are a lot healthier now, that's for sure," I said, reminding him that the Saudi life expectancy until recently was forty-five years.

"Here we are," said Tom, as we drew up to the front of a house that looked very similar to Mel's. Tom's wife, Tricia, was a gracious Southern lady in her fifties, with a ready smile and hazel eyes which sparkled as she spoke. She was tall and slender and her tanned skin bespoke the many years she had spent in Saudi Arabia. She appeared from the very beginning to be a happy, vivacious woman.

"Welcome to Aramco," she said after Tom had introduced me. "We're having roast pork for lunch in your honor." She laughed. "Mary Gilbert told me it's one of your favorites." Her voice was musical and her Deep South accent a delight.

Tom then asked me whether I would like "brown with water or white with water." When I looked puzzled, he explained that the "brown" was sadiki which had been aged in oak kegs and tasted somewhat like bourbon.

"The first time I went back to the States," Tricia said, "I asked for 'brown and water' and nobody knew what I was talking about."

"I'll try the brown and water, please," I said.

They told me that they made brown sadiki by fermenting concentrated orange juice with sugar, molasses, and yeast. The procedure was called "starting a run" and took three weeks. It was then poured into the kegs and stored for up to a year. The white sadiki was much less choice, took less time to prepare and tasted somewhat like vodka.

"We imported the oak kegs under the guise of 'kitchen stools' in order to get them through customs," Tricia said, laughing.

In the early years of Aramco, beer and liquor had been permitted on the compound but were rationed and carefully controlled so that none would fall into the hands of the Saudis. However, the Ulema had been warning King Ibn Saud that he was risking Paradise by allowing the importation of liquor to Aramco. Finally, in 1952, a year before he died, Ibn Saud prohibited all alcoholic beverages at Aramco to ensure his admission to Paradise. As if to compensate for this prohibition, the King shortly thereafter granted women the right to drive automobiles inside the compound.

"A car made life much easier," Tricia said. "The other big event for us was the opening of a beauty parlor in 1954. Before then, we had to cut each other's hair, and you know how women are about beauty shops!"

Tricia said that when she arrived in Saudi Arabia in 1948 the few women who had arrived earlier were still wearing the very short dresses which had been out of fashion for two years.

"In general," she said, "we were two years behind the rest of the world. Whenever I went back to the States, I bought two years' supply of clothing for my three children and often brought back fifty to sixty pairs of shoes. We later set up a clothing exchange."

"What about the food in those days?" I asked, helping myself to the hors d'oeuvres.

"Frozen meat and poultry were available then as they are now in Riyadh," she said. "Fresh vegetables came by boat and were scarce. When they arrived, there was a mob scene at the commissary which looked like bargain day at Macy's! Food was not flown in until years later.

"And we were obliged to sign at the commissary for all bacon and ham to be sure it didn't go to the Saudis," she added. "They were very strict about that."

"There were really no serious shortages," said Tom, "and we shared whatever we had with our friends."

"Everyone was invited to our parties in the early days," remarked Tricia with animation. "I would merely say, 'Tonight's my night,' and everyone would come. We borrowed each other's servants and paid them extra, so we had plenty of help."

"We often had music and dancing at our parties," Tom said. "The music was supplied by the locals in our area or by a pickup orchestra of Americans from the air base at Dhahran."

While Tom went out to replenish the drinks, Tricia said that living here really wasn't very difficult but that it took some time for the women to adjust to a new way of life. When the air conditioning failed, for example, they went to the swimming pool with their children to escape the 140-degree heat. Movies were shown three times a week and the women organized bridge clubs, sewing circles, tennis clubs, and even flower shows. Tricia added that she had founded the first Girl Scout troup in Saudi Arabia and started a Sunday school for children of all denominations, which was held in a schoolhouse.

"Churches are not permitted, even at Aramco," Tom said, as he handed me another brown and water. "At first we held outdoor church services but they were discontinued because the Ulema feared that the Saudis might attend. Church services were later held in auditoriums or private homes, and ministers of various denominations were brought in as 'teachers.' The Saudis were aware of all this and made it clear that no Moslem was to attend a Christian church service."

"They just didn't want the Moslems to learn anything about Christianity," said Tricia. "In fact, I had to smuggle my Bible into Saudi Arabia by hiding it in my purse."

"And no customs officer in the world could find anything in Tricia's purse," Tom added. "She also hid some playing cards in that purse, because the Wahabis considered them idolatrous. The same applied to dolls. I hid our little girl's doll in my briefcase to avoid difficulty."

They said that their children went to schools run by Aramco until the ninth grade. There were Arabic-speaking teachers from Lebanon and Egypt for the Saudi children and American teachers for the others. Then the children went on to boarding schools in England, Switzerland, or the United States. Aramco paid for their education and also financed the college education of promising Saudi students.

We sat down to a delicious luncheon, consisting of shrimp cocktail, roast loin of pork (which Tricia had promised me), applesauce, tossed salad, and fresh pineapple for dessert. Afterward, we went out to the terrace, where the houseboy served us iced tea and a variety of cheeses.

"You have been here about thirty years," I said, to Tricia. "Would you do it again, if you had your life to live over?"

"I enjoyed every moment of it," she replied, "and the children loved it, too. We had a wonderful life here."

"Some women are of another opinion," I said, remembering my conversation last night with Betty Mason.

"It depends on the individual," said Tricia. "Some women just can't adjust to living in Saudi Arabia. Others wouldn't be happy anywhere."

She went on to say that some women who had little to do took to drinking excessively out of sheer boredom. Later Aramco offered them jobs, which helped the situation.

Tricia told me that when she went to an Arab party at Aramco she would first go to see the Arab ladies and their children in the back of the house and then return to the parlor up front to join the men. The Arab host would offer her a drink and the men and women mingled freely, but the Saudi women never appeared.

"The status of women has changed very little in the past thirty years," Tricia said, "but we have been educating them and there is bound to be a change for the better."

"Speaking of education," said Tom, as the houseboy refilled his glass with iced tea, "formal education in this country, before Aramco arrived here, was conducted according to Islamic tradition and was available only to a small percentage of the male population. It consisted primarily of memorizing the Koran under the direction of an *imam* [religious leader]. Schooling at the *kuttabs* [Islamic elementary schools] began when a boy was six years old and ended when he had memorized the Koran at the age of ten or twelve.

"The need for modern educational facilities led us to develop a modern school system in the Eastern Province. In the past twenty years we built fifty-five schools for both boys and girls in this area and later turned some of the schools over to the government. We also brought closed-circuit television into the schools in the Eastern Province and initiated for our employees the most advanced system of vocational training in the Arab world."

Tom sipped his tea and looked out into the distance. "In the area of industrial relations," he said, "we were the first in the Middle East to institute comprehensive retirement programs, termination awards, and workmen's compensation. Our welfare and educational facilities benefited many thousands of Saudis outside of Aramco and set a standard for the government to follow.

"You know, the Saudi government has adopted many of our programs. And, of course, the huge revenues derived from the oil helped to implement them."

"I wonder whether the Saudis appreciate all you have done for their country," I said. "They have been gradually acquiring Aramco and will control the remainder of it shortly, according to the newspapers."

"Yes," replied Tom, "but we will still do the planning, transporting, and marketing of the oil production as before. Formal acquisition means everything and nothing.

"We can now produce twelve million barrels of oil a day, and we are working on a program to increase the production capacity to fourteen million barrels. We are also starting a new project to recover and utilize the natural gas in the Eastern Province. Aramco will be here for a long, long time."

It was now two-thirty. The afternoon session was scheduled for three o'clock. On the way back to the library building, we passed an oil derrick marking Aramco's first strike.

"I've been wondering where the oil wells are," I said. "I expected to see a forest of drilling rigs, derricks, and pumps all over the place."

"They are all around you," said Tom, laughing, "but they're not very conspicuous. There is one right in front of you." He pointed to a collection of intertwining pipes, wheels, valves, and gauges standing about eight feet above the ground, known as "Christmas trees." He explained that, in order to control the flow of oil rising through the shaft under extreme heat and pressure, each well was capped with one of these Rube Goldberg contraptions. Since the oil was already under great pressure, pumps were obviously unnecessary. The oil dispatcher simply turned a wheel and the oil flowed into an underground pipeline, which carried it to a separation plant, where the gas was removed. From there it went to a stabilization plant to eliminate the poisonous hydrogen sulfide. It then passed through a double pipeline to Ras Tanura, which has the largest oil port and refinery in the world. The oil was piped as crude oil into some of the world's largest tankers, standing by some fifteen miles out in the gulf, or it went directly to the refinery at Ras Tanura, which could process up to a half million barrels of oil a day.

The wells hidden under the unobtrusive Christmas trees were all but forgotten, said Tom, except by the dispatchers who watch the constant flow of oil on the dials of a faraway control center. As we drove along slowly, I spotted another Christmas tree three hundred yards away, and then another and another.

"It's amazing," I said. "The Christmas trees at home will never seem the same."

The meeting presided over by the King Faisal doctors adjourned at six-thirty. Mel, Ron, and I returned to the Gilberts' home to freshen up for the party that night. Mary told us that it would be held outdoors on the estate of the chairman of the board and that she had invited Tom and Tricia Frazier to sit at our table.

We arrived at eight o'clock. It was a clear, balmy, moonlit evening. The driveway to the massive two-story mansion was lined with tall palm trees dramatically lighted from below. We left our car in the parking area and proceeded to the garden, which was illuminated by multicolored lights strung from the treetops. Tables set for dinner were arranged on the extensive lawn, in the center of which was a rectangular swimming pool. At the periphery of the garden in the distance were palm trees, yellow-blossomed acacia trees, and brilliant red and purple bougainvillea. The garden was at the back of the house, which had a broad terrace for dancing. Overlooking the terrace was a second-floor balcony, where an orchestra was playing softly. Indian men in native dress circulated among the guests, serving drinks and hors d'oeuvres.

Mary found the table she had reserved for us near the pool and we made ourselves comfortable.

Nobody was living in the big house at present, Mary said. It was used mostly as a guesthouse for visiting dignitaries and their entourage. The gardens were frequently available for large parties such as this.

"We're expecting about 150 people," she said.

A young Indian servant approached us with a tray of drinks. Mel explained that we had the choice of adding soda water, lime, or ginger ale to the sadiki. Most of us ordered "brown and water."

A Saudi, about forty years old, came over to greet Tom. He was dressed in Western clothes and spoke excellent English. When he returned to his table, Tom told us that he was an administrator who lived in the Aramco compound not far from him. He was a graduate of Cal Tech and an engineer.

"Do any of the Saudi employees leave Aramco and go into business on their own?" I asked.

Tom told us that, when Aramco needed Saudi Arabian contractors, they selected a few men already working for Aramco, gave them six-month leaves of absence and then contracted them to do specific jobs. "Some of them fail and return to Aramco, but a few have succeeded and are now billionaires," Tom said. "One Saudi named Suliman Olayan started out with us as an oil dispatcher and is now one of the richest men in the world. His investments in the Chase Manhattan Bank are second only to Rockefeller's. His Olayan Saudi holding company in Riyadh earns $300 million a year and he owns an insurance company which nets an equal amount. He's a brilliant entrepreneur."

"How did he get started?" I asked.

"In 1947 we asked Olayan to become a contractor," Tom said, "and gave him a leave of absence. He borrowed money, bought four trucks, and began to haul pipe for Aramco on our Trans-Arabian pipeline. After that, he bought company after company, and now owns or controls thirty-five corporations involved in chicken farming, water desalination, and construction work. And a third of his holdings are in bank stocks in the United States.

"We're proud of Olayan," Tom said, "and he in turn calls Aramco 'my university.' He had no formal education beyond high school. His American wife was one of our secretaries at Aramco, and the man in charge of his U.S. operations is William Simon, formerly Secretary of the Treasury."

That surprised all of us. More sadiki was passed around as Tom told us another success story. "Ali Tomeemi, a friend of mine, used to work in Abqaiq as a gang pusher in the labor pool. Then he started hauling pipe for us as Olayan did. When he'd saved some money he went into the transportation business. He now owns a fleet of five hundred Mercedes Benz buses, and has the exclusive dealership for Peugeot cars in this country."

"But where does the big money come from?" asked Ron.

Tom hesitated. "He's a manufacturer's representative," he said quietly.

"It would take fifteen minutes to name all the companies he represents, beginning with General Electric."

Tom proceeded to tell us that when Aramco made a purchase of gas turbines from an American company for approximately $300 million, Ali was paid his usual 3 percent or $9 million as the company's representative in Saudi Arabia, and he wasn't even in the country at the time of the transaction.

"There's probably more to this than meets the eye," I said.

"No," Tom said, emphatically. "It's just the way business is carried out in this country."

One of Aramco's managers, a friend of Tom's who was in charge of auditing, had joined our table with his wife. Henry Simpson was a graduate of the Wharton Business School in Philadelphia. He had been listening attentively to Tom.

"Let me enlarge on that subject," he said. He proceeded to tell us about a Saudi sheikh in Riyadh who acted as an intermediary between an English company negotiating for a desalination plant and the Saudi ministry involved. When the contract for $500 million was signed, the English company paid the sheikh $15 million, the usual 3 percent.

"An American friend of mine, an engineer, who works for the sheikh, told me the story," said Henry. "The question is, how much of his $15 million commission did the sheikh pay a royal or a government official as a kickback to help him get the contract? The amounts are staggering when you consider that some of these contracts involve billions of dollars. The agents themselves are sometimes Saudi princes whose close relatives run the ministries which parcel out these huge sums of money.

"Corruption is endemic in this country although the Saudis may not think of it as such," he concluded.

"They just consider the agent's commission as an ordinary part of the business transaction," explained Tom. "The role of the agent and his usefulness in buying 'influence' has been recognized since biblical times. This system is traditional in the Middle East and has been going on for two thousand years. It won't go away easily.

"The Western concept of corruption is meaningless to the Saudis," he added. "If the agent performs his brokerage successfully, he is indispensable in their view, and they are willing to pay for it.

"Moreover," Tom added, "the French and the English do not hesitate to pay these excessive fees. They just add the commission to the price of the contract paid by the foreign customer."

"In fact, an American hospital-supply company paid $5 million in such fees to get a $50-million contract to equip your new King Faisal Hospital," Henry said to me. "It was before the present management took over. The payoffs went to people of power in the Saudi government, and the American supply company allegedly compensated for the payoffs by marking up the price of the goods sold to the hospital under the equipment contract."

"I remember reading about it in the newspapers," Tom said. "It's a common practice in Saudi Arabia."

Dinner was superb. It began with shrimp from the Arabian Gulf and was followed by hamour, a fish which tasted like salmon, served cold with mayonnaise. The main course was filet mignon. There was fresh fruit for dessert, followed by cheese and crackers.

We took turns dancing with the ladies, who fortunately were expert. I like to dance and am always grateful and relieved when I have a good partner. Since we had more men than women at our table, we had plenty of opportunity to continue our conversation after dinner.

Henry told us of several Saudis who had amassed great fortunes by taking advantage of their family connections with the royals. "Two were doctors' sons," he said. "One is Adnan Khashoggi, whose father was a physician and confidant to the fabled King Ibn Saud, and the other is Ghaith Pharaon, whose father was a physician and a close advisor to King Faisal, and now to King Khalid. Both were educated in the U.S., both made great fortunes through their fathers' influence, and both now have world-wide financial empires."

"And both have controlling interests in some U.S. banks," Tom added. "Ghaith Pharaon has contracted for much of the construction work on the roads and sewers of Mecca, Riyadh, and Jidda, and is engaged in world-wide construction engineering. His other operations as chairman of the Saudi Research and Development Corporation include insurance, steel, shipping, and banking. He travels in his Boeing 707 to the companies' branch offices in London and Paris, making lavish new deals with large international consortiums."

Khashoggi is the more flamboyant of the two according to Henry. He owns a Boeing 727 with its own apartment and offices, to symbolize the new Arab wealth, and a magnificent yacht, which he puts at the disposal of his clients. He has made billions by acting as agent for companies selling military equipment, such as French tankers, British helicopters, and American combat planes. He became an agent for Lockheed at twenty-six. In the 1970s, Lockheed's sales of military equipment to Saudi Arabia were about $1 billion a year, and they paid Khashoggi $100 million to "influence" the right people in the Saudi government. Later there was a scandal when it was learned that Lockheed was paying him an additional $200,000 per aircraft for "under-the-table compensation," agents' fees, and "commissions."

Then Henry told us that Northrop, in 1975, had a $1 billion contract with the Saudi air force. Khashoggi, as their agent, received $50 million. However, the Pentagon learned that he had in turn paid almost a half million dollars to two Saudi generals in the air force, and tried to intervene, but Khashoggi eventually won the dispute. He depicted himself as a bridge between two cultures and two concepts of morality. It was a situation, Khashoggi told the Pentagon, of a highly organized industrial bureaucracy confronting a resourceful representative of feudal princes. "You cannot transport American morality," he insisted.

"Amen to that," Tom said.

"But eventually the U.S. won the argument," Henry said. "When Raytheon sold $1.5 billion of HAWK air-defense weapons systems to Saudi Arabia, with Khashoggi as the agent, the Saudis decreed that there would be no further agents' fees for the sales of arms.

"And speaking of using influence in high places," he continued, "Aramco hired the famous British Arabist Harry St. John Philby to use his influence with King Ibn Saud to give them the original oil concession. Philby was an advisor to the King and a close friend for many years."

"I used to see Philby driving around the compound in an old, broken-down Nash automobile," said Tom, laughing. "Aramco probably paid him one hundred dollars and a skin of goat's milk as a commission.

"Another family which benefited from a 'friend at court' was the Juffali family," he said, "close friends of King Ibn Saud. The firm, Juffali and Brothers, had contracts to bring electricity to Mecca and the telephone system to Jidda, and it started the country's cement industry. It acts as a sales agent in Saudi Arabia for about three hundred major international companies, such as IBM, Volkswagen, Borg-Warner, Michelin, and so forth. You can imagine their profits."

"And they pay no income tax," added Henry.

It was approaching midnight. We had been drinking, dining, dancing, and discussing for almost four hours. The people about us were beginning to depart.

As we rose to leave, I said, "There's one more thing I would like to do tonight."

"What's that?" Mary asked.

"Swim in the Arabian Gulf," I said wistfully.

There was a dead silence, following which the ladies politely told me they thought I was insane.

"Maybe it's the sadiki," I said, "or the climate."

"It's probably the full moon," Tricia offered.

"It may be difficult to get out of the compound at this hour," Mel said, "but I may be able to arrange it; and I have some extra swim suits at home."

Ron enthusiastically endorsed the idea. The ladies, however, announced that they would wait for us at the Gilberts' home.

We drove back to Mel's house, put on our bathing trunks, and were on our way.

In about ten minutes we arrived at the gate. As Mel had predicted, the security guard hesitated to allow us to pass, but Mel knew or had treated a number of them. The guard made some phone calls and finally opened the gate reluctantly. A few miles further on we came upon a great inlet of the Arabian Gulf, which had been named Half Moon Bay by some nostalgic Californian. It was only ten miles from Dhahran. We could see miles of beach and soft sand dunes sloping downward to the sea.

In the brilliance of the full moon, the water appeared highly phosphorescent. As I plunged into the warm sea, my body was outlined by a flickering blue-white light, which turned on at the slightest movement as though controlled by an electric light switch. As the other men swam about me, the motion of their arms and legs made a swirling circle of glistening droplets. I saw Mel and Ron swim by, surrounded by nimbuses of white-blue light, leaving behind them wakes of whirling sparks like those from a meteor.

The water was so salty I seemed to remain on the surface indefinitely and probably could have gone to sleep without fear of sinking. I floated on top of that warm, gently swaying bed of water, gazing up at the stars, which seemed close enough to reach out and touch.

We were engulfed in heavy silence except for the quiet, rhythmic lapping of the sea against the shore. I felt again the sense of timelessness and mystery which I had experienced in the desert. Here the sea, bathed in moonlight, seemed to conjure up romance and adventure.

In the distance, I could see the glowing gas flares reaching toward the sky. There, from deep within the earth, flowed the energy which nurtured the Western world and kept it alive. Here I am, I thought, only a few miles away from where it all began.

◇ *18* ◇

THE KINGMAKER: HOW RICH IS RICH?

I WAS SITTING in my office at the hospital when the phone rang. It was John Barrow, the assistant to the Executive Director and a troubleshooter for the royal family.

"Seymour, we have another crisis," he began. "Frank Taylor asked me to call you."

"What is it this time?" I asked. If Barrow was involved it meant that the patient was a royal, and that it was probably a relatively minor problem. I was well aware by now that every time a Saudi prince coughed it was deemed a crisis.

"This is a very important patient," Barrow assured me. "We have an appointment to examine him at his palace this afternoon."

"Why can't he come to the hospital?" I asked. "According to the regulations our doctors are not supposed to examine patients outside the hospital."

"This is a special request from the King himself. The patient's name is Prince Ibrahim Mugrin el-Kabir. Does that mean anything to you?"

"He's one of the royals," I shrugged.

"He's one of the *original* royals who helped King Abdul Aziz conquer the Nejd," said Barrow, trying to impress me. "El-Kabir means 'The Great.' The prince happens to be one of the most politically influential men in the kingdom and is probably one of the richest. If I told you how much money he has you wouldn't believe me."

"Try me. I have a pretty vivid imagination."

"All right. He owns Haradh."

"What do you mean?"

"He owns the town of Haradh. As a young man, he fought side by side with the King, who later gave him the town of Haradh as a present."

I began to laugh. "You're right. I can't imagine it."

Barrow chuckled. "I'll come by and pick you up at two o'clock. We can talk football on the way out."

Barrow was a football fan. What he missed most about America was football, and he loved to talk about it. Whenever we met, he insisted on reporting all the football news, which he had gleaned from the *International*

Herald Tribune and from a copy of *Sporting News* that a friend regularly sent him from the U.S.

That afternoon, he picked me up in a hospital car and drove me out toward the Mecca Road to the palace of Prince Ibrahim. Barrow had established himself as the liaison between the royal family and the hospital, and although he was sometimes sycophantic when dealing with the top royals he was genuinely interested in people. He served as a public-relations man for the hospital and was the official greeter. Barrow had been in Saudi Arabia for a number of years, and spoke enough Arabic to get around and develop valuable friendships among the Saudis.

For the first several miles we talked football, or rather Barrow talked while I nodded and stared out the window. Then we began to discuss the patient. Barrow knew almost nothing about his medical condition. However, he knew the prince's political and financial condition very well indeed.

"The prince is rich beyond imagination," he told me. "He's worth about $30 to 35 billion, but that is only a guess. His holdings are so extensive that nobody really knows how wealthy he is and probably won't know until he dies and they add it all up for his estate."

With my encouragement, Barrow began to outline the prince's background. Prince Ibrahim had joined King Ibn Saud during the long and grueling wars between 1901 and 1926 that ultimately enabled the House of Saud to conquer and unify all of Arabia. Although overshadowed by the charismatic King, Ibrahim had been a valiant fighter and was a key member of the small inner circle that dominated the Saud family and Saudi Arabian politics. In fact he was a member of the council which had selected Khalid as King.

Ibrahim had distinguished himself in the conquest of the Nejd and the Eastern Region. When control of Saudi Arabia was achieved, the grateful Ibn Saud rewarded him with an area around the Al Hasa Oasis which included the town of Haradh. Although the area did not amount to much at the time, some twenty years later it proved to be in the center of rich oil and gas deposits, and made Prince Ibrahim a tycoon.

Much of his wealth, however, was derived from his own efforts in developing Haradh. In the early days the town was little more than an oasis for herders and Bedouins and much of it was uninhabited desert land. In the next fifty years, Ibrahim turned the area into the breadbasket of Saudi Arabia. He pioneered the initial phases of the Haradh land-reclamation project. Artesian wells were dug and extensive irrigation undertaken. Electricity was introduced, and so was modern mechanized farming.

"Today," said Barrow, "Haradh is a rich agricultural center cultivated by tenant farmers. The prince still owns most of his land, and you know how real estate has increased in value the last five years. It's out of sight!"

After a few minutes we approached Prince Ibrahim's palace. I was surprised by the curiously nondescript appearance of the surrounding area. In contrast to the green, landscaped lawns which often herald the approach to palatial homes, the palace was surrounded by a cluster of shabby, crumbling mud-brick houses, cluttered with rubbish. There were no roads leading to or from these huts, only dirt paths which wound across the hard, rocky ground. What people I could see looked poverty-stricken. It was hardly the sort of neighborhood that one envisioned for the richest man in Saudi Arabia. It reminded me of the decaying inner cities in the U.S. which were crying out for urban renewal.

Later, I learned that some of the people in the grimy mud huts were former slaves of Prince Ibrahim, who had left the palace in 1962 when slavery was abolished in Saudi Arabia. The destitution that surrounded the palace served as a reminder for the numerous ex-slaves who chose to remain with the prince and who lived on the palace grounds in relative comfort, content with their lot despite their meager pay. The old prince was obviously not a charitable man.

The palace itself was surrounded by a high, impressive stone wall. As we approached, two servants dressed in guardlike uniforms swung open the ornate iron-grillwork gate, and Barrow drove slowly into the compound. The palace itself was very old, and its overall dimensions were enormous, as big as the largest castles in Europe. The palace compound contained separate servants' quarters, a wing for the prince's four wives, small villas for his secretary and for his private physician, and a private mosque, where the highly religious prince performed his daily prayers. Although the scale of the compound was impressive, its condition was not. The buildings in Saudi Arabia deteriorate quickly, and the palace had not been well maintained. The cement was cracking, and in places the edges of the buildings were beginning to crumble. The elaborate flower gardens surrounding the palace were overgrown and unkempt, and seemed to belong to another era. In all, the palace appeared antiquated and in disrepair, reminiscent of our great old deserted mansions in the South after the Civil War. Somehow, *Gone With the Wind* came to mind!

The servants greeted Barrow, who had been there before. One of them led us into the palace while another took our car around to the garage. The interior of the palace was of typical Saudi design, with high ceilings to keep the rooms cool. The walls were the ubiquitous Islamic green, but the paint was badly faded and it underscored the drab, rundown feeling of the place. Because of the Islamic injunction against adornment, the walls were bare, and the furnishings were of an ornate French style that managed to be large, heavy, and lifeless all at the same time. The whole ambiance of the palace seemed empty and desolate.

Prince Ibrahim's secretary soon joined us, speaking fluent English in a crisp British accent. He impressed me as one of the most efficient Saudis that I had ever met. Later, I learned that he was more of a business manager than a secretary, and that his job was to supervise all the prince's properties and business affairs. A few minutes later Dr. Ghandour arrived. He lived in the compound and was the physician in charge of the prince's ménage—the wives, children, and servants, involving a total of about 500 people.

Dr. Ghandour and the secretary had both noted a change in the prince. Not only was he becoming more forgetful, but he seemed to be unable to express himself. This speech difficulty had appeared only recently and was of great concern to both the prince and his family. He apparently knew what he wanted to say but could not say it or write it. He was still able to walk about and function normally, but he was forced to gesture in order to express himself, and his speech had become garbled. Dr. Ghandour added that the prince's blood pressure was higher than usual. The prince refused to go to the hospital for an examination, and since he was one of the King's closest advisors on family and Saudi political matters the King ordered the hospital to come to the prince.

I had brought the prince's medical record with me from the hospital. He had been examined by a urologist six months earlier. The only complaint of this ninety-year-old prince was that of "decreased sexual prowess." According to the report the prince had not fathered a child for about five years, since he was eighty-five, and he wanted something done about it. He was suffering from "feelings of inadequacy," according to the urologist.

As we were discussing the prince's physical condition, a small elderly man wearing glasses walked into the room. We all stood up: it was Prince Ibrahim. The prince was dressed in the typical white Saudi thobe, over which he was wearing an incongruous English tweed jacket. He was smaller than I had expected, for most of the men in the royal family stand well over six feet tall, and the prince was at most five feet seven. Later I would decide that he probably suffered from "short man's syndrome," a series of aggressive, stubborn personality traits that are associated with people who resent their physical stature. It did not surprise me that the prince liked John Barrow: John was even shorter than he was.

Dr. Ghandour introduced me to his royal highness. The prince sat down in a tall armchair, and a servant immediately appeared with a pot of cardamom coffee, which was quickly followed by a serving of the traditional tea. The prince sat silently, staring into his coffee cup as if indifferent to our presence. Hesitantly, Barrow asked him a question about his health, but the prince dismissed it with a shrug and a wave of his hand. He tried to speak but his words lacked coherence. This put an effective silence over everyone, and we sat wordlessly sipping our tea.

At length, I turned toward the secretary, and said that I would like to perform a physical examination. The secretary obsequiously broached the matter to the prince. He nodded, then rose and walked through the doorway, while the secretary motioned for me to follow.

Down the long hallway we walked until we arrived at an old ornate gilded elevator. The prince was obviously proud of this very modern contraption in his very old palace. He glanced at me to see if I was impressed. It reminded me somewhat of the cagelike gold lift at the Connaught Hotel in London.

"Magnificent elevator," I murmured. Barrow translated with an ingratiating smile. The prince looked pleased.

We took the elevator to the second floor, proceeded down another gloomy long hallway and finally entered a huge room carpeted with beautiful Chinese rugs. Here the secretary translated my instructions for the prince to disrobe and then discreetly withdrew to an adjoining room. While the prince was removing his tweed jacket and thobe I wandered about the room inspecting the very ancient furnishings, some of which were inlaid with gold. The room was more like a museum than a bedroom except for the presence of a huge ornate bed, which made the short old man atop it appear pitifully small and impotent.

With Dr. Ghandour serving as an interpreter I examined the prince, keeping in mind the very real possibility that a stroke was imminent, in view of his age, high blood pressure, and speech difficulties. The prince submitted grudgingly to the examination. After it was completed, I called the secretary and discussed my findings with him and with Dr. Ghandour: the prince's inability to speak was probably a form of expressive aphasia, caused by an injury or small stroke in the speech center of the brain. The prince understood written or spoken words and knew what he wished to say but could not utter the actual words.

"There is no weakness in his limbs, and his reflexes are normal," I concluded. "I doubt that he has had a major stroke, but he is certainly a candidate for one."

"What do you suggest?" asked the secretary.

"Have him admitted to the hospital," I stated bluntly. "He should have a thorough battery of tests and a brain scan to determine the cause of the speech difficulty."

The secretary shrugged uncomfortably, indicating that it was a decision that remained with the prince. At my urging, he asked the prince to reconsider a visit to the hospital. The obdurate prince shook his head, rejecting the proposal with a series of vigorous gestures and grunts.

"If he insists on avoiding the hospital, then he must limit his activities and get plenty of rest," I advised. "What is his schedule during the day?"

"He has a council meeting with the King scheduled for this evening," answered the secretary, "and a ministers' meeting tomorrow. Then there is a *majlis* in the early afternoon, and a meeting with government functionaries later."

I looked at him, shaking my head. "He'll never make it," I said. "Tell him that if he doesn't slow down now his body will make him slow down."

The secretary said nothing.

Outside, the prince led us on a tour through his gardens, pointing silently to certain flowers and trees that, according to the secretary, had been specially imported for the prince.

At the end of the path the prince shook our hands and then left to pray in his private mosque on the east side of the palace compound. While we were returning to our car I told the secretary that I would send back a diet and some medicine to help lower the prince's blood pressure. Dr. Ghandour approved, and offered to arrange for a nutritionist. The secretary said he would dispatch a car and a courier to the hospital to bring back the medication.

I left the palace with the sense of frustration that every doctor experiences when a patient refuses to follow sound medical advice. The prince, I was sure, would be visiting the hospital soon enough, but by that time it would be a real "crisis." Worse, I had a feeling that because of his age his next visit to the hospital would probably be his last.

Five days later, while making my rounds in the hospital, I received the emergency call that I expected and feared: Prince Ibrahim had collapsed at home, apparently suffering from a massive stroke. He had lost his power of speech completely and the right side of his body was paralyzed. Incredibly, the prince still refused to come to the hospital, and only upon the insistence of the King did he consent to a brief visit for laboratory tests and x-rays.

Prince Ibrahim arrived by special ambulance that evening at 9 P.M., accompanied by Dr. Ghandour and three black limousines carrying his immediate entourage. The prince was agitated and cantankerous, indicating with wild grunts and gestures that he was being forced to do this against his will and that he wanted to return to the palace immediately. His agitation was so severe that I felt it necessary to administer a sedative by injection. The prince was then taken to the x-ray and laboratory areas, where a brain scan revealed a blockage of one of the major blood vessels in the brain.

Obviously he could not leave the hospital. I called the neurologist and neurosurgeon in consultation and arranged for his hospitalization. An area on the third floor was set aside for the prince, and it was quickly transformed into a suite that befitted the richest man in Saudi Arabia. Furnishings were brought in that reflected the prince's taste for French décor, and cushioned chairs and sofas were installed in the hallway for his visitors. Each day fresh flowers arrived in quantities surpassing those sent to Princess Sultana. When the prince was allowed visitors, the number quickly grew so large that the corridor outside his room had to be cordoned off like a popular exhibit in a museum.

Among the prince's daily visitors were King Khalid and Prince Fahd. They usually arrived before the midday prayers, visited Prince Ibrahim very briefly, and then sat down to talk with his family, most of whom were cousins. As the convalescence stretched into weeks they began to come singly on alternating days, but either the King or Prince Fahd always appeared for the daily visit. Two or more of the prince's twenty-three sons were in constant attendance upon their father. Curiously, no women ever visited the prince, not even his wives. When I asked about this, the sons simply said that the women were not permitted to visit him. There was no further explanation until much later.

As the horde of visitors grew larger, I attempted to limit the number of visitors and the visiting hours, hoping to give the prince a respite. In this effort I was totally unsuccessful, for the visitors included the most eminent men in the kingdom. Tactfully but insistently, the royals let me know that this was their hospital, and that nobody was going to keep them from paying their respects to the prince. They did, however, agree to keep the visits short and to come within certain specified hours of the day. Actually I had a feeling that they came primarily to visit with each other and to demonstrate their fealty to the family. Since the prince could not speak they spent no more than five minutes with him, just to put in an appearance.

Although the prince had two male nurses in constant attendance, his sons established a twenty-four-hour vigil, which they operated as efficiently as a military guard. The sons took turns according to a fixed schedule, rotating every six to eight hours, with two sons present at all times. At first I was impressed by this show of family devotion, but I learned later that there might be another reason for the round-the-clock watch. Prince Ibrahim had not written a will, and if he died without drafting one then the estate would be divided according to Koranic law and everyone would receive a share. However, if the prince decided to draft a will, then some family members might be deprived of inheritances worth literally billions of dollars. Thus, it appeared to me that the vigil was designed to "protect" the prince from people seeking favorable treatment in his will.

As the prince's stay stretched into weeks and months, I began to discern the fractious and divisive schisms that lay beneath the placid surface of the Saudi royal family. It seems that the sons were suspicious of each other and of the prince's wives, particularly the youngest wife, who was allegedly a "schemer." I noticed that the two sons in attendance were usually of disparate ages, one older and one younger, and I soon learned that they were paired so that they represented different mothers and different branches of the family. Keeping the women away from the prince and keeping a strict two-man rotation was their way of ensuring that the status quo was maintained within the family. It was a Saudi solution to the problem and a very effective one.

Still, I felt more and more sympathy for the prince. Apparently because of family jealousies he was being put under a virtual quarantine and was denied visits from his wives and daughters. It seemed like a sad and cruel fate for an old man, and particularly ironic for someone who could legitimately claim to be one of the richest men in the kingdom. I didn't like the strange and subtle games that were being played with my patient, and yet I felt powerless to stop them. All I could do was provide good medical care and keep a sharp eye on everything that was going on.

Because of his genuine concern for the prince's health, the King requested that we call in some consultants from the outside to make certain that everything possible was being done. Our neurologist, an Englishman, selected the most distinguished neurologist in London, who was flown in by special jet. He checked the x-rays and the laboratory reports, examined the prince at great length, and then agreed with the diagnosis and the course of treatment. I selected an expert on strokes from the Massachusetts General Hospital in Boston, and a visa to enter the country was arranged through the Saudi Arabian embassy in Washington. The specialist, a friend of mine, arrived after a long, grueling flight, slept for two days, then devoted a full day to examining the prince and reviewing all the data. He then spent another day reassuring the family that he concurred with the diagnosis and treatment, and that nothing further could be done. Although these consultations were exorbitantly expensive, they were worthwhile because they gave the royal family a sense of security and confidence in the new hospital. At the same time, it was gratifying to me that there was no talk of flying the prince to London for treatment. In fact, they told me afterward that they preferred the American consultant because he had spent much more time talking to the family.

A few weeks later there was an emergency call from the prince's nurse. The prince had suddenly developed a cough, severe chest pain, and shortness of breath.

"His lips are blue, and his breathing is labored," she added. "He looks terrible."

"Sounds like a pulmonary embolism," I said. "Give him some oxygen, order an emergency portable chest x-ray and an electrocardiogram. I'll be right over."

Pulmonary embolism is a common and often fatal complication in elderly people who are bedridden or inactive. The patient develops inflammation in the leg veins, where small clots develop (thrombophlebitis). The clots (emboli) may break off and travel to the lungs, obstructing the circulation. We had done everything possible to prevent this complication, such as mobilizing the prince as much as possible and having him perform leg exercises.

We had considered treating him with anticoagulants to prevent the clots from forming but decided that this was too great a risk because the anticoagulant might produce hemorrhage in the stroke area of his brain. Actually we had discussed this problem with the consulting neurologist. Now our hand was forced. In spite of the risk, we had no choice but to administer an anticoagulant to prevent extension of the clots and further embolism to the lungs. The dose of anticoagulant was regulated carefully, and the blood's ability to clot was measured daily. Too much anticoagulant might produce hemorrhage and too little might result in further pulmonary embolism. We were on the horns of a dilemma.

The prince responded well to the anticoagulant medication, which was given daily at 4 P.M. Within a few days the chest pain and shortness of breath disappeared, and he appeared to be on the road to recovery from his pulmonary embolism. The plan now was to keep him on this treatment indefinitely to prevent further complications.

Then, one afternoon at 4:15 P.M., about a month later, there was another urgent phone call. It was the medication nurse on the prince's floor. She was almost hysterical.

"Please come over right now," she cried. "Something *terrible* has happened."

Rushing to the floor I found the nurse standing in the hallway, wiping tears from her eyes. "The prince was given an overdose of anticoagulant," she sobbed. "It's all my fault."

She went on to give me the details. The hospital shifts had changed at 4 P.M., and the previous nurse had administered the anticoagulant just before going off duty. Unfortunately, she had recorded it at the bottom of the medical chart, and the page had accidentally folded so the entry was not visible. The nurse coming on duty saw no record of treatment, and had proceeded to give the prince a second dosage of the anticoagulant. When she went to record it she found the first entry. She was well aware that an overdose could produce a fatal hemorrhage in an elderly patient who had suffered a stroke.

"Don't panic," I said. "Since the anticoagulant was given orally we have a few hours before it takes full effect. There is an antidote which counteracts the anticoagulant very quickly and effectively and returns the blood coagulation to normal. It is vitamin K_1 and can be given by mouth or by injection."

I went on to explain that the trick was to give the right amount of vitamin K_1. If we gave too much it would completely counteract all the anticoagulant effect, but the prince would be faced again with the clotting hazards and pulmonary embolism which existed prior to the anticoagulant treatment. If we gave too little vitamin K_1 he would bleed for sure.

"Thanks to you," I said, "we know the exact amount of anticoagulant you just administered. There is a formula for the dose of vitamin K_1 necessary to make the correction, without restoring the conditions which originally permitted the embolism to occur. Now where the hell is that formula?"

The library did not yet exist, but I had shipped a trunkful of books from Boston. In fact, I had sent pencils, rulers, rubber bands, dictionaries, etc., which amused my secretary because the hospital was well stocked with all the newest office equipment and supplies. I walked quickly to my office, pulled out the books which might have the necessary information, and within ten minutes I found the appropriate dose of vitamin K_1 necessary to correct the excess anticoagulant administered.

I phoned the hospital pharmacy and ordered the vitamin K_1, which was delivered directly to the prince's floor. By the time I arrived back at his bedside the antidote was waiting for me. I administered it to the prince at about 5 P.M., a little more than an hour after the accidental overdose. We closely monitored his condition the rest of the night, and by morning the blood coagulation test was exactly where we wanted it to be. While the nursing staff and I had a restless night, the prince slept blissfully through it all.

Medicine is not an exact science, although it is becoming more laboratory-oriented and scientific every year, particularly American medicine, which leads the world in its scientific approach. Sadly the laboratory advance is often at the expense of the humanistic dimension and the clinical art of medicine. Yet science and the laboratory probably saved the prince's life that afternoon. Since all went well, I saw no reason for reporting the accident to the family at that moment, but I did tell the whole story to his sons months later.

It was my responsibility to report the incident to the medical director and to the nursing office, although I was reluctant to do so. In the report I made a special effort to commend the nurse highly for her professionalism and integrity. If she had not brought the matter to my attention promptly her error would never have been discovered, because the prince would have died from a brain hemorrhage which would have been considered natural for a ninety-year-old man who had suffered a stroke and had high blood pressure. It is often said that doctors bury their mistakes. Mistakes in judgment and in treatment are inevitable. Rectifying this human error promptly had demonstrated that the entire hospital organization could react efficiently and competently in an emergency situation. The hospital was young, multilingual and multinational. It was maturing very quickly indeed.

The hospital administration thanked me for the report and adjusted the format for recording medications. No further action was taken. I was still very proud of that nurse! She completed her two-year tour of duty and returned to the United States.

As the weeks slowly turned into months, Prince Ibrahim showed signs of improvement. Although the right side of his body remained paralyzed, he began to develop some garbled speech and a limited ability to communicate. Gradually, he recovered sufficiently to "talk" with me during my daily visits. As his speech improved, his old arrogance disappeared; this irascible old man seemed to have mellowed from the experience. At times he would try to answer my questions with garbled Arabic. When this proved too difficult he would simply smile and squeeze my hand.

As his health improved, the prince became restive and wanted to return home. He took small trips outside the hospital by wheelchair and by automobile, always accompanied by two of his sons and a male nurse. Somehow, he never made it back to the palace. With the prince's improving health, the family vigil grew more complicated, for his activity seemed to increase the possibility that he might write a will after all. The sons began to approach me, one by one, stressing the confidentiality of our conversation and inquiring whether their father was "mentally competent." I assured them that at this point he was probably competent, an answer that did nothing to assuage their anxieties. I learned later that they had put the same questions to the neurologist from the U.S.

At length, after six months had passed, I suggested to the family that the prince might be happier if he was discharged from the hospital and sent home. The nurses could go with him, and the laboratory tests could be brought to the hospital each day by limousine. Besides, his treatment in the hospital now consisted primarily of physiotherapy and the anticoagulant medication, which he took orally. This treatment could be given at home just as easily as at the hospital. However, the sons were dismayed by my suggestion, and were adamant in their resolve to keep their father in the hospital. Clearly they intended to keep the old prince under constant surveillance.

I was troubled by the situation, and I began to make discreet inquiries to the top officials in the hospital as to whether I had the power to discharge the prince on my own. Their answers were uneasy and ambiguous: I did, but at the same time I didn't. Like everything else in Saudi Arabia, hospital policy often took a back seat to the wishes of the royal family. The administration decided that, since the prince arguably still needed the care available in the hospital, they could not discharge him against the family wishes, no matter how long it took.

I thought that Barrow would side with the prince, who now appeared very anxious to go home, but he went along with the dictum of the family. Although he visited the prince daily and appeared genuinely interested in his welfare, he spent a good deal of time with some of the prince's sons.

I was particularly impressed by a young man named Ahmad, who had spent four years at the Colorado School of Mines and spoke English fluently. He seemed genuinely concerned with his father's welfare.

"Young people in the U.S. do not really appreciate their country," he remarked one day when we happened to meet outside the prince's room. That remark, of course, endeared him to me. Over the months we spoke frequently, and he gave me considerable insight into his father's life and into his own.

"My father has been a fighter all his life," said Ahmad with pride. "He lived in the shadow of King Abdul-Aziz, and he had to fight to maintain his own identity." Ahmad described his father as a very religious man, and one who believed in the Wahabi principles. "As a father he was a strict disciplinarian, and when we misbehaved he would not hesitate to give us a beating. But he also took very good care of us. When I went to the United States to study he bought me a two-acre estate in the best section of town. I lived in a bigger house than most of my professors."

"Your income is much bigger than theirs," I said.

"All the princes throughout the country get $5,000 [U.S.] monthly when we become eighteen years of age, and this increases as we get older," he volunteered. "My father gave me the money to buy the estate, and it was a good investment."

"Your father is very wealthy," I said, "and that is the understatement of the year. Does he also receive a stipend from the government?"

"In a way my father is a kingmaker," said Ahmad. "He serves on the Royal Cabinet, and the government pays him about $30,000 a month."

Ahmad emphasized that his father demanded respect from everyone, particularly from his family, and that he always preached family unity. Consequently the children had their meals together, and were attended by all four wives so that the half brothers and sisters would have a feeling of a strong family affiliation.

"There is no difference between any of us," said Ahmad. "We are all brothers, we are all our father's sons."

A year had now passed and the prince was still in the hospital. I asked Ahmad one day whether the family was being fair to his father.

"You know," I said, "that the Saudis prefer to die at home, the Bedouin and royal family alike. Your father craves to go home, and he is a very old man. He has now been here for more than a year. Do you want him to die in the hospital, away from his palace?"

Ahmad tried to explain the intricacies of the family, and the reason that they wanted to keep the prince in the hospital.

"The wives would drive him crazy if he went home," he said. "They would bicker over who got what share of his property, and he would never have any peace. The youngest wife is only thirty-five and she would be the most demanding. It is a difficult situation. We are doing this for his own good."

It appeared to me that it was also in the sons' self-interest to keep the prince isolated from his wives or from anyone else who might make financial demands upon their father.

I could not resist remarking that the level of family unity seemed a little strained, given the suspicion that seemed to motivate the family vigil. I expected Ahmad to deny this; instead he shook his head sadly.

"Yes, it is true that we have distrust and jealousies in the family. My father tried to teach us differently, but he was not entirely successful." Ahmad shrugged. "There are some things that even a great man cannot do in one lifetime."

Prince Ibrahim remained in the King Faisal Hospital for almost fourteen months. Although he was taken on numerous outings, he never returned home.

On a sunny morning in November he suffered another massive stroke on the left side of his brain, and he died quickly and quietly in the hospital, which had become his second home, the hospital he had hated and feared. The family was in attendance but only the male part of the family.

Prince Ibrahim's death I thought would be an occasion for national mourning and ceremony, to pay homage to a man of his stature who had contributed so much to the founding of the nation. But this would not be appropriate according to the ultraconservative Wahabi tenets. Death is only a state of transition. Once a person dies his body is of little consequence. Burial was quick and simple. There were no tombs or monuments. There was nothing to distinguish the grave of this prince from that of the simplest Bedouin. Only rough stones marked the head and foot of the grave, which would soon be obliterated by the blowing sands. The wives merely secluded themselves at home for four months and ten days—no more, no less.

The prince left no will and so his estate, valued at about $32 billion, was settled according to Koranic law. One-eighth of the estate—some $4 billion—was divided among his four wives. The remaining $28 billion went to his twenty-three sons and eleven daughters. According to the law the male offspring received twice as large a share as the female offspring. Thus, each son inherited about $980 million. The daughters, who had not seen their father during the last sixteen months of his life, had to make do with roughly $490 million each. Of course, much of this was in the form of land and other properties not readily negotiable.

Ahmad told me that the wives would not be able to remove any of their billions from the country and that their lifestyle would not change significantly. Their children, in turn, would be the beneficiaries.

"What is the inheritance tax?" I asked.

"Saudi citizens pay no inheritance tax," he answered, "lucky for us."

"How do I become a citizen?" I said, laughing.

I was surprised to learn that no part of this huge estate went to charity. Ahmad explained that the Koran requires Moslems to give alms to the poor, particularly during the holy month of Ramadan, when everyone is obliged to give food, clothing, or money to the needy each year. Ahmad said that his father as a religious man had already fulfilled this obligation.

"Charity is accountable only to God," he said. He told me that the only tax, called *zakat,* was a small, traditional religious tax of 2.5 percent on income and property. It was a nominal tax which the government collected and distributed to its needy citizens. In these days of affluence, however, the tax was not enforced very vigorously.

And so this ninety-year-old prince, a pioneer, a maker of kings and a builder of his own immense empire, simply passed from the scene without applause or accolade. He died a pathetic and isolated old man, prisoner to his wealth and to the family he had raised so carefully.

Barrow fared very well. He was appointed by the Saudi government to head a Swedish consortium which had contracted to build and manage a number of Saudi Arabian military hospitals throughout the country.

Kings, these days, must stick together! The King of Sweden came to visit King Khalid and shortly thereafter the costly projects were announced. Within a few months, Barrow moved from his tiny nondescript apartment to a magnificent villa replete with servants, limousines, and a chauffeur.

◊ *19* ◊

A ROYAL PARTY

THE BIRTH OF A SON in Saudi Arabia is a happy event, and the arrival of the first male, particularly if he is a royal, is a most auspicious occasion. On the wedding day, friends traditionally wish the young couple "many sons," and the bride prays for one because her marriage depends on it. A man's standing in the community often depends upon the number of sons he has sired. The older generation of royals frequently had twenty or more.

In the Arab world, the double standard for men and women begins at birth. Centuries ago female infanticide was practiced although Mohammed preached against it. Girls were tolerated as a first-born but the tolerance diminished with each successive female birth. The disappointment at a girl's birth soon changed into apprehension that she might bring further shame and disgrace upon her father by infringing upon the moral code. In some instances a daughter could be put to death by her father if she brought dishonor upon the family.

I first met Prince Khalil when he was a patient in the hospital. Over a period of time we became friends, and he invited me to his home to celebrate the birth of his first son.

It was a celebration for all of us because the delivery of his son at the King Faisal Hospital had precipitated a crisis which was resolved happily. When the hospital had first opened, Dr. Jonathan Warren, the highly respected head of the Department of Obstetrics, had delivered Prince Khalil's first child, a daughter, by Caesarean section. Two years later, Khalil's wife was again pregnant and wished to have Dr. Warren as her obstetrician, but he had returned to London at the expiration of his contract. Khalil had considerable confidence in Dr. Warren and furthermore felt he wouldn't dare deliver two girls in a row. When he told the administration that he wanted Dr. Warren to deliver his second child, they objected on the grounds that Dr. Warren was no longer on the staff and therefore not qualified to use their facilities.

Prince Khalil then had the choice of either sending his wife to England for the delivery or selecting another hospital in which Dr. Warren could deliver his baby. He investigated available hospitals in Riyadh and Jidda and found them unacceptable. The prince then pulled rank and demanded that Dr. Warren be reinstated so that he could deliver the baby at the King Faisal Hospital. A stormy meeting of the Medical Advisory Board ensued over the issue. The administration felt that allowing a physician who was no longer on the staff to deliver a baby would open the door to many unqualified physicians; and this was a closed hospital.

I favored making an exception in the case of Dr. Warren because he had only recently left the staff and had been treating the patient during her pregnancy. The Associate Director of Medical Affairs threatened to resign. Finally, the Minister of Health overruled him and allowed Dr. Warren to be reinstated for one month so that he could deliver Prince Khalil's baby. When the due date drew near, Dr. Warren flew in from England, was reinstated, and delivered by Caesarean section an eight-pound boy.

Prince Khalil was thrilled. He reimbursed Dr. Warren handsomely for the delivery of his first son and sent gold watches to the obstetrical team involved: nurses, technicians, and anesthesiologists. Bending regulations again, the prince brought photographers into the hospital to make moving pictures of his son for posterity. Meanwhile, the Associate Director, who had resigned out of pique, was reinstated by the Minister of Health. A celebration was indeed in order.

The evening of the party, Philip Westbrook, Ron Lambrie, and I set out for Prince Khalil's home at nine o'clock. With us was an obstetrician named Trevor Evans, whom the prince had also invited. Trevor was a short, red-headed Irishman with a red mustache and an amusing tic which made him sniff through his nose and twitch his mustache at the same time whenever he became excited. He was an intelligent fellow but a bit eccentric.

Prince Khalil's mansion was in an exclusive residential area northwest of Riyadh, not far from the palaces of the King and the Crown Prince. We were met by servants in a walled-off courtyard, where they parked our car and then directed us to the entrance. The party was held in a separate wing of the mansion, which consisted of a large drawing room, three beautifully appointed bedrooms with colorful satin drapes, and a long, ornate dining room, with heavily carved French furniture and a chandelier centered over a long table with thirty high-backed mahogany chairs.

The drawing room, where the party began, was lined with heavy, carved Italian armchairs, interspersed with large velvet-and-gold cushions. There were bright Chinese rugs on the floor, and the walls were covered with textured carpeting. Ornate gold-framed mirrors reflected the light from another magnificent chandelier. The main attraction was the large

TV console, flanked on either side by elaborate video players, which occupied a third of one wall of the room.

No women were present, of course. Presumably, Prince Khalil's wife was in another wing of the house with her newborn son and servants. Prince Khalil greeted us warmly and directed us to the bar. We thought it was a mirage. The bar was stocked with everything from Chivas Regal, Courvoisier, and Benedictine to Dom Perignon 1959. Sudanese servants resplendent in turbans and white robes circulated among the guests serving drinks. Although alcohol is strictly illegal, it seems to find its way into some royal homes. Nobody knows for sure where it comes from but it is said that three times a year it arrives from Italy in zinc containers marked "office supplies."

The room rapidly filled with Prince Khalil's friends—all royals and look-alikes. Wearing their long white thobes, beige mantles lined with gold, polished black shoes, white ghutras and black circular headbands they almost flaunted their conformity. This was enhanced by their height, single-style mustache and beard, and their youth. They appeared to be between thirty and forty years old, and they were all cousins.

Our host introduced us to his friends. Many of them were, like Khalil, deputies in the various government agencies. Their education too was almost identical. After finishing the equivalent of high school in Saudi Arabia, they attended college in California for four years or more, and then returned to work in the ministries. This was the generation who would someday govern Saudi Arabia.

I expressed surprise when one prince told me he had recently completed his education in the United States. "You look much older," I said.

Khalil laughed. "Our headdress makes us look older than we are. How old do you think I am?" he asked as he removed his ghutra, exposing his pitch-black hair. "You see, I'm only thirty and you probably thought I was forty."

I admitted that the national dress often made the men look older because the ghutra covered their hair completely and obscured the contour of the face.

The guests continued to arrive at all hours, greeting each other effusively with handshakes and embraces that sometimes went on for minutes. Cousins kissed each other on the nose or cheek or on the lips. Baroque politeness seemed to be their tradition.

Khalil continued to circulate among his guests, receiving them with ritual and drama and making sure they all felt welcome. At one point he introduced us to a late arrival named Sam Stark, a young, pimply-faced

American who worked in the U.S. Consulate in Riyadh. He was inarticulate and unattractive and spoke not a word of Arabic. And he seemed to know very little about Saudi Arabia. I wondered how in the world he got his job.

Khalil seemed to read my mind. "Sam is probably a CIA agent," he said quietly with a half-smile.

I nodded. That would explain it. He simply couldn't be as insipid as he appeared.

The TV had been turned on. A taped English documentary was showing how Saudi soccer players, under the tutelage of the English, are selected and trained. The documentary closed with clips of a game between Oman and Saudi Arabia which the Saudis won. It was boring and most of the guests ignored it. The next program was a live question-and-answer period on religion, followed by a round-table discussion. Ten-minute prayer sessions were interspersed between programs.

After a while, Khalil turned off the TV and announced that he had a movie to show us. The lights dimmed and we stood around or sat on pillows facing one of the large screens. His pictures were of good quality. They showed a beaming Prince Khalil in the hospital corridor holding his newborn son, then other male members of his family similarly holding the infant. Then there were more pictures of the baby taken at home, again in the arms of his father and various men, including the servants. Not a single picture of the mother or the women in the family appeared, nor was Khalil's wife mentioned. Ron Lambrie and I had treated her and knew her quite well, but obviously Khalil would not put her on exhibit before his friends, even though all of them had already been exposed to Western culture.

TV has had a stormy history in Saudi Arabia. The Koranic injunction against making a graven image or likeness of any living thing is taken seriously in Islam, particularly by the Wahabis. They consider these images to be similar to the idols deified by other religions and therefore oppose photography. Originally King Ibn Saud assured the Ulema, the Council of Religious Scholars, that photography was actually good because it depicted Allah's creations without violating them. Aerial photography was crucial at the time in the search for oil deposits.

When television was introduced in 1965, there was a riot and the first transmitter was torn down by the fundamentalists. King Faisal finally convinced the Ulema that television was another means of spreading religious doctrine. At first, TV time was spent in the reading of the Koran or in other forms of religious programing. Although religious themes still predominate, there are now live quiz shows and cartoons. In the late hours Egyptian orchestras and singers appear quite regularly.

Few films are shown on Saudi television and public cinemas are banned in Saudi Arabia. The Wahabis feel that cinemas are contrary to Islam because the Koran states that when a man and a woman are in the same room the devil is between them. All the worse if the room is so dark that the faces cannot be seen. By contrast, cinemas abound in nearby Islamic Bahrain and Kuwait, once again demonstrating the powerful influence of Wahabism upon Saudi Arabia.

What followed next, therefore, came as a surprise, It was about eleven o'clock and still no food was in sight. Voices were becoming louder as our drinking continued without the beneficial effect of food in slowing down the absorption of alcohol. Prince Khalil announced that he "had a surprise for us in honor of Dr. Gray." With great ceremony he led me to a large, colorful tufted cushion in front of the video screen. Two smiling Sudanese servants brought in a large video cassette and inserted it into the video player before me and turned it on. It was the unexpurgated version of *Deep Throat!*

I was shocked, never having seen a pornographic film before. "I don't believe what I'm seeing," I said to Khalil, who had seated himself at my side. "I just can't believe it. I can't believe it," I kept repeating.

Everyone around me laughed and Khalil was delighted with my disbelief. "You see," he said, "you must come to Saudi Arabia to see things like this. It's an education for you."

I learned later that the Saudis are great cinema enthusiasts. There are more private film projectors and video tape recorders and players per capita in Saudi Arabia than in any other country. Private film libraries flourish and clubs have been organized which rent films and video tapes. Membership in these clubs costs $350 per month. A video player sells for $6,000 or more. The films are pirated from American television by American or Saudi students in the United States and brought to Saudi Arabia, where there are no copyright laws. A black market in Riyadh is open from sunset until three o'clock in the morning. Here one can buy or rent projectors, movie cameras, lenses, and all types of film. In some places a Saudi can obtain pornographic films or tapes without any direct confrontation with the seller. The transaction is carried out through a window located above the head of the purchaser, but within reach, so that the money and the film can be exchanged in complete secrecy. This arrangement is reminiscent of the speakeasy and the days of bootleg liquor during Prohibition in the United States, but the Saudis have yet to learn that Prohibition doesn't work.

By midnight, when *Deep Throat* mercifully ended, everyone was pretty much in his cups and the party was getting boisterous. The Deputy Minister of the Interior raised his drink and called for attention. "Do you know the difference," he asked in perfect English, "between Socialism, Communism, Fascism, Newdealism, Nazism, and Capitalism?"

"What's the difference?" we all asked. When he felt he had our undivided attention he took a paper from his pocket, carefully unfolded it, and read:

Socialism—*If you have two cows, you give your neighbor one.*

Communism—*If you have two cows, you give them to the government and the government gives you some milk.*

Fascism—*If you have two cows, you keep the cows and give the milk to the government and the government sells you some of the milk.*

Newdealism—*If you have two cows, you shoot one, milk the other one, and pour the milk down the drain.*

Nazism—*If you have two cows, the government shoots you and then keeps the cows.*

Capitalism—*If you have two cows you sell one and buy a bull.*

"But what happens in Saudi Arabia?" someone asked after the laughter had subsided.

"In Saudi Arabia, if you have two cows, the government gives you money to buy more cows, and doesn't charge you interest or expect you to pay back the money. You then sell the cows, buy a farm, and the government gives you more money to develop the farm. Then you take this money and buy another farm," one of the prince's cousins said.

I later asked the deputy minister if I could have a copy of his list and he pulled out the paper and presented it to me with a flourish. I still have it to this day.

Discussion of religion or politics is generally taboo at a social gathering, but the drinking had been going on for almost four hours and our inhibitions were approaching an all-time low. The trouble started when Prince Khalil asked me what I thought about Saudi Arabia. "After all," he said, "you have lived here for more than a year."

"I am amazed," I said, "at the contradictions in this country. You are modernizing Saudi Arabia with the speed of jet propulsion and are embarking upon the most ambitious building program ever seen in this part of the world. You have begun what might be called a 'modernization' revolution, but you are in the dilemma of adjusting to the present without compromising the past. You still subjugate your women and hold on to your orthodox traditions a thousand years old. It's an astounding paradox!"

"The foundation of our country is built upon Islam and the family," said

Khalil. "That's what keeps us together. Religion and the family are the true arsenal of Islam, which will defend us against the corruption of the materialistic modern world."

"We already have plenty of corruption among us now," one of the deputy ministers said. "I could give you some examples—"

Khalil interrupted him. "Say you're sorry. Say you're sorry," he shouted, pointing a finger at him. "Don't condemn the whole country because of the greed of a few. They should be imprisoned."

"Some of them are in prison now," said the deputy from the Ministry of Justice, "including members of the royal family—very young and very foolish."

"There are always a few bad apples in every family," I said. "There is no shortage of corruption in the Western countries."

"How long can the devout puritanical Moslem society, the Wahabi, hold out against the impact of Western technology and thinking?" asked Ron Lambrie. "Particularly when large numbers of your young people are studying in the U.S. and elsewhere?"

"As we educate our children both here and abroad, the fundamentalists may lose some of their influence," said the deputy from the Ministry of the Interior. By now everybody was listening to our discussion. "Rapid change will produce problems and tensions between the new and the old, but it may take a generation for the present material revolution to bring about significant social change."

"I disagree," said Prince Khalil. "The Wahabis are fanatical in their religious beliefs, and they won't give up without a fight. In fact, they are now more powerful than ever, and the King upholds them. Our kingdom has strong ties with the Wahabis which go back two hundred years. They are violently opposed to the breakdown of the Islamic tradition, the modernization of our country and the destruction of our cultural heritage, but they are loyal to the King and he is loyal to them. I doubt their relationship will change in the foreseeable future. Don't forget, our roots are a thousand years deep."

"We all know what is going on in Iran," Philip said in his best Oxonian accent. "How stable is the monarchy here? Will the growing middle class and the students educated abroad want a greater role in running the government?"

Khalil became very angry at this question and his ghutra swung back and forth on his shoulders as he talked, his eyes blazing. "In the West you talk about royalty from your own peculiar background without understanding the Islamic character of our government. All Moslems are equal regardless of origin, color, or economic status. Our royal family is always accessible to the poorest Bedouin at the *majlis*. We are in contact daily with the common man and we relate to them."

I tried to stop the argument by telling them I was impressed to see how easily a poor Bedouin, who fell off his camel at the camel races, could speak personally with the King. But Khalil had more to say.

"Intense religious feelings are bound up in our social and political life in a manner you in the West can scarcely begin to understand. The Saud family provides the kingdom with religious, social, and political cohesion.

"The royal government will be stable because there is no separation between the mosque and the state. They are one. Islam is the state." He went on to point out the vast differences which exist between Iran and Saudi Arabia. The King in Saudi Arabia is titular head of the religious community. The royal family claim descent from the Bedouins and subsidize them. The King and Crown Prince are unpretentious and do not flaunt their wealth within their own country (although they may make up for it when they go abroad).

"There is no Peacock Throne here in Riyadh," said Prince Khalil, "and nobody here displays the arrogance of the Shah of Iran.

"There are practically no political prisoners in Saudi Arabia as there were in Iran, and we do not execute or murder political dissidents. We are mostly Sunni Moslems. Our country is the home of Islam. The Iranians are Shiites, whom we regard as heretics.

"As you can see, Iran is completely different from us! The Shah and his small family were lost in a population of 38 million. We in Saudi Arabia have only 6 or 7 million people, the population of Chicago, and our 4,000 princes can relate to them more closely."

"Do you think," I asked, "that you will eventually have a free and open society in the Western sense? Once you educate your people, they may demand it. There is at present no electoral machinery, no political party, no constitution, and no legislature."

"Yet our government has been impressively stable for the past fifty years," said the Deputy Minister of Education. "Our people have been illiterate until very recently and unable to assume legislative responsibility. The fact that we don't have a Congress doesn't necessarily mean that our system is archaic. We have a welfare program for the elderly which does not institutionalize them but gives them subsidies and decreases their costs for water, electricity, and food. We are building 200,000 new housing units, schools for a million students, and universities to educate our students. The approximate cost for all this is about $10 billion. Our people have the highest per capita income in the world. We subsidize those who help develop and modernize our country. We give our people the best money can buy, and Saudi citizens pay no sales tax or income tax."

"Speaking of the democratic process," I said, "reminds me of a story I heard about King Faisal. He was asked, 'When will the men get the vote in Saudi Arabia?' and replied, 'When the women get the vote,' which was probably another way of saying 'never.'"

"Time will tell," said the Deputy Minister of Education, putting an end to that subject.

It was now one o'clock in the morning. Trevor Evans and several other guests had disappeared. Those of us who had survived sat about drinking more slowly, but keeping a watchful eye on the door to the dining room.

We all turned to Philip as he cleared his throat. "Why are no religious services other than Moslem allowed?" he asked. Prince Khalil gave a long sigh of disapproval.

"Because," said the deputy for the Justice Department with some discomfort, "this is a Moslem country and Islam is the only official faith. You must understand that any other faith is 'unconstitutional' in the Western sense, because the Koran alone is our constitution.

"Our official Saudi Arabian flag bears the legend 'There is no god but God and Mohammed is his Prophet.'"

Sam Stark told me later that the American Embassy in Jidda held P & C "Welfare Service Meetings" on Sunday mornings. *P* stood for Protestant and *C* for Catholic. The bulletin board stated that private interviews (confessionals) could be scheduled with the "lecturer," who was a priest or a minister. I told him of the well-attended Catholic services that were held out in the open on Friday morning at Aramco. The Saudis were aware of this, but did not interfere.

While we were on the subject of religious freedom, I decided to broach a very sensitive subject. Everyone now was three sheets to the wind and they might, I hoped, forget the discussion by morning.

"What about the Jewish situation?" I asked, pointing out that Saudi Arabia does not even acknowledge the existence of Israel. Saudia Airlines, owned by the government, deletes Israel from all of its maps, and the Saudi censors cut out the state of Israel from maps appearing in the *International Herald Tribune*. Companies doing business in Israel, like Coca-Cola, are not allowed into Saudi Arabia.

"This boycott against American companies has aroused a great deal of animosity in the American Congress," I said.

Much to my surprise, they answered very calmly.

"We oppose Zionism, not Judaism," said the deputy from the Information Ministry. "We Arabs recognize all monotheistic religions and there are no proscriptions against Judaism in the Koran. King Khalid himself recently conceded Israel's right to exist, and there are Jewish businessmen working in Saudi Arabia and consulting with us."

"King Faisal was fanatically anti-Communist," he continued, "and opposed Zionism because he originally feared a Zionist-Communist plot. Our main concern is Communism.

"Saudi Arabia does not oppose the Jews as such," he concluded, "but we oppose Israel because of the Palestine issue. We are members of the Arab League and we uphold Arab unity."

"Are there any Jewish citizens in Saudi Arabia?" Philip asked, reminding him that it was the Jews who offered Mohammed a haven in Medina when he was forced to flee from Mecca in A.D. 622.

"No," he replied, "but there are no Catholics either. Nobody can become a citizen in this country unless he embraces Islam."

Prince Khalil joined in the conversation, once more the gracious host. "Speaking of Jews," he said, "Shelley Berman is one of my favorite entertainers. I went to hear him perform in California whenever I could, and I have a collection of all of his records. I'll play some for you later."

The Deputy Minister of Foreign Affairs told us that Russian Communism, not Israel, was the principal enemy, and that they had given billions of dollars to countries which opposed Communism. In fact, King Faisal's price for the Saudi support of Egypt during the October war with Israel was Sadat's repudiation of his Soviet connection.

"We have given Egypt about $11 billion since 1973, and we were instrumental in getting the Russian military out of Egypt. We now give them about $2 billion yearly and we don't know what happens to the money. The more we give them, the more they want, and Egypt's population gets bigger and poorer every year.

"We are subsidizing North Yemen with billions to maintain their independence from the South Yemen Marxist government. We don't want the radical forces to win in Lebanon and have supported the Lebanese Christian right to crush the radical elements there."

It was clear that the Saudis strongly condemned Iraq and Libya because of their Soviet connections. They were very suspicious of the Palestinians because of their radical leanings, but supported them financially in an effort to wean them away from the Communists. The foreign policy of the Saudi Arabian government, they said, was to oppose Communism throughout the Middle East and to prevent radicalization of the region at all costs. The government was dedicated to promoting stability and moderation in the region and to remaining neutral in inter-Arab conflicts.

"Is there a possibility," I asked, "that Saudi Arabia, like Egypt, might someday initiate a dialogue with Israel to help maintain stability in the Middle East and strengthen the opposition to Communism?"

"When the Palestine issue is settled and when women get the vote," replied the Deputy Foreign Minister, as he drained his glass.

About one-thirty in the morning dinner was finally served. Prince Khalil explained that the Egyptian chef, a recent arrival in Saudi Arabia, had occasioned the delay. Those of us who were still ambulatory staggered glassy-eyed into the large formal dining room. The prince sat at one end of the long table and asked me to sit at the other end, as the guest of honor. The Saudis respect seniority and I had more gray hair than anyone else.

The Sudanese servants brought in huge decorated trays heaped high with steaming rice and baby lamb stuffed with nuts and raisins surrounded by pieces of sautéed chicken, eggs, tomatoes, cucumbers, and onions. Another main dish was *kabsa*, chicken sautéed with onion, garlic, fresh tomato, grated carrots, and orange rind, then seasoned further with cloves and cinnamon. It was garnished with raisins and almonds and served on a bed of hot rice.

The aroma of cinnamon, cloves, onions, and turmeric greeted us with each tray. Smaller plates of cooked pumpkin, apricots, and melon surrounded the larger trays. Then there were platters of dates stuffed with almonds, apricots, grapes, figs, and pomegranates from the fruit-growing area of Taif. A large tray placed before me held the head of a lamb and the eye, a delicacy reserved for the guest of honor.

Knives and forks were placed before us in deference to the foreigners, but we ate with our fingers like everyone else, pressing the rice and meat into small balls with the fingers of the right hand and popping them into our mouths. I ate the eye of the lamb and thanked Prince Khalil for the honor. It was soft and tasted like gelatin. I gulped it down quietly and sipped my wine. The food was superb and we ate in silence—a compliment to the host.

It is proper to leave shortly after a meal, but Prince Khalil wanted to talk some more, so we all remained seated. Nobody had yet sobered up completely.

"Dr. Gray," he said, "I won't ask Sam Stark because he is a CIA agent, but I will ask you how we Saudi Arabians impress you as human beings."

"I have found you are a very gentle people," I said, "much different from the fierce Bedouin tribesmen I've read about who conquered the Arab world for Islam. That's another contradiction—instead of belligerence there is kindness, gentility, and warmth. Saudi Arabians seem to be a peace-loving people."

"Don't count on it," said the prince, but I could see my reply had pleased him. I recalled an incident at our hospital, where an English doctor was making teaching rounds and couldn't talk above the noise of a vacuum cleaner. He asked the workman to turn off his machine, but when the man, who did not understand English, continued his work the doctor pulled the electric cord out of his hand. This was considered an act of violence by the Moslem worker, who reported the doctor to his superiors. The doctor was forced to make a formal apology, lest he be asked to leave the country. We had been warned beforehand never to touch or push a Saudi because it would be construed as a hostile act.

After the servants passed the hand censer (*mabkhar*), heavy with vapors of frankincense, we decided the time had come for us to leave.

We thanked Prince Khalil for a memorable dinner party and returned to our car. We had noted the disappearance of Trevor Evans earlier in the evening and assumed that he had had too much to drink and gone home by taxi. Before leaving, however, we discreetly searched the bedrooms, but he was nowhere to be found.

There was plenty of room in Peter's Landcruiser so Peter, Ron, and I sat up front on our way home. We were about halfway to our Petromin apartment when we heard a loud voice from the back of the car.

"I'm starving! When the hell do we eat?" It was Trevor, who had gone to sleep it off in the Landcruiser.

We informed him that dinner was over and that we were on our way home. At that pronouncement he broke out in song. His selection of bawdy English ballads and his raucous singing indicated that he was still in his cups. As the Landcruiser sped through the Nasseria area, the quiet of the Saudi Arabian night was broken by his performance of such classics as

The Virgin Sturgeon

"Caviar comes from the virgin sturgeon,
The virgin sturgeon's a very fine fish,
The virgin sturgeon needs no urgin',
That's why caviar is my dish.

"I gave caviar to my girlfriend,
She was a virgin tried and true,
Ever since she had that caviar,
There ain't nothing she won't do."

Trevor was still in good voice when we arrived at Petromin. As we helped him up the stairs to his apartment he broke out into a loud rendition of "The Sexual Life of the Camel."

> *"The sexual life of the camel,*
> *Is stranger than anyone thinks,*
> *At the height of the mating season,*
> *He tries to bugger the sphinx,*
> *But the sphinx's posterior sphincter*
> *Is all clogged by the sands of the Nile,*
> *Which accounts for the hump on the camel*
> *And the sphinx's inscrutable smile."*

Trevor's repertoire seemed endless. Lights appeared. All the women in the complex came out of their apartments to see what was going on and to greet their errant husbands.

Trevor was so entertaining that everyone joined in chorus after chorus of "Clementine," "The Maid of the Mountain Glen," and others, much to the amusement of the Saudis who also had apartments in our complex.

Finally, as the women in their night clothes stood side by side with their husbands along the circular three-story stairwell, we sang "God Bless America" and "It's a Long Way to Tipperary," followed by "Rule Britannia" and "Be It Ever So Humble, There's No Place Like Home."

At 4:30 A.M. we closed with "Good Night, Ladies," turned off the lights, and went to bed.

◊ *20* ◊

THE WOMEN'S DILEMMA

ALL-NIGHT HOSPITAL DUTY is a chore generally relegated to the junior doctors, but in our hospital it was a must for everyone. The beepers had not yet arrived, and in cases of emergency the telephone was the only means of reaching a physician. This presented a problem because the doctors on call at night were scattered all over Riyadh, and some of the apartment houses had only one phone for all the occupants. The time lag between the appearance of a patient in the emergency clinic and the arrival of the physician was considerable. Consequently an on-call schedule was drawn up for medicine and surgery, so that a physician would be available within the hospital from 7 P.M. until 7 A.M.

At first each physician was on call every seventh or eighth night. Later, when the beepers arrived, the physicians living in Gerrin Village or in the Campus Villas within the hospital complex remained on call at home. All others, living outside the complex, slept in the hospital. As departments increased in size, and as the intern and residency program developed, the on-call duty came only two or three nights a month.

Much to my surprise, some of the younger English physicians loudly objected to remaining in the hospital overnight. I pointed out that I hadn't been on call for thirty years, and that if I could sleep in, they "jolly well could too." This seemed to satisfy them. The older English doctors were cooperative and conscientious from the outset. The Americans were generally agreeable, although the younger physicians, I must admit, were somewhat less gracious about it.

Actually I looked upon the all-night vigils in the hospital as a retreat, during which I could contemplate life: where I had been and where I was going. I enjoyed the hushed silence, the symphony of people in deep sleep, the smell of disinfectants, the dimly lit corridors, the sight of nurses bent over their charts and orderlies quietly checking the supplies.

A hospital is a living entity, and there is something special about a hospital at night. It pulsates quietly, resting from the frenetic activities of the day while it prepares for the morrow. A hospital harbors warmth and love if you look beneath the surface. It is the stage for the whole human tragedy: the joy of birth, the sorrow of death, the challenge of pain, the suffering, and the sense of fulfillment. There is no reward equal to the satisfaction derived from healing the sick. Medicine is an amalgam of art, science, devotion, commitment, and faith. The physician, in my view, is a high priest.

A room on the medical ward of the hospital was set aside for the physician on call. Late at night I would open the drapes and gaze upon the desert outside my windows. Sometimes when there was a full moon the sand glistened white like snow, and the stars appeared almost close enough to touch. I liked to recall my younger days as a resident physician at the University of Chicago hospital, where I started at a salary of $50 a month, plus room and board. The interns and residents all lived on the top floor of the hospital adjacent to the animal quarters, which housed a variety of animals used for experimental purposes, including an old horse who was kept to supply immune horse serum. All that stood between the animal farm and the interns' quarters was a large door. The barrier between us was broken on a New Year's Eve when the neurosurgical resident took the old mare out of her stall and rode her up and down the corridor of the interns' quarters. Some of the doctors welcoming in the New Year thought they were hallucinating, but almost everyone eventually rode the horse. Nellie herself was feted with lumps of sugar and apples, and finally was returned to her stall no worse for wear, and probably grateful for the exercise.

In addition to allowing me time for reflection, the "duty" also gave me an opportunity to catch up on my correspondence. In writing home, I took pleasure in telling of a country with the lowest crime rate in the world, a sharp contrast to the mayhem which I had left behind in the United States. My own story concerned a beautiful alligator billfold I had lost recently in the Jidda airport. It contained my passport, several credit cards, and about $150 in cash. When I arrived in Riyadh I went to see Moussa in the Travel Department.

"I'm desperate," I said, as he looked up in alarm from all the papers on his desk. "I must have lost my billfold while passing through customs and reclaiming my luggage. The airport was a mob scene because of the *hajj* [the pilgrimage to Mecca]. Is there anything I can do, like posting a reward?"

"Not to worry," Moussa said, picking up the telephone. "There is no need for a reward. I'll call customs in Jidda and ask them to return your billfold. It may take a few days," he said apologetically.

"You must be kidding," I said. "There were thousands and thousands of poor pilgrims milling around there. It was absolute chaos, and you tell me that my wallet will be returned in a few days."

Moussa and I were old friends. "That's the trouble with you infidels," he said with a smile. "You don't have faith. You should become a Moslem! Of course your billfold will show up." I shook my head in disbelief.

About ten days later Moussa called me. "Come pick up your wallet," he said.

When I went to his office Moussa handed me the billfold. I couldn't believe my eyes. Nothing had been removed, not even the crisp $10 and $20 bills.

"That's Saudi Arabia for you," he said. "Now, if this were Egypt, they would steal your billfold, your luggage, and the coat off your back as well."

Just as I had finished a letter home, at about nine o'clock, the nurse in the Emergency Room called and asked me to see a patient who was complaining of pain in the lower right quadrant of her abdomen.

"It may be appendicitis," she said.

The patient was an Egyptian nurse named Nassara. She had a long record of repeated episodes of pain in the right side of her abdomen, which peculiarly enough always appeared whenever she was about to go on night duty. Blood tests in the past were always normal; she never had fever; she always recovered after a good night's sleep in the emergency bedroom.

I examined her and found nothing abnormal. The laboratory tests were again normal and she had no fever. I asked her if she was scheduled for night duty in the hospital.

She said, "Yes," and produced a paper for me to sign excusing her from working that night.

I left the room and returned with the nurse carrying a shiny metal instrument called a sigmoidoscope. Nassara recognized the instrument immediately. I told her that before signing the paper, I wanted to perform an examination which involved inserting the twelve-inch-long rigid instrument into the rectum and lower colon.

"The x-rays have all been normal in the past," I said, brandishing the vicious-looking instrument. "This examination might help locate the cause of your pain, which seems to come on before your night duty."

She looked at the instrument and then at me. "My pain is gone," Nassara said, taking the paper from my hand.

After she had dressed, I sat down with her and explained that whenever she absented herself from night duty she imposed a hardship on the other nurses. Moreover, she was not fair to herself, I said, because someday she might really have appendicitis and nobody would believe her. Then I related the story of "Cry Wolf." She had never heard it.

Nassara started to cry and told me how unhappy she was in Saudi Arabia. She felt like a prisoner, she said. Moslem nurses were much more restricted than American or English nurses. She felt discriminated against because the Egyptian nurses were housed in separate and inferior quarters and were not allowed in the Recreation Center with the Western nurses. And, because men and Moslem women are forbidden to swim together, they were not permitted to use the swimming pool, nor could they go out with non-Moslem men.

"Life is bad enough for Western nurses, but for us it is impossible," she said. "I miss my family and friends and don't know whether I can stay here for the full two years."

"Why did you come here?" I asked.

"For the money," she said, still weeping. "My family is very poor and they depend on me."

"Something must be done," I said, "to give all nurses equal privileges and opportunities. The Saudi officials are probably responsible for your predicament. They want to protect Moslem women from foreign influences, and, as you know, they restrict and segregate their women particularly when Western men are present."

I then suggested that she and other Egyptian nurses draw up a letter of complaint, which I would present to the Medical Advisory Board on their behalf. I promised to discuss the matter with the Nursing Office and with the Director of Medical Affairs.

She thanked me and left with a glint of hope in her eyes.

It was midnight. I was sound asleep when the phone rang. It was the nurse covering emergency admissions. She told me that a patient would be arriving at the airport in about an hour. She was a royal and was flying in from Jidda with her doctor. That was all the information she had. The nurse had notified transportation to send an ambulance to the airport.

"The ambulance will pick you up at the hospital entrance in half an hour," she said.

"We're fortunate to have somebody like you in emergency," I said admiringly. "I wouldn't have known how to handle a situation like this. Do you want to come along for the ride to the airport? I haven't been in an ambulance since I was an intern, and that's a long time ago."

"You know very well that I can't leave," she reminded me, "but thanks awfully."

The ambulance arrived ten minutes late, and the Saudi driver made up for lost time by driving eighty miles an hour and blasting the silence of the night with his sirens. I sat up front with him, and could see that he was enjoying every moment of it, particularly when he turned the corners on two wheels.

"*Shwayy, shwayy* [slow down]," I pleaded, closing my eyes. My reaction only encouraged him to drive faster.

"All ambulance drivers are alike," I remarked to the two medics who were sitting in the back. "When I was an intern the ambulance man drove like crazy whether there was an emergency or not."

"It's part of the profession," said Jim Simpson, who had served as a medic in the army in Vietnam, Iceland, and the Philippines. With him was a young medic from Lebanon, whom Jim had trained as his assistant. Two medics always accompanied the ambulance drivers because it was against Saudi tradition for the driver to do heavy manual labor, such as carrying a patient on a litter.

By some miracle we arrived at the airport without mishap. After making several inquiries, we drove to an area set aside for cargo. There we saw a large camouflaged military plane marked "Royal Saudi Arabian Airforce."

Jim identified it immediately. "It's a Lockheed Hercules HC-130," he said, "which is used for transporting cargo."

We entered the huge belly of the plane. By the light of a single small electric bulb we saw two shadowy, black-veiled, black-robed figures fluttering about like ghouls, attending to a nondescript figure in black who was lying on the floor of the plane. A man, whose features we could barely distinguish, came forward and introduced himself. He was the Egyptian doctor who had been treating Princess Lulwa, one of King Saud's many ex-wives, who had been discarded by Saud years ago. She was now eighty-two years old, he told us, and was suffering from diabetes and pneumonia. The doctor gave me a handwritten summary of her medical history and treatment, and thanked us for taking her off his hands.

I could barely see the princess in the semi-darkness because she was heavily veiled and covered completely in black. The doctor made an effort to introduce me to her but she did not respond. Jim and his assistant put her on the ambulance litter and carried her to the ambulance. The doctor thanked us again, and took his leave, saying that he was returning to Jidda in the morning.

When we arrived at the hospital, Lulwa fought to keep her face covered and refused to be examined. Her attendants who had accompanied us in the ambulance were as frightened as she was. Lulwa had never been in a hospital before, and expressed her terror by striking at anyone who approached her. When she bit the nurse trying to take her temperature, I decided to try a new approach.

I asked Nassara, whom I had examined earlier in the evening for "appendicitis," to interpret for me. Then Nassara and I sat down and tried to explain to Lulwa that she was seriously ill and we could not make her well again unless she helped us. I promised her that no men would attend her except me, and that she could keep her veil on at all times, even when the nurse took her temperature. I explained the importance of the blood tests and x-rays and promised to give her some medicine immediately if she cooperated.

Then I stood up, leaned over her, and said, "If you don't follow our instructions, you may die, and we don't want you to die." I repeated, "We don't want you to die." And then added, "We want to make you well again. Do you have any questions?"

"Yes," she said her voice muffled by her heavy veil, "when can I go home?"

"When you get well," I said, "maybe in two or three weeks."

She grudgingly allowed me to examine her, but kept her face completely covered. I drew some blood from her arm for a blood-sugar determination and told her that a woman from the laboratory would do this every day for a while until we could get her diabetes and pneumonia under control. I then started an intravenous infusion of fluid because she was badly dehydrated.

The eighty-two-year-old Lulwa would have died without hospitalization. She not only had pneumonia and uncontrolled diabetes, but her kidneys had begun to fail because of her severe dehydration. In situations like this only a sophisticated physician with a good laboratory to back him up can reverse the process and save the patient's life.

The princess improved slowly. She responded to the intravenous penicillin and to the insulin injections, and her kidney function gradually returned to normal as her body chemistry and fluid balance were restored. I visited her once or twice daily. It was obvious that she was illiterate and completely ignorant of the outside world. That a man would be interested in a very old woman was beyond her comprehension.

The princess slowly grew to trust me and carried on simple conversations with me during her convalescence. Then one day she paid me an extreme compliment: she removed her veil voluntarily and gave me a big smile. Most of her teeth were missing, but there were two fangs front and center. Lulwa seemed ugly at first glance, but her smile made her appear almost beautiful. Every time I entered her room thereafter, she quickly removed her veil and smiled broadly. It became an intimate ritual, which pleased her immensely.

After she left the hospital, she remained in Riyadh with her family for several months. Whenever she returned to the clinic, we again went through the veil ritual with much laughter. If I was not available in the clinic, she refused to see another doctor, and patiently awaited my return. She had grown to trust a man—but not mankind.

On another night I was called to the emergency room to see a young woman who had taken an overdose of sleeping pills in a suicide attempt. The patient was comatose, cyanotic, cold and clammy. Her blood pressure was barely obtainable, and her pulse was very rapid and thready. Her father said she had been depressed recently. He showed me the empty medicine bottle which he had found next to her bed. Fortunately, she had not taken a lethal dose of the drug, and she gradually recovered with the help of stimulants and supportive intravenous treatment.

Her name was Samira. She was twenty-two years old, the daughter of a well-to-do Saudi merchant, and very attractive. During her convalescence she told me that she had been studying at the University of California for three years and planned to be a teacher. She had been about to return to southern California to complete her education when a royal decree was issued which banned all Saudi women from traveling abroad for education, even though accompanied by members of their immediate family or by their husbands.

"Why did they do that?" I asked.

"The religious leaders, the Ulema, are exerting a great deal of pressure to tighten the restrictions on women," she said. "It's the usual battle between modernization and Islamic tradition. King Khalid is not as progressive as King Faisal."

Samira said she became terribly depressed at times by the difficult situation women face in Saudi Arabia, particularly the educated women.

"Why couldn't you finish your education at the University of Riyadh, where one-third of the 16,000 students are women?" I asked.

"Because," she said, "the women in this country are educated within the framework of Islamic tradition and the old code of ethics. The religious leaders are in control. A lot of time is spent teaching the Koran, the teachers are all women, and the students have no contact whatever with men or with the outside world."

I pointed out that women had come a long way in the past twenty years. There were 500,000 girls now attending primary and secondary schools, and there was a college for women in Riyadh, and another nearing completion in Judda.

I drew my chair closer. "What's the real reason you took those pills, Samira?" I asked softly.

Samira burst into tears. She had fallen in love, she said, with an American. They both knew it was an impossible situation. Her family would never accept him. Samira said she was very close to her family, and felt that she could not bring disgrace upon them. Moreover, the government had recently decided that such marriages were illegal.

"And now I will never see him again," she sobbed.

"You are a very attractive woman," I said, "and you have your whole life ahead of you. Perhaps you will meet someone else."

Samira said that was very unlikely. Her family had already selected a cousin for her to marry, but she had decided against the match because she did not know the man, and "refused to marry a stranger."

"Besides, he was very shy," she added, "and I never could communicate with him."

"What about the telephone?" I asked. "I understand that most courtships in Saudi Arabia are carried out by telephone." I recalled the importance of the telephone during Sultana's courtship.

"That didn't seem to work for us," said Samira, "but many Saudi women are now calling men who are outside the family.

"You know," she added, "it is forbidden to talk to such men face to face, but they are doing it over the telephone. Sometimes they call men at random, men they have never met. All they have is a telephone number."

"You see," I said, trying to be encouraging, "the newer generation is becoming more liberal. You have the right to reject the man chosen for you. And the religious leaders have decreed recently that a man may now see his intended wife's face before the marriage. That's certainly a step forward!"

"It could be a catastrophe for the woman," said Samira with a smile.

"I think you're getting better," I said as I rose to leave. "Your sense of humor is returning. I'll see you tomorrow."

When I returned the next day, Samira had two visitors: her sister, Wasisa, whom I had met before, and a cousin, Basama. Both women reached for their veils when I knocked on Samira's door, but now laid them aside while we talked.

Wasisa was six years older than Samira, married with four children. She could read and write, had the equivalent of a junior-high-school education and was traditional in her thinking. Her husband was a shopkeeper. She and Samira seemed to have little in common.

Basama was a few years older than Samira and employed by the government as a social worker. She was a graduate of the University of Riyadh and was married, but had no children. She worked in an agency that took care of orphans and illegitimate children. She told me that if an illegitimate child was born in a hospital the police were notified, and the mother was flogged publicly according to Islamic law. Consequently the infants were often abandoned at the mosques.

I told Basama that I had not met, until now, a Saudi woman who worked because our hospital employed no Saudi nurses, technicians, or secretaries, although we hired Moslem women from Egypt and Lebanon for these jobs.

Basama explained that Saudi women serve as social workers, teachers, doctors, and nurses only in institutions run exclusively by women and for women. "For example," she said, "we have a bank in Jidda for women only, and even the janitor is a woman. However, if a boutique or restaurant run by women is patronized occasionally by men, the business may be closed down by members of the Society for the Preservation of Virtue and the Prevention of Vice." She shook her head sadly as she smoothed the veil beside her.

"You have almost two million foreigners in your labor force," I said. "If more women worked, Saudi Arabia might become less reliant on foreign labor. Do you think that will ever happen?"

"Not in the near future," Basama said. "The men don't want us to work. They say that working women neglect their husbands and children and weaken the family structure." She rose and started pacing Samira's small hospital room. "My husband says educated women argue too much and don't take care of the house. He's really afraid that we have learned to think for ourselves. As more women become educated they will think as I do, but it will take a long time." She stopped speaking and I could tell she had been through these arguments before at home.

"Let's face it," said Samira, her eyes flashing, "women in this country have very few rights. Less than 10 percent of women work, and a woman cannot go into business without the written approval of her husband or a male member of her family.

"Legally, a Saudi woman is a half person. She inherits half of what a man inherits; it takes the testimony of two women in court to equal that of a man; and even the blood money paid for the accidental death of a woman is half that paid for a man."

Basama had settled herself at the foot of Samira's bed as if to align herself with her young cousin. Wasisa had retreated even farther into her chair and looked as if she would prefer to be wearing her veil. Samira continued, "The veil protects our bodies, it does not imprison our minds. The issue of sexual equality is not the veil, but what's behind it. There is a growing interest among Saudi women of my generation for equal rights. We are in the middle of a cultural revolution and we're caught between the heritage of our past and the modern world outside." As she spoke of the world outside her face softened and I thought she was going to cry. But she was too angry to cry.

Wasisa, who had listened intently to the conversation, now spoke up angrily, her hands busy with the hem of her veil. "The question of equality of men and women has no meaning. It is like discussing the equality of a rose and a jasmine. Each has its own perfume, color, and characteristics. Men and women are not the same." Basama tried to interrupt but Wasisa held up her hand for silence as the oldest of the three women. "Women are not equal to men, but neither are men equal to women. But that's not an issue because they're not competing. They complement each other, according to Islam.

"The man is responsible for the support of his family even if his wife is rich. A woman in traditional Islamic society does not have to earn a living. She can always find a place in the larger family structure if her husband leaves her. The man often supports not only his wife but members of her family, if necessary. Then why should she work?" She spread her hands as if the answer were obvious. I was fascinated to hear these Saudi women debating the issues and recalled similar opinions expressed by Sultana long ago.

"I don't want to be *just a housewife*," Basama said to Wasisa, and then to me, "I want more out of life."

"What's wrong with being a housewife and taking care of your family?" Wasisa asked. "I am in charge of my home and my children. I don't care about politics and going to war. These are things that shouldn't concern us, as women. My only responsibility is to my home, my children, and my family. This is my world." She drew herself up as if she were about to depart, and Basama just shook her head.

"And the Saudi men in turn revere their mothers," I said to Wasisa, trying to smooth things over. "Many have told me that they never let a day go by without speaking to their mothers. The royals seem to be particularly attentive."

"My marriage, like most Saudi marriages," Wasisa said, "was arranged by my family, and is a happy one. I didn't have to sell myself and put myself on display to get a husband. There was no need for singles bars, computer dating services, desperate flirtations, or trial marriages. There was no anxiety of having to find a husband, or of missing the opportune moment by not submitting to one-night stands or live-in situations. To me the Western mating system is barbaric. A marriage based on the sentiments of the moment is doomed from the beginning."

I was impressed with Wasisa's logic although she was obviously biased. Samira meanwhile was thinking of her friend, perhaps her lover, left behind in the United States. She closed her eyes as Wasisa continued talking.

"Our families take a long time in making a decision. The Saudi woman can sit at home and await the match arranged by her elders, who are experienced in such matters. These marriages are often successful."

"I'm not so sure about that," Basama said, softly. "My marriage was arranged and is not a very happy one, from my viewpoint, but I make the best of it. The life you describe sounds very boring for the woman. All she can do is watch television, or a movie on a videotape machine at home if she can afford one, or she can meet occasionally with other women in the family if her husband or son will drive her. It's an empty existence."

I was deeply moved by Basama's honesty in describing her marriage to her cousins, and to me, an outsider. Although only a few years separated her and Samira from Wasisa, they were truly a generation apart in their thinking. We were silent for a few moments and then I tried to change the mood by telling of one of my own experiences.

"Let me tell you how bored the women can get in this country," I said. I went on to tell them of an afternoon in December shortly after I had arrived in Riyadh. The telephone operator called me at five o'clock in the afternoon and said that Princess Fatima had called and asked if I would please come to the Intercontinental Hotel to treat her for a severe headache. Her hotel was on the way to my hotel so I picked up my black doctor's bag containing equipment for such occasions, and took the hospital bus to the Intercontinental Hotel. I didn't know at the time that outside visits were against hospital regulations.

When I arrived I found two beautiful young women about thirty years old elegantly dressed in colorful long gowns. The woman with the "severe headache" was gracefully reclining on a divan reading a magazine. The other woman was her sister. They both lived in the Eastern Province and were the wives of two very prominent Saudi princes, whose names I recognized immediately. They told me they were in Riyadh to visit their family. Neither woman wore a veil.

I took the blood pressure of Princess Fatima, the young woman on the divan, and checked her eyes and reflexes. Everything was normal. Her sister then came forward and said that she also had headaches, and could I please take her blood pressure. Again, everything was normal and the sisters sighed dramatically. A few minutes later there was a knock on the door and a cousin arrived, completely veiled and wearing a black abeyya over her long, beautiful gown. She was older and moderately obese. Her husband, also a prince, was a patient of mine. She removed her veil and joined the group just as I was putting my instruments away in my bag. She too said she had headaches and wondered whether I would take her blood pressure. Her rings flashed in the dim light as she held out her arm.

It suddenly dawned on me that this headache epidemic was a ruse. These young women were bored and just wanted to talk to someone different, like an American doctor, for example, with whom there could be no question of breaking the Islamic rules. After I assured them there was no cause for concern, they invited me to stay for tea, calling for their servants before I even had time to accept.

While we had our tea they asked me again what caused their headaches. I looked around at the opulence of their suites, at the beautiful clothes thrown over the bed, the jewels on the tables, the latest fashion magazines on the floor.

"Boredom," I said bluntly. "You ladies don't have anything to do."

"What can we do?" Princess Fatima asked helplessly.

"We need interpreters at the hospital," I said. "Why don't you work as volunteers?"

"What time do you start?" Fatima asked, her eyes wide.

"At eight o'clock," I said.

"But we don't get up until noon," replied Fatima's sister from the divan.

I knew full well that they would not be permitted to work in the hospital, where men were present. Woman's place was in the home, just as Wasisa said. A woman's duty is to her husband and to her family, not to herself.

As I finished telling my story, Basama said, "Headaches!" We all smiled. Soon she and Wasisa put on their veils and said goodbye to Samira. Our discussion certainly hadn't settled anything for now. Samira was right: the woman's issue was not the veil itself, but the way of life behind it.

LIFE AND DEATH
ACCORDING TO ISLAM

MAN'S INHERENT biological instinct is to survive. This instinct is essential to the preservation of the species and prevails throughout the animal kingdom. Although man recently has been intellectualizing the quality of survival in the event of a choice between life and death, the physician is committed to the concept of human survival regardless of how it is threatened and at whatever cost. He does this instinctively, yet with forethought, planning, and skill. He is a crusader against death.

During his professional life, the physician encounters death many times, and he comes to look upon it as an old and familiar adversary. I was a twenty-four-year-old intern when my first patient died. I had never seen anyone die before and the memory remains indelibly seared in my mind. My patient was a beautiful six-year-old boy with blue eyes and blond, curly hair. He had pneumonia complicated by a bloodstream infection. His physician, an excellent pediatrician, and I had been up all night treating him with a special serum, which proved ineffective. Penicillin was not yet available.

The young Scandinavian parents stood near the bed of their only child, clutching hands in an effort to support each other and sobbing uncontrollably. The pediatrician cried openly as he watched the boy die, and I too couldn't hold back my tears.

Then the distraught father leaned over, kissed his son on the forehead, and clipped a blond curl from the boy's head as a keepsake. This act just fractured me! I remember it vividly after almost forty years. I also remember some questions. Why? Why this boy? Why these parents? If there is a just God, how does He justify this? I am still asking these questions.

Penicillin became available a year later and would have saved this child's life. In my sorrow and frustration, I concluded that maybe God has nothing to do with all this. Later, I would learn that such a concept was far different from the tenets of Islam.

Another difficult experience I had faced as a doctor might be termed "death by appointment." It involved a forty-five-year-old woman with inoperable cancer of the breast, which had spread to other organs, including her bones. Radiation therapy offered little hope and chemotherapy was not yet available. She was in constant pain and knew she had cancer and was going to die. However, she desperately wanted to stay alive until her oldest son had graduated from college. "How much time do I have?" she asked me one day after an examination. "Can you keep me alive for three months?"

I promised to do my best. "Maybe you will have a remission," I said, not too persuasively. "Such things sometimes happen."

In the next three months I did what I could to make her comfortable and to maintain her body fluids and nutrition, but her cancer spread rapidly. Watching this elegant, gracious woman deteriorate day by day was almost unendurable, and after a month I had to steel myself to enter her room. Her mental clarity made it more difficult for me to accept her approaching death as she talked about her life, her husband, and two children. She discussed funeral arrangements, her burial, and the effect her death would have upon her family. Her immediate goal was to stay alive each day until June 15, her son's graduation day.

She also talked about immortality, the life hereafter, the soul, and her faith in God. The Catholic chaplain visited her several times a day and gave her extreme unction. By June first, she was barely able to speak and then only about graduation day. Her indomitable spirit alone seemed to keep her alive. Finally her son arrived in cap and gown after his graduation ceremonies, and the family gathered around her bedside to share her joy in his accomplishment. She died quietly two days later. She had kept her appointment with death, gallantly and graciously.

As I look back, it seems to me that the devout Catholic faces death more calmly and more peacefully than members of any other faith in the Western world. The Catholic accepts the inevitability of death with dignity and inner strength. In Saudi Arabia I learned that not only does the Moslem accept death graciously, he almost welcomes it. That's the difference!

Time passed quickly. After a year, my good friend, Philip Westbrook had left the hospital to return to London, and I was selected to succeed him as chairman of the department. Philip and I had shared many memorable experiences and his departure left a void in my life. Lifelong friendships can be made quickly in a foreign environment where interdependent strangers with a common interest are suddenly thrown together.

The hospital now was always filled to capacity except during holidays. The physicians competed with each other to have their patients admitted. The most common problems in the Department of Medicine were parasitic diseases, infectious diseases, tuberculosis, cancer, and diabetes. Amoebic and bacillary dysentery were common because of poor sanitation facilities, the abundance of flies, and the use of human excrement as fertilizer. The same factors contributed to the high incidence of virus hepatitis, a severe infection of the liver which often leads to cirrhosis and cancer. Typhoid fever and undulant fever caused by contaminated water or food were not as prevalent as we had anticipated, even though many Saudis drink unpasteurized goat milk.

A large number of patients in our clinic had a mild form of diabetes. Intermarriage among cousins was probably responsible for the high incidence. We encountered very little venereal disease, which was more likely to be treated in the military hospitals.

Many patients with cancer came from all over the kingdom because of our highly sophisticated methods of treatment. Malignancies of the esophagus, liver, blood-forming organs, and small intestine were particularly common.

All of us were impressed by the scarcity of high blood pressure, coronary heart disease, and peptic ulcer among the Saudi population. Whether this is related to the lack of stress and their avoidance of salt is unknown. The Egyptians, Lebanese, and Palestinians, whose salt intake and exposure to stress, however, are simliar to those of Westerners, seemed to have the same incidence of these diseases as the Americans and English. I wondered what effects "civilization" would have upon the Saudis ten years hence.

In the hospital dining room once, I was asked to join six visiting Saudi doctors for lunch. All were dressed alike in the traditional thobe and ghutra. During dessert I surprised them by pointing to two of the doctors and saying, "You cannot be native-born Saudi Arabians."

They were amazed and admitted that they indeed were Egyptians who had become Saudi Arabian citizens when they were about thirty-five years old. "How could you tell?" one asked.

"Because you were the only ones who poured salt on your food," I said, "the two of you and I."

Among the most important departments in the hospital was the Admissions Office, which had the responsibility of selecting patients for hospitalization each day. It was also the most difficult to administer because of the constant demands by staff physicians to admit their patients and by royals requesting hospitalization for people they were sponsoring. In addition, outside doctors were sending in "emergencies" as a subterfuge to get their patients admitted.

Life and Death According to Islam ◊ *279*

The Medical Advisory Board tried to formulate a system of priorities but it failed because the demand far exceeded the supply of 250 available beds. The admitting officer had to have the patience of Job, the wisdom of Solomon, and a light touch to keep everyone happy. Such a person was Julie Northrop, a young, attractive, vivacious woman with a cheerful disposition and a ready smile. Julie and her newly-wed husband, an athletic instructor in the Recreation Center, had come from the Midwest. To me, she typified all that is admirable in women bred in the wide-open spaces of Middle America: integrity, beauty, and a sincere dedication to humanity.

One of my responsibilities was to visit the Admitting Office almost daily to check on the patients scheduled for hospitalization. I always looked forward to exchanging pleasantries with Julie, but this time she burst into tears when I entered the room.

"It's terrible," she said, dabbing at her eyes with a handkerchief. "I've never seen anything like it."

"What's this all about? Where's your beautiful smile?"

"Look at that man outside the door," she said. "I can't get anyone to take care of him."

In the waiting room sat a Bedouin, about twenty years old, beside an older man. Both wore soiled, bedraggled thobes and worn sandals, and both looked exhausted. I went closer and saw that the younger man sat motionless, staring in front of him as though hypnotized. His right eyeball was bulging from its socket. It was severely inflamed and protruded so far out that the eyelid was barely visible. A fly sat on his feverish right brow over the bulge, attracted by the moisture. The man could not blink and seemed too apathetic to brush the fly away. He just sat there in utter hopelessness and despair. No wonder Julie was upset.

Fortunately, Nabil, the Lebanese interpreter, was on duty. The patient's name was Sattam. Nabil told me that Sattam and his father had come a long distance from the Nafud desert in the North, partly by camel and partly on foot. Someone in the vicinity of Riyadh had then driven them to the hospital and deposited them here. Nabil talked to them for a few more minutes and then said that they had never been to a physician before and weren't sure why they had been brought here. Sattam had been ill for more than three weeks.

"His pain must be agonizing," I said, "and he could lose one eye or both, if we don't act fast. Tell him that his condition is very serious and that he is in a hospital and that surgery may be necessary to save his sight."

As Nabil explained his situation to him, Sattam maintained his stoic calm and resignation. "God gave and God may take away," he said in Arabic, "*Allah akbar* [God is great]."

I returned to Julie's office. She told me that Sattam had no money and there was no prince to sponsor him. The usual procedure in such situations was to apply for funds from the Central Hospital Committee, but it would take several weeks.

"I'm sure they will approve his hospitalization," I said, "but meanwhile Sattam is suffering and may lose his sight. Let's call Dr. Schiller."

Dr. Schiller, our only eye surgeon, was a superb ophthalmologist from West Germany who had studied in eye clinics all over the world.

"He's in surgery now and will be there all afternoon," Julie said, "and he has more patients than he can take care of for the rest of the week. But I can't just send that man away." She began to cry again.

"First of all," I said, trying to comfort her, "I have the right to admit him as an emergency, with or without money. If no beds are available, we can put him in the outpatient clinic overnight and admit him into the hospital tomorrow. The main problem is to get Dr. Schiller to see him. He's a stickler for following regulations, and I know he'll be upset by my admitting a patient to his service without his knowledge or consent."

"Particularly when he's already swamped with patients," Julie said sympathetically. "Meanwhile I'll try to locate a bed." As Julie began checking through her admitting lists, she was almost her old self again. I left orders for some blood tests and x-rays of the skull and sinuses, then waited until Schiller had completed his surgery.

At about five o'clock, I located Schiller in the doctors' dressing room and told him the story. In his thick German accent Schiller said that he still had six patients waiting for him in the clinic. "There are only so many hours in the day," he added, shaking his head.

As he finished dressing I tried appealing to his professional ego. "Schiller, you're the best damn eye surgeon in the Middle East so you have only yourself to blame for being so busy." I went on to tell him that I honestly thought that he could hold his own with the best in Boston, including the Massachusetts Eye and Ear Hospital.

That did it! He could see that I meant every word. "Let's go," he said, picking up his bag of instruments. "The other patients will have to wait."

After an hour of examining Sattam and reviewing his x-rays, Schiller arrived at a tentative diagnosis. The cause of the dramatic protrusion of the eyeball was a fulminating infection of the right maxillary sinus, a cavity situated between the nose and the eye. The infection had spread to the tissue of the right orbit, the bony cavity containing the eyeball. The swelling caused by the infection was pushing the eye out of its socket, and according to Schiller would produce blindness by its pressure on the optic nerve.

"There is a real possibility that he may develop a bloodstream infection [septicemia] or brain abscess, which will kill him unless we act fast," Schiller said. "He must be in terrible pain. I'll need Dr. Thomas to help me with the surgery." Dr. Thomas was the expert on maxillofacial surgery.

While Nabil interpreted, we explained the situation to Sattam.

He seemed stoic as ever. "*Allah karim* [God is merciful]," he murmured. "*La ilah illa' llah* [There is no god but God]."

Throughout the following weeks, Sattam suffered with his characteristic resignation. He was treated with antibiotics to combat the virulent staphylococcus infection and then underwent extensive and very painful surgery. But he remained undemonstrative and indifferent. As far as he was concerned, his fate was sealed. He was in Allah's hands and his submission to Allah's will was complete.

His father slept on the floor next to his son's bed and also showed no emotion. He prayed almost constantly during the critical period of surgery and immediately after.

As was true with Sattam and his father, the name of God is constantly on the Saudi's lips throughout his lifetime. He invokes God's name on every possible occasion. "Praise be to God," "In the name of God," or "God protect you," are said in reverence. It is quite different from such exclamations in the West as "For God's sake," "Thank God," or "My God!," which often have little true religious connotation. The word "*Inshallah* (God willing)," which all of us had adopted because the Saudis used it so frequently, is added to every plan for the future, such as "I'll see you tomorrow, *Inshallah*." Hearing or seeing something surprising brings forth "*Wallah* (By God)," and to ward off evil: "*Staghfir Allah* (God forbid)." In all, there are more than twenty such invocations to Allah, emphasizing that God is always in the Saudi's mind.

Sattam improved dramatically. His eye gradually returned to normal, although the vision on that side was slightly impaired. Julie came to visit Sattam and one day brought him some sweets. He rewarded her with a rare smile. She left his room with a broad grin on her face, her triumph complete. Just as he was about to be discharged from the hospital, the committee's approval for his hospitalization arrived, as we knew it would.

I had a strong conviction that Sattam attributed his recovery entirely to Allah. "*Alhamdu lillah* [Praise be to God]," he said to us solemnly as he prepared to leave the hospital. "All is divine plan!" I was glad that Schiller was too busy with other patients to hear Sattam's departing words!

In Saudi Arabia, illness is traditionally regarded as a manifestation of God's will, which is unchangeable. In this context, there is no point in trying to interfere with what Allah has already ordained. This complete submission to fate was exemplified to me by a fifty-year-old Saudi princess who had arrived at the hospital from Jidda with her Eygptian physician and several attendants. She was deeply jaundiced, had a high fever, and was in severe pain. Tests showed that she had gallstones, some of which had blocked her bile ducts and produced severe colic and jaundice. Her medical condition was further complicated by a severe gall-bladder infection, and the bacteria had invaded her bloodstream, producing septicemia. Shortly after she arrived, she went into shock and almost died. I treated her intravenously with a special antibiotic called Gentamicin, which was specific for her type of infection, and she recovered over a period of several weeks. I then explained to her that it was essential to remove her infected gall bladder because the jaundice and colic would probably recur and another bloodstream infection might be fatal.

"Man proposes, God disposes," she said in Arabic. "I want to go home. *Tawakkalna Al Allah* [We put our trust in God]."

Three months later, the Egyptian doctor called me from Jidda on a Sunday night. "The princess is very ill," he said. "The family wants you to come here for a consultation. She is too sick to travel. It's an emergency."

"I'll take the next plane," I said.

I arrived in Jidda the following day shortly after noon. The princess's physician met me at the airport. "The princess died early this morning," he said. "It was very sudden. The family is quite upset, particularly the women."

That was an understatement! When we arrived at the princess's villa, I heard screams and shrieks of agony. There, in a large room, about twenty grief-stricken women were dressed completely in white, the mourning dress. Their heads and faces were also covered with white scarves and veils. Some of the women were crying, others were screaming and beating their breasts as they flung themselves about the room. Several were in convulsions probably caused by hyperventilating (overbreathing) from grief or hysteria. A Hindu physician in a sari passed among them, placing spoons in their mouths to prevent them from swallowing their tongues and strangling. She injected some with sedatives to control their convulsions and contortions. Two of them collapsed and were carried out of the room by servants.

A tall prince, a minister high in the government, passed among them, flapping his arms under his white mantle like a huge bird, as he tried to restore calm. "*Ahda ahda* [Quiet, quiet]." Some of the servants were also tearing their hair and beating their heads to show their grief. I was told later that the respect for a bereaved woman rises in proportion to the amount of grief and emotion she displays. Some of the exhibition was real, but part of it appeared feigned or hysterical. I wished that their emotion had been channeled into persuading the princess to undergo surgery, which would have saved her life. It was a scene I won't forget.

Peculiarly enough, these manifestations of grief are common in the Hejaz region paralleling the Red Sea Coast, where Mecca, Medina, and Jidda are located, but are forbidden in the Nejd, the heartland of the country and the site of Riyadh. In the Nejd, the women merely seclude themselves, but in Hejaz the bereaved family must open their homes to receive friends who come to offer their sympathy, and to renew the weeping and mourning. Refreshments are served in a bleak and bare room outfitted only with carpets. A professional reader may recite from the Koran. It is, however, against the strict Wahabi tenets to mourn the dead, or to display grief, as I learned when Prince Ibrahim died. Why an exception is made in the Hejaz region is unknown. In all areas the dead are washed, shrouded in white, and buried as soon as possible. Monuments and headstones are forbidden everywhere.

Sattam and the princess demonstrated the complete resignation of the Saudi to his fate and his acceptance of whatever might befall him, on the thesis that it is preordained by Allah and irreversible. However, this passive, fatalistic attitude to illness is not shared by all Moslems. There are various nuances and degrees of faith among Moslems as there are among all religions. The Lebanese, Palestinians, and the more educated and sophisticated Saudis have more confidence in modern medicine than they had in the past, particularly as medical facilities become more available and their efficacy is demonstrated.

Thus, the less-orthodox Saudi reacts differently to his illness. He fights for his life, although his faith in Allah remains resolute. An example of this was a patient named Radifa, a thirty-five-year-old Saudi woman with three small children. Her husband was a Palestinian who worked in a bank in Riyadh. She was a Saudi by birth.

Radifa had been operated on in the hospital for a malignant tumor of the small intestine called a lymphoma, which is a common form of cancer in this part of the world. Afterward, she was unable to absorb food normally because a large part of her small intestine had been removed. When I first saw her, she weighed seventy pounds and looked like a skeleton. Her surgeon asked me to see her. He felt that in spite of the success of her operation, she could not survive much longer because of her malnutrition. Her appetite was fairly good but she didn't have enough absorptive surface left in her intestine to keep her alive.

Radifa and her husband were desperate. "You must help me," she said. "I have a husband and three small children who need me. I'm losing weight every day even though I eat well."

I told her about a special dietary supplement called Portagen made in the United States for just such a condition. It is a powder that when dissolved in water can easily be absorbed into the body. "It's made just for you," I said. "If you drink six glasses of the mixture daily, you should gain weight. However, it will take some discipline on your part to drink it because it isn't very tasty."

"When can we start?" she asked.

I called the pharmacist. He knew all about the medication but did not have any on hand. I explained Radifa's problem and asked him to call Mead Johnson in the United States and have it flown to Riyadh by Saudia Airlines.

Within a week the powder arrived in sealed metal containers. Radifa was so anxious to begin treatment that in the beginning she took too much of the mixture and it made her sick. But, once she organized her dietary program, she was able to absorb fifteen hundred calories from the Portagen in addition to her food. Over a period of four months, she gained twenty pounds. She came to the clinic with her husband every two weeks to check on her progress. On one such visit, she brought her children for me to meet and cried with joy. Her husband tried to thank me as he comforted his wife, but he too broke down and cried.

"It was American medicine that helped you," I said. "Don't thank me, thank the country I come from." As they left, all four of them waving goodbye, I thought to myself that Radifa might also thank God for her positive attitude. It certainly helped her to survive.

The Saudis, like most Moslems, want to go home to die. Marwan Al Hamad, a sixty-eight-year-old Bedouin from the Eastern Province, was tall and lean, with sharp facial features and dark brown, penetrating eyes. His skin, at first glance, appeared to be tanned by the sun, but the creases of his palms were deeply pigmented and the "whites" of his eyes, the sclerae, appeared yellowish brown. A second look told the story: Marwan was intensely jaundiced. He sat calmly in a comfortable chair in his hospital room, and two men sat across from him. They were all dressed alike in white thobes, which accentuated the yellow in Marwan's skin. Their beards were well-trimmed and pitch-black, but Marwan's was turning gray. The skin of all three men was creased and weatherbeaten. They had been talking intently but quietly, looking deeply into each other's eyes as they spoke.

They rose as the nurse interpreter and I entered the room. Marwan introduced me to his son and to his brother. They were the eldest men in his family, he explained, and they had come to discuss his illness with me.

"What did the tests and examinations show?" asked the brother.

I told them what I had already disclosed to Marwan, that he had a cancer of the liver which had already spread to other parts of his body. It was causing jaundice and pain, and was very serious. Surgery might help lessen the jaundice but would not cure the disease. The cancer could not be removed by surgery.

"Would medicine help?" asked the son who had been listening intently, his eyes never leaving mine.

"Treatment with chemicals or radiation therapy might slow down the growth, but would not cure the cancer," I told him. "It could prolong his life somewhat."

"For how long?" asked his brother.

"Maybe months," I answered. "I really can't be sure."

"Will the treatment make him sick?" asked the brother.

"Yes, it might make him sick," I answered.

"How long can I live without treatment?" Marwan asked from his chair.

"I really don't know," I answered, turning to him. "Maybe six months, maybe longer. Nobody can be certain."

"*Allah karim* [God is merciful]," Marwan said quietly.

As the three men looked at each other and nodded, I realized that the discussion was over. I was impressed with the dignified way they had asked such difficult questions. I stood up and shook hands with each of them. As I clasped Marwan's hand, he said simply and with dignity, "*Shukran* [Thank you]. I want to go home to die. It is God's will. We are from God and to God we shall return."

That was the last time I saw Marwan. He was surrendering himself to the will of God according to Islam, with the blessing and understanding of his brother and son.

The Saudi's belief in predestination is as old as Islam itself. Allah predetermines the fate of each person individually. According to the Koran, "every small and great thing that a person does is recorded *in advance* in God's books" (54:53). The individual cannot alter his character or his destiny. Hussein, my Bedouin friend, had already told me of the concept of *maktub* (it is written) when we had dinner with him in the desert, but I did not realize that the devout Moslem theoretically has no control whatever over his fate or destiny. He believes in God's absolute decree of every event in his life, both good and evil.

Marwan faced death with fortitude and graciousness. He was in the hands of Allah and looked forward to Paradise. His belief in fate, called *qisma* and known to us as *kismet,* endowed him with calm and equanimity in the face of the inevitable.

His decision to go home to die was probably wise. There was no effective treatment for his disease. If there had existed even a remote chance for a cure, I would have tried to influence Marwan to remain in the hospital, but at best he would have survived a few months longer and with great suffering. The treatment is often worse than the disease. The end, in many instances, does not justify the means.

When Marwan dies, he will be buried lying on his side, facing Mecca. His eyes will not be closed, as in the West. Marwan can look forward to Paradise, where it is always spring, with plentiful and permanent green grazing, and where the water flows freely. There is no disease or hunger. Food is in great abundance. Pleasure is perpetual, and a man can enjoy the services of many houris, the eternally young, beautiful, and virginal maidens. All of a man's tribe live together in green pastures with their friends and relatives. No one grows old. All live forever. Should a woman have children who died in this world, she will meet them in Paradise grown to the age they would have been if they had lived. The children will welcome and greet their parents as at the end of a journey. The sun, moon, and stars always shine. Allah keeps in close touch with the inhabitants of Paradise and sometimes allows them to visit in dreams their loved ones still on earth.

Hell is just the opposite. There is a perpetual hot and blistering summer. There is no green grass or springs of water, and the camels and sheep will be short of grazing. Food is scarce. The inhabitants must forever break their backs drawing water for thirsty family and flocks, from wells which are deeper than any in this world. They will be bondsmen indefinitely and servants to an "inferior" tribe without honor.

Marwan, I felt certain, would be in Paradise.

I try not to get emotionally involved with my patients so that I can remain completely objective while treating them. Sometimes I fail, as in the case of Dr. Ghandour, the seventy-five-year-old physician whom I had met at Prince Ibrahim's palace shortly after the prince had suffered a small stroke. Dr. Ghandour had been a professor in a medical school in Egypt for years and then had come to Saudi Arabia to serve as physician to the fabled Prince Ibrahim and his family. This tall, bearded physician in Saudi dress, who spoke English, French, and Arabic, impressed me with his urbane manner and his wit. I saw him frequently during Prince Ibrahim's long hospitalization and we became good friends.

I was appalled when a year later Dr. Ghandour developed a cough, and an inoperable cancer of the lung was found. The biopsy indicated that it was the type of cancer which would not respond to radiation treatment. The cancer specialist tried x-ray therapy but said it would probably not be effective and that chemotherapy would be useless. (Dr. Ghandour, I might add, was a nonsmoker.)

I went to see him in the hospital twice daily, and every afternoon about five o'clock I met with him and his family for tea. His wife, who was twenty years his junior, was Egyptian. They had met in Cairo while she was doing graduate work under his direction at the university. Dr. Ghandour, I learned, was born and schooled in France, in Marseille, and came from an old, affluent Moslem family. He and his wife had lived in Riyadh for twenty-five years and Dr. Ghandour had become a Saudi citizen. Their lifestyle, however, was European. As a Saudi, he wore a thobe and ghutra and his wife wore a veil, but they did not live separate lives. Mrs. Ghandour told me that her Saudi friends, including the wives of the prince, envied her close relationship with her husband.

"I feel very sorry for them," she said. "They are very lonely."

"That's because their husbands do not treat their wives as well as I treat mine," said Dr. Ghandour.

"Wife—not wives," corrected Mrs. Ghandour. "Don't forget that." We all laughed.

Dr. Ghandour and his wife liked to reminisce over the "old days" in Riyadh. They said there had probably been more change in the past twenty-five years than in the past two hundred years since the Wahabis gained control.

"The abolition of slavery in 1962 had a tremendous impact on life in Saudi Arabia," Dr. Ghandour said, "and the discovery of oil revolutionized this country."

"Did you have any slaves?" I asked them.

Mrs. Ghandour said that she and her husband went to the slave market once to buy a servant. "But I refused. I wanted a slave to serve me, not to service my husband."

Dr. Ghandour went into a paroxysm of coughing at that remark.

Mrs. Ghandour went on to say that a slave who was not very young and beautiful cost the equivalent of $6,000 (U.S.), but a young and beautiful one was very expensive—about $10,000 (U.S.). The young ones served mainly as concubines. "Life was simpler and more gracious in the old days," she said, shaking her head sadly. "The wives knew that their husbands were sleeping with the concubines and they had some control over the situation. Now, the men pay for their sex wherever they can find it, in Riyadh or elsewhere. The women have no control. Most of my friends are Saudis and the women are not satisfied with their lives because of their husbands."

"Why did you leave Cairo?" I asked.

"The Saudis are honorable people and are more cultivated than you think," Dr. Ghandour said. "They don't lie, they don't steal, and they don't kill each other."

The Ghandours had two sons who usually joined us for tea. One was nineteen and a student at the University of Riyadh. The other, Dalal, was an entrepreneur, who took frequent trips to Jidda and returned telling his father how much money he had made. Dalal was twenty-two years old, very mature and worldly for his age. He explained that slavery in Saudi Arabia never was a racial issue as in the United States. The slaves were all Moslems from the Middle East, often sold into bondage by their own destitute families, who couldn't support young daughters. Slave dealers sometimes kidnaped ten-year-old girls, brought them up, taught them how to serve, and then sold them at a huge profit when they were thirteen or fourteen years old. "It was just a business," said Dalal. "The slaves came from everywhere—Syria, Sudan, Yemen, Ethiopia, Iran, Afghanistan, or Iraq. It was no disgrace at all for the Saudis to marry them if they produced sons. Even the royals married them. So you see it was an economic problem, not a racial or social one."

During these afternoon teas, we did our conversational best to distract Dr. Ghandour from thoughts of his impending death. I brought a tape recorder to his room to tape our discussions and to play classical music. There were attempts at gaiety, but they were forced. Dr. Ghandour began to cough up blood. He was dying and he knew it. I called the National Cancer Institute at Bethesda, Maryland, to see if anything further could be done, but they had nothing new to offer. All I could do was make him as comfortable as possible and wait for the inevitable. We continued the radiation treatments primarily to give Dr. Ghandour a faint ray of hope.

One evening, he called me at home and said he wanted to talk to me alone. When I arrived, he was coughing uncontrollably. I called the inhalation therapist, who administered to him, and soon his coughing subsided.

"I want to go to Paris," he said, his face drawn and white. "I have a friend there who is a cancer specialist. He has a new treatment which may help me."

"I'm glad for you," I said, because my first inclination was to believe it. "Hope springs eternal in the human breast" is a cliché but it is true. Maybe there was a new treatment in France. I had read recently of a radioactive isotope which concentrated in cancer tissue.

"But I won't go unless you come with me," he added. "It would be too dangerous for me to travel alone. I'm bringing up blood when I cough."

I told him I'd talk to Dr. Compton in the morning, that I should be able to get away for a few days, and in fact had some vacation time due me.

"Thank you," he sighed. "I knew I could count on you."

On the way home, cold scientific reasoning replaced my initial burst of optimism. The National Institutes of Health know what's going on all over the world. Dr. Ghandour didn't have a chance, but I would go with him anyway. There is a spark of immortality in all of us, and as long as it was glowing in him, I wanted to keep it alive. I understood Dr. Ghandour perfectly—it is difficult to conceive of yourself as nonexistent. I've tried, in the dark of night many times, but found it quite impossible. This indefinable link of eternity between man and the cosmos is the best argument I know for some sort of Supreme Order.

Dr. Compton at first was hesitant. "Suppose he dies on the plane. We'll be responsible."

"You owe me a favor," I replied, reminding him of Prince Yusef, my first patient. "I'll take emergency equipment along and several units of blood. Saudia Airlines can supply a special attachable bed and an extra attendant. A prince has reserved the entire first-class section of the plane for him. Dr. Ghandour realizes the risk and is willing to take it."

"Be sure he signs a release," Dr. Compton said.

Mrs. Ghandour flew ahead to Paris with her younger son to make arrangements at the cancer hospital. Dalal stayed behind to travel with his father and me.

We left Riyadh at midnight. I had given Dr. Ghandour a mild sedative before we left the hospital. Dalal and I both noted that he coughed less during the flight than in any night in recent memory, although the sedative and other medications were the same. He slept very little and was awake during the flight comments of the pilot and the instructions of the stewardess. We stayed close to his bed to be near him when he wanted to talk. He said he was happy to be "going home." It was the first time in forty years.

Dalal hovered over his father, lovingly wiping his brow and tending to him as a father might tend his child. He fed him, brought him fruit juice, held the urinal for him, and washed his hands afterward. Throughout the night he kept asking anxiously, in French, *"Ça va? Ça va?"* Are you all right? Finally, toward the end of our long journey, when his father fell asleep, Dalal sat down next to me.

"I love my father," he cried. "He is going home to die."

I tried to comfort him by asking him questions. "Do you usually speak French to your father?"

"When the family is alone, we always speak French," he said. "You know, he had an unhappy marriage in Marseille. That's why he left France and went to Cairo, where he met my mother several years later. He has been very happy with her. The prince for whom he worked in Riyadh was very envious of my father because of his happy married life. The prince had many wives and concubines but he envied my father, who had only one wife."

"I hope you remember this, Dalal," I said, "when you return to Riyadh to take up your life again there."

"Most men of my age now have only one wife," he replied. "Only the very rich can afford to marry more."

We arrived in Paris the next morning. Mrs. Ghandour was waiting with an ambulance and we drove directly to the hospital. It was a small private cancer hospital. The director, who was Dr. Ghandour's friend, greeted him warmly at the door. Somehow I sensed immediately that no great cancer cure would emanate from this hospital. It looked more like the Holy Ghost Hospital we used to have in Boston for the terminally ill. After Dr. Ghandour was settled in his room, which was very old but immaculate, I went to the director's office to show him Dr. Ghandour's x-rays and hospital records. After reviewing them carefully, he told me that he had nothing to offer except continuation of the x-ray treatment.

"After all," he said, *"entre nous,* Dr. Ghandour really came here to be near his home in Marseille. I am happy to be able to provide him with that."

"He looks better already," I said, thanking him for his sincerity.

When I returned to Dr. Ghandour's room, he was having lunch. He coughed but looked jubilant. "It's good to be home," he said. Then he looked lovingly at his wife and two sons and sighed. "I am a fortunate man," he whispered.

Several days passed in much the same routine we had followed before—quiet conversation, tea. Finally, it was time for me to return to Riyadh, and I went to Dr. Ghandour's room to say goodbye. His wife and sons were there. After some small talk, I rose to leave. Our eyes met briefly in understanding before we embraced each other in silence. He kissed my cheek as I turned away and tears welled up in his eyes. I knew I would never see him again. He knew it, too.

I never did.

◇ *22* ◇

SEX

THE SAUDIS HAVE a voracious appetite for sex. When the clinic first opened, we were inundated with Saudis complaining of "impotence." The condition could not be attributed to age because most of them were between thirty and fifty years old and seemed otherwise in perfect health. When the complaints began to assume epidemic proportions, the genitourinary clinic evaluated all its records and found that the Saudis considered themselves impotent if they could not indulge in sexual intercourse more than two or three times a day. All admissions to the clinic for "impotence" were thereafter sharply curtailed.

"I hope I become that 'impotent' when I turn fifty," said the urologist fervently. He was an American.

We soon learned that sexuality is rife in Saudi Arabia at all ages. It is part of the Saudi tradition. King Abdul-Aziz, the founder of modern-day Saudi Arabia, married his first wife when he was fifteen and he was said on good authority to have married approximately three hundred women in his lifetime, but never more than four at one time. This number did not include the innumerable concubines and slaves with whom he consorted. According to the records, King Abdul-Aziz, in 1930, told Harry St. John Philby, the English explorer, that he had married 135 virgins and more than 100 others but had decided to limit himself in the future to two new wives a year. He lived an additional twenty-three years, which would have brought his total close to the three hundred mark, assuming that he could remember those to whom he was married for only a few days and whose faces he never troubled to unveil.

The Saudis, as a nation, consider sex the greatest of all worldly pleasures. King Ibn Saud once said that what was most worth living for was to put his lips on a woman's lips, his body on her body, and his feet on her feet, which would be no ordinary accomplishment since the King was six feet three inches tall.

As time went on, it became apparent that many of the Saudi men were obsessed with sex. A general with a drinking problem tried to explain it to me. He was a handsome man in his forties who had attended a military academy in England and later married a Saudi woman. She was his only wife. They had four children. The general was admitted to the hospital with convulsions brought on by the abrupt withdrawal of alcohol upon his return from a trip to England. While he was recovering, he talked at length about his problems: sex and alcohol. He attributed most of his difficulties to his preoccupation with sex.

"How do you explain it?" I asked.

"The segregation of the sexes in this country, the veiling of the women, and the very limited contact between men and women during my childhood and adolescence made sex a prime compulsion," he said. "The taboo of sex for as far back as I can remember created a fixation on the subject."

"What about the women? What part do they play in this sex ethos?" I inquired.

The general told me that the segregation of the sexes is based on the concept that Saudi women cannot resist the temptation of sex and will submit automatically to the overtures of any erotic Saudi male.

"We are all oversexed," he said, "but a woman's lust is greater than a man's." This was a typical Saudi statement which I'd heard before. "It is taken for granted," he added, "that a woman is a sex symbol and that a Saudi man and woman left alone together will engage in sexual intercourse even though they are strangers. The mere sight of a woman will arouse a man."

"You think, then, that this uncontrollable sexuality is the reason for segregating the sexes in this country?" I asked, wanting to be sure I had heard correctly. "A few moments ago you said that the segregation of the sexes created the fixation."

"Yes," said the general, nodding his head gravely, "but the cure is probably worse than the disease."

"How do you mean?" I asked.

The general told me that the only way he could satisfy his erotic drive was to have sex with foreign women working in Saudi Arabia, like the airline hostesses or nurses and technicians, preferably non-Moslem.

"We have no real prostitutes, as such," he said, "but we usually give the foreign women expensive gifts and it takes a lot of time and trouble to seduce them. I prefer to go to England. It is much easier. But this time I drank too much and landed here in the hospital."

"Did you ever have sex with a Saudi woman other than your wife?" I asked.

"Never," he replied. "It would be too dangerous, because I am well known, and it would bring disgrace on her family and even death to her if it were discovered. Some of my friends take a chance, however, and have sex with Saudi women, usually divorced ones."

I tried to be helpful. "Since you have these sexual compulsions, why don't you marry two or three more wives?" I suggested.

"It's too expensive and too much trouble," he said. "Besides, I love my wife and children." He showed me their pictures. "My compulsion is to have sex with many different women. Sometimes I pace the floor at night thinking about it."

He went on to tell me that Islam admits that man is polygamous and that lifelong sexual fidelity to one woman is against human nature. When a man marries, he is not expected to be faithful to his wife. Even if he has four wives, he is allowed to have sex with concubines, prostitutes, or with unmarried women.

"I told my wife about having sex with women in England but that I loved her," he said. "She was unhappy about it but tried to understand me."

"But, general," I said, "you told me that Saudi women are more lustful than the men. Why can't they have affairs, too?"

"A Saudi woman," snapped the general, "must be a virgin when she marries, and must remain faithful to her husband. The honor of her family is at stake. The worst sin she can commit is to permit her sex to be enjoyed by anyone but her husband. Adultery, for a woman, is a crime. If she wants a lover, she must ask her husband for a divorce.

"The Christian world," added the general, "does not understand the Moslem marriage laws permitting polygamy and our harsh punishment for adultery. The Moslem world cannot comprehend your legally enforced monogamy or your very permissive attitude to adultery."

"You may not understand our liberal view on adultery," I said, "but you certainly take advantage of it."

The general laughed. "Many of us develop a dual personality," he said. "We lead exemplary and abstemious lives within our restrictive society at home until we can't tolerate it any longer. Then we go to England or to the United States, where we can get drunk and have all the women we want. The orgies may go on for months."

"Yes, I know," I said, recalling the brothel-like scene I chanced upon at the hotel when King Saud was in Boston some years ago. "And many of you end up in the hospital to recover."

The general gazed out of the window into the distance. "It was worth it," he said softly.

Shortly after my first patient, Prince Yusef, had left the hospital, Dr.

Hugh Compton phoned me. "This time," he said, "I have a pleasant assignment for you, one you'll enjoy."

"What is it?" I asked.

"I have a new intern here in my office whom I would like to assign to you for a while," he said, with a smile in his voice. "You have had a great deal of experience as a teacher and can be very helpful in directing and supervising this young doctor."

"I'll come over," I said. "We really need another intern on the medical service."

When I arrived at his office, Dr. Compton introduced me to a voluptuous young woman with fair skin, blue eyes, and red hair. Her name was Madeleine Yamine. Dr. Compton picked up her folder and gave me some vital statistics. Madeleine was twenty-three years old and had just graduated from a medical school in Belgium. They would grant her the M.D. degree after she completed her first year of internship under the tutelage of a qualified physician. She was also obliged to write a thesis under his direction.

Dr. Compton went on to say that Madeleine's father was in the import-export business and that Madeleine had lived for the most part in Morocco and in the Middle East.

"I speak French, of course, and Arabic," announced Madeleine, with a thick French accent, "but very little English—*un petit peu.* I must learn English."

"I speak French *un petit peu aussi,*" I said. "You teach me French and I'll teach you English."

"The first thing I'll teach you," said Janet, who had just entered the room, "is how to dress properly in Saudi Arabia. You can't go about with those bare arms and a short dress."

"But it is so hot," said Madeleine in French. *"Il fait très chaud."*

Dr. Compton came to the rescue. "Janet will take you to some dress shops. Meanwhile, you can wear a white coat," he said, "and with long sleeves," he added to placate his secretary.

I assigned some hospital patients to Madeleine, mostly women to begin with, and also arranged for her to work with me in the clinic. The language barrier presented problems but we got along fairly well with the help of an English-French dictionary. Her knowledge of Arabic more than compensated for her deficiency in English.

Hospitals tend to spawn gossip and our hospital was particularly susceptible. The word went around that I was having a fling with a beautiful young lady and a European one at that. Actually, our relationship was friendly but entirely professional. It was at first that of teacher and student and later that of a father and daughter. In fact, when the dentist was about to extract a wisdom tooth, Madeleine insisted that I go along with her and hold her hand. We just laughed at the gossip and the knowing glances.

The Saudis, however, viewed Madeleine from a different, more challenging point of view. A woman with red hair and blue eyes was rare in this country and would be a choice conquest. The first bidder for her favors was the manager of the dilapidated Al Yamama Hotel, where I was staying. I had complained to the Saudi manager several times about my room, which was intolerably hot because there was no air conditioning. At first he said that they had turned it off because it was not necessary in my part of the hotel. The second time he said that it was in need of repair. The third time I complained he said that the air conditioning was beyond repair and that no other rooms were available. Then one evening he called me into his office, asked me to sit down, and offered me a cigarette. I declined with thanks, saying I didn't smoke cigarettes.

"I may be able to get you an air-conditioned room," he said. "They are very scarce but I will try." He had attended the hotel school at Cornell and spoke perfect English. "It all depends on you," he continued, as he exhaled a cloud of cigarette smoke.

"What do you mean?" I asked.

He stamped out his cigarette and stood up. "There is a beautiful young doctor working with you at the hospital. I would like to meet her," he said. "You could arrange it."

I told him that her social life was her own and that she had very little free time because of her work. "Besides," I said, "you are married. I have seen your children." The manager lived in the hotel with his family.

"What difference does that make?" he asked. "Your friend is not a Moslem, so there is no problem." I already knew that the Saudis were constantly trying to seduce non-Moslem women because they had little or no opportunity for sexual contact with young Saudi women.

"The room is a very choice one," said the manager. "It's up to you."

I thanked him and said that there was nothing I could do. He was very disappointed, he told me. "Maybe you will change your mind," he said hopefully.

I didn't change my mind and I didn't get the air-conditioned room.

The next in line to court my favor was the headwaiter at the Intercontinental Hotel.

"Let me choose your dinner," he said one night when I was there with my good friend Ron Lambrie. Our wives had not yet arrived and we had decided to treat ourselves to a good meal in the posh dining room, the best Riyadh had to offer.

The dinner was excellent. It included shrimp cocktail and a superb sirloin steak, which the waiter sliced and weighed on a special scale brought to our table. The steak and the fresh raspberries which followed were flown from France, the waiter told us. The hotel, Ron reminded me, was owned by Pan American Airlines. Throughout the dinner we sipped non-alcoholic "champagne," which was served with all the ritual accorded the finest real champagne, including the popping of the cork, the preliminary taste testing and inhaling the bouquet of the "wine."

"Wait until you see the bill," said Ron. "Only the royals and people with large expense accounts eat here."

I called the headwaiter, congratulated him on the dinner and asked for the bill.

"The dinner is with my compliments," he said, much to our surprise. "I am glad you enjoyed it.

"I hope you will bring the red-haired doctor from the hospital to dine here as my guest," he added. "I would like very much to meet her."

I made some noncommittal remark and thanked him. As we left, I noticed that there was only one woman in the large dining room, which was filled to capacity. She was having dinner with an American, presumably her husband. I was reminded again that in Saudi Arabia the men never take their wives out in public. This does not apply to foreign, non-Moslem women, whom the Saudis entertain in any manner that suits them.

I told Madeleine about all the excitement she was creating among the Saudis. "That's because I have red hair," she said, "and am a foreign woman. We are in great demand."

"For one purpose only," I remarked.

She continued to work in the clinic with me, getting the medical history from the patients in Arabic and recording it on the patient's chart in English. Then she would present the history to me and I would perform the physical examination and make the recommendations for diagnosis and treatment. She was an excellent student and progressed rapidly. Soon she took responsibility for the complete history and physical examination, the pertinent parts of which I repeated just to make sure.

One morning, several months later, she asked me to see a patient she had just examined. It was Prince Khalil. He too, apparently, had heard about Madeleine, while visiting his wife and new son in the hospital. He was more ingenious than the other Saudis, however, and arranged an appointment with me in the clinic for a "checkup," knowing that Madeleine would see him first to get his medical history.

"All is fair in love and war," he said when we were alone. "I knew you wouldn't arrange a meeting with her so I took matters into my own hands. She's a gorgeous woman!"

"Anyone who has *Deep Throat* in his video library at home is capable of anything," I said, recalling his all-night party.

"That was a great party," said Khalil, laughing.

Within a month, Madeleine moved from her austere accommodations in the single women's quarters in the hospital compound to a spacious apartment on the outskirts of Riyadh, which the immensely wealthy Prince Khalil had purchased for her. A chauffeured limousine brought her to the hospital each morning and remained there for her use. Everyone at the hospital knew of her affair with the prince, and some were envious. Madeleine continued her duties without interruption, however, but gradually withdrew from the social life of the hospital.

When she returned from her first week's post leave, which she had spent in Iran with Khalil, I thought that a talk with her was in order. Compton had placed her under my tutelage and I was in a sense responsible for her. My wife had met Madeleine and liked her. Ruth felt that my responsibility, however, did not include interference with Madeleine's sex life.

"If it weren't Khalil, it would be some other Saudi," she said. "She's a very attractive woman and the Saudi men are starving for women, particularly young women."

Madeleine had brought me an antique hand-painted Iranian pencil box as a gift. This gave me the opportunity I had been waiting for.

"You know," I said, "that Prince Khalil already has two wives and has no intention of marrying you. Besides, it's illegal to marry a non-Moslem woman."

"Maybe I'll become a Moslem. Then I can be his third wife," she said, trying to provoke me.

"Your whole relationship is based on sex and you know it," I said.

"They're very good at it," she replied. "This isn't my first Saudi lover."

"What would your family think of all this?" I asked.

"They would probably be unhappy about it but would not pass judgment upon me," she answered.

"Are you doing this for the sex or for the jewels and the gold?" I asked.

"Both," she said. "You don't understand European women."

I made one last desperate attempt. "How would you react if you had a daughter who behaved the way you do?"

"I would not interfere with her life," she said angrily.

"Well, I won't either," I said, "but the generation gap is too much for me."

"You sound exactly like my father," said Madeleine. We both laughed.

When I returned home that night, I told my wife about Madeleine and my naïveté. "By the way, what did you do with all your free time in London?" I asked.

"Don't be ridiculous," said Ruth, laughing, "but I am glad you asked."

The Saudi seduction campaigns continued. The American and Canadian nurses, technicians, secretaries, and dieticians later moved to the Gerrin Village apartments, where visitors were permitted. The Moslem women, however, were kept in the restricted, single-women's quarters, into which no men were ever allowed. Security was strictly enforced there on a twenty-four-hour basis.

Liaisons between the Saudis and foreign women were common knowledge. One American technician, a divorcee, had a display in her apartment of the gifts bestowed upon her by her Saudi lovers. They included Persian rugs, gold bracelets, and fine jewelry. A Canadian nurse lived openly with one of the Saudi employees. When she returned home, he subsequently had an affair with her roommate, an American nurse. He apparently admired the nursing profession.

Prince Bhadir, one of Khalil's young cousins, began making overtures to an American nurse. He was engaged at the time to a Saudi princess, with whom he carried on his courtship over the telephone. He caught glimpses of her on occasion, he told me, when she went shopping with her maid, as prearranged by telephone.

"She's always heavily veiled," he said. "I've never had a real good look at her, but I'm told she's beautiful." He promised to invite me to the wedding.

Meanwhile, he was toying with the nurse, buying her gifts and courting her favor. He was a handsome devil and immensely wealthy. The nurse was taken with him and began to consider his advances seriously.

One of my missions in life was to prevent pain and suffering. I called the nurse into my office. "This is none of my business," I said bluntly, "but if you expect Prince Bhadir to marry you, forget it. He is already engaged to marry his cousin."

Tears welled up in her eyes. "Thank God," she said, "nothing has happened between us and nothing will." She gave me a peck on the cheek, thanked me, and left.

Prince Bhadir married his princess three months later. It was a very fashionable wedding. I was not invited.

The Saudi administrators did not seem to be seriously concerned when adultery involved a non-Moslem woman, but woe to the Moslem woman who associated in any way with an infidel. A young Egyptian secretary fell in love with an Englishman, who wanted to marry her. There was nothing illicit in their relationship, she assured me, but she was warned by Saudi officials that she would be discharged from the hospital and returned to Egypt if she ever saw the Englishman again.

"My family is very poor," she said. "I send most of my salary home for them to buy food. I cannot afford to lose this job."

The Saudi administrators were sympathetic, but they discharged the Englishman and sent him home two weeks later. As far as I know she never heard from him again.

Sex is the "supreme joy of life" among the Saudis. Men and women alike enjoy its pleasures. The Bedouin bride usually shows great modesty on the first night by trying to keep her face as well as her body covered. She resists with all her strength, in a proper show of modesty, when her husband uses force to remove her veil or various parts of her clothing. In some tribes, where the women wear the *burqa* or mask (made of coarse silk with slits for the eyes) they try to keep it on for ten days out of modesty but usually don't succeed.

In some areas, it is considered good form for the bride to struggle and fight off her husband in a vain effort to save her virginity. She may scream as she bites and claws her husband until he forces her to surrender. The more violent and prolonged the struggle, the more credence to the modesty and virginity of the bride. The next day the husband displays his battle scars to the family with pride, and shows them the bloodstained bedsheet or undergarment of his bride, extolling her family with "God whiten your faces; you have indeed kept your daughter pure."

This required proof of innocence may present problems for those who may have lost their "virginity" by natural means without ever having indulged in sexual intercourse. The girl may then resort to such subterfuges as cutting herself or smearing a little chicken blood on the sheet to satisfy her husband. The men are on the lookout for such trickery, and if the girl is caught she may be taken away and killed by her male relatives to vindicate the honor of the family, even though she was, in fact, a virgin.

Sometimes, the bride and groom overindulge in the joy of sex or in the seduction rituals on the wedding night and then celebrate the next day in the hospital. A young Bedouin bride was brought into the clinic by her proud husband, whose face was covered with scratches. She had fractured two ribs on her wedding night while trying to protect her virginity or while enjoying her submission. They both seemed very happy, however.

Later they told me that, according to the precepts of Islam, both the man and the woman must have a complete bath after sexual intercourse. There is a special prayer for the pious woman to recite while performing her ablution. Women are forbidden to have sexual intercourse for seven days during the menstrual period and must bathe all over before resuming their sex life. This is called "washing the hair" by the Bedouins. During the thirty-day feast of Ramadan, sexual intercourse is forbidden by day but not by night.

Virility and fecundity are Saudi Arabian hallmarks. The Saudis of the older generation pride themselves on the number of sons they have produced and the number of wives they have married. It was not unusual for a man to have thirty or more wives in his lifetime in addition to his concubines. Prince Yusef had twenty-five sons and Prince Ibrahim twenty-three.

The sexual prowess of the older Saudis is legendary. Many in their eighties continue to marry and produce children. When he was ninety Prince Ibrahim complained constantly of impotence, although he allegedly sired three children after he was eighty.

One afternoon, an elderly Saudi appeared in the clinic with his son. I was impressed by the appearance of the old man. He was tall, erect, and sinewy. His thick hair was silver in color and his beard white. There was a broad smile on his face. His only problem, according to his son, was the appearance of a small lump in his right groin, which was painless and had been there for about six months. It had not increased in size.

On physical examination, I found him to be in excellent condition except for a small hernia in his groin. It was only about one inch in diameter and easily reducible. I told them that it was nothing serious and could be repaired easily.

"How old are you?" I asked.

"Seventy-five," he said, still smiling.

"Eighty-five, at least," corrected his son. "I'm nearly sixty years old myself."

The son appeared to be almost as old as his father. The Saudis usually understate their age by five to ten years.

"Does he still work?" I asked.

"Oh, yes," said his son. "He has a small business."

"Well, he probably should have the hernia repaired sometime," I said, "but since it is painless and has not increased in size during the past six months, there is no hurry."

"Oh, yes, there is," said the old man with a grin. "I must have it fixed immediately. I'm getting married in two weeks!"

"Who is the bride?" I asked out of curiosity.

"An eighteen-year-old girl," said his son proudly. "He likes young women."

The eighty-five-year-old man had already married thirty-two women. He had twenty-eight sons and sixteen daughters.

"We better have that hernia repaired now," I said. "It may get larger after he is married."

Dr. Ghandour's words came back to me: "There are no old men in Saudi Arabia."

Although the Saudi Arabian men were unusually libidinous by nature, they had no monopoly on lust or licentiousness. The men and women of the Western world did not lag far behind. Fornication flourished within our small modern oasis of advanced technology but with less obsession and compulsion than in the old Arab tradition. It went on quietly, consistently, and graciously with little fuss or bother. The young women of the West contributed generously and more than made up for the Saudi women, who had no opportunity whatever to participate in the sex games.

A fair number of recently divorced and remarried physicians and other personnel were among the early arrivals at the hospital. Some looked upon the Saudi Arabian experience as an opportunity for a clean break from their old environment. Their conduct seemed consistently exemplary, as was the behavior of all those who had been married a long time to one partner.

There were two groups, however, who contributed to the sexual over-activity and promiscuity. One consisted of the unattached men and women who were either divorced or legally separated from their spouses and going it alone in Saudi Arabia. The other was made up of men and women between twenty-eight and thirty-five who had not yet married. There were many in both of these categories, however, who apparently did not indulge at any time. A few who did married later on.

I don't have statistics but I suppose the inhabitants of "Hospital City" followed the same sexual patterns as might be anticipated for any California suburb of equal size and constituency. It was the flagrant violations of the code that made the deepest impression. For example, there was a chemist from Texas in his thirties, who lived in one of the Campus Villas with his wife and five children. Both spouses had been divorced previously and had been married to each other for about ten years. The Texan first had an affair with an English secretary. It became an open secret in the hospital. Everyone seemed to know. After six months, he transferred his affections to one of the American technicians in the laboratory. His wife finally learned about the affair and left Saudi Arabia with her three children. He continued to live in the villa with his two children, and the young technician moved in with him. When the administration learned of it, they discharged her forthwith. To their relief his contract expired a few months later and it was not renewed. Nobody seemed to know what happened to them afterward.

Then there was May-Ellen, a tall, well-built, attractive thirty-year-old brunette from Alabama who was separated from her husband. She was a laboratory technician and was good at her job. She was also very good in bed, she told me one day, when she appeared in the clinic with hepatitis. Since we had seen very little hepatitis among the Americans, English, or Europeans, I was anxious to determine the source of her illness because hepatitis could become epidemic in a closed community like ours.

May-Ellen was very helpful. She told me that her sex partner at the moment was a Saudi who also had become jaundiced. I explained that hepatitis could be transmitted by sexual intercourse.

"Too bad," she said. "I found out about his jaundice too late. I better tell him about it before he infects his wives."

"The wives should be injected with immune serum right away," I said. "Hepatitis is common in this country."

During the next month, she told me about her sex life. "Next to the Saudis, the Greeks are the best," she said. She went to Greece whenever possible, even though she could only get away for ten days at a time.

"Those ten days are unbelievable," she said, "but I can't take more than ten days at a time. I'm a wreck when I come back."

"What about the Italians and the French?" I asked.

The Italians, she told me, ran a close third. The English and the Americans were only fair but there were exceptions. I expressed my regrets. "You must try to be more patriotic," I said sympathetically. "Do you have a lover in Greece?"

"No," she said, "I just play the field. The men there are all gorgeous. I usually go to the island of Mykonos. There's a nudist colony there."

"One of these days you may come back with a venereal infection," I warned her.

Several months later, May-Ellen's roommate called me from their Gerrin Village apartment. "May-Ellen just came back from Greece," she said. "She looks terrible, she has a high fever, and I think she needs to be hospitalized."

Sure enough, May-Ellen had a severe venereal infection, and I transferred her to the gynecology service.

"Please get me fixed up quickly," she pleaded. "My husband is coming here next month. We've been reconciled."

"There's an old proverb I learned in college," I said. "Beware of the Greeks bearing gifts."

"Oh, you doctors!" she said. "You think you know everything!"

The behavior of human beings is sometimes unaccountable, as in the case of Cynthia Watson, a strikingly attractive secretary in the Department of Medicine. She was twenty-eight years old and was engaged to be married to an engineer in her home town in Wisconsin. Her family owned a dairy farm and she often brought me generous samples of cheese which her parents had sent from home. Sometimes, after I finished my dictation, she would prepare some cheese and crackers and we would have coffee in my office. She liked to talk about her family and her fiancé, who was working for an advanced degree at the University of Wisconsin. They were planning to marry, she said, in about two years, at the expiration of her contract in Saudi Arabia. She shared an apartment in Gerrin Village with another secretary and an American nurse.

As time passed Cynthia seemed withdrawn and preoccupied. The cheese supply dwindled and she rarely spoke of home. Then one afternoon she invited me to a dinner party.

"What is your apartment number in Gerrin Village?" I asked her.

"I won't be in Gerrin Village," she replied. "A car will be waiting for you at the hospital entrance at eight o'clock."

"It sounds pretty posh," I said, thanking her for the invitation.

A specially designed Cadillac limousine drew up at the hospital entrance precisely at eight o'clock. The Saudi chauffeur, who spoke little English, asked for me at the front desk. He introduced himself in Arabic and explained that my host's name was Sheik Majid Toonsi. He spoke slowly and was pleased that I could understand him. We drove to the exclusive Nasseria area not far from where Prince Khalil lived.

A servant met me at the entrance of the sheik's palatial villa and directed me to the drawing room. Cynthia, bedecked in jewels and wearing a long flowing mauve gown, greeted me and introduced me to the sheik. He was an elegant, rather portly man in his fifties. It soon became apparent that Cynthia was the hostess and mistress of the house. She introduced me to the other guests and their wives. They were all businessmen or bankers from various parts of the world: England, the U.S., Belgium, West Germany, Korea, and Japan. Majid Toonsi was a Saudi from the Eastern Province, who had made a fortune in oil. He was a self-made man of humble origin and had educated himself, he told me. He spoke four languages. Cynthia told me later that he had only one wife and she was illiterate. She lived with their five children in Dhahran.

I learned that Cynthia had been living with Toonsi for the past six months and managed his home and servants. Her lifestyle was somewhat similar to that of Madeleine. She maintained her apartment at Gerrin Village for appearance's sake, continued to work in the hospital as before, and commuted by chauffeured limousine.

"It keeps me busy," she said, as she showed me around the villa, which included a lovely garden room with a small pool and a fountain in the center.

After a sumptuous dinner, which included superb vintage wine and champagne, I thanked my host and hostess, said goodbye to the guests, and went home in the Cadillac limousine shortly after midnight.

Before leaving, I congratulated Cynthia on the superb meal but couldn't refrain from adding, "I was hoping for some Wisconsin cheese for dessert."

"I'll bring you some tomorrow," she said, laughing.

After fulfilling her contract with the hospital many months later, Cynthia returned to Wisconsin and married her engineer.

One of my memorable patients in the clinic was a technician who had been working in the hospital since it opened in 1975. Khasna was a tall, attractive woman in her thirties, who wore long, beautifully tailored, colorful gowns. She had a heart murmur, which required periodic examinations. What intrigued me about her was that she was a Moslem and a blonde, which is a rare combination in this country. She explained that she was not a Saudi but was of Russian and Iraqi extraction. Her ancestors came originally to Mecca and Medina from Russia and Iraq to make the pilgrimage and settled in the area. There were a number of such small foreign minority groups in the Hejaz area, who were never assimilated into the Saudi culture and never became Saudi citizens.

"We are considered outsiders," she said, "although we are Moslems, of course."

She was the only Moslem woman patient who ever invited me to her home. "You must come and have tea with us," she said.

I was flattered but politely declined. I didn't feel like driving to the Batha Apartments where she lived (overlooking the open sewers) and where parking a car was impossible. She took the hospital bus, she told me.

Several months later, she invited me again. "You should meet my parents," she urged. I declined once more.

One day after Dalal, Dr. Ghandour's son, returned from France he pointed to Khasna as we were walking down the corridor of the hospital.

"She's a prostitute," he said. "She gets as much as 4,000 riyals ($1,300, U.S.) a night!"

"That's incredible," I said. I told him that Khasna had invited me to her Batha apartment to meet her parents.

"Her parents are in Mecca," he replied. "You can be sure."

"My wife will be as surprised as I am," I said, shaking my head.

"Maybe one day I'll tell you things about some of our women that you couldn't possibly know and probably won't want to believe," Dalal said, laughing.

"I'll keep you to that promise," I replied.

◇ 23 ◇

LIFE BEHIND THE PALACE WALLS

A MONTH LATER Dalal and another young man came to my office.

"When we were in Paris," Dalal said, "my father talked about you frequently. He knew you would write a book one day about our country and asked me to help you in every way possible. He really loved you. So here I am with my friend Jamil. We came to tell you everything."

He introduced me to Jamil, a tall, slender, handsome man, about twenty-four years old, with sparkling brown eyes, a black mustache, and glistening, porcelain-white teeth.

"Jamil and I grew up together," said Dalal. "For most of our lives we have lived in adjoining houses right on the palace grounds within the shadow of the palace itself." Jamil's father was chief of staff in charge of Prince Ibrahim's vast estates in the Nejd and Haradh regions.

"You see," explained Dalal, "the prince wanted both his physician and the manager of his estates to be close at hand."

"First," I said to Dalal, "tell me about your father. The last time I saw him he was in the Paris hospital."

Dalal told me that his father had left the hospital after a few weeks and gone to his family home in Marseille, where he died. He was buried in the family plot.

"He just wanted to go home to die," said Dalal softly.

"He was a wonderful man. Our family is very grateful to you for what you did for him."

"I wish I could have done more," I said. "I felt very close to him. His passing must have been very difficult for your mother. Will she be able to get along financially? Your father took care of Prince Ibrahim and his family for twenty years. I hope the prince remembered him in his will."

Dalal told me that Prince Ibrahim left his entire estate valued at $32 billion to his immediate family. There were no other beneficiaries or bequests to charity.

"My father had no pension or retirement benefits," said Dalal, "but the King took care of everything for us. He paid the hospital bills in Riyadh, the air fare to Paris, and all the hospital expenses in France.

"And he gave my mother a generous monthly allowance for the rest of her life," he added. "My brother and I will also get an equal amount until we are twenty-six. We are obliged to the King for all this."

"Who actually contacted the King about your father?" I asked.

"A friend named Dr. Rashad Pharaon gave my father's letter of petition to the King and the King gave my father the money and the allowance for our family," said Dalal. "Dr. Pharaon was the advisor to the late King Faisal and is also an advisor to King Khalid. He and my father were friends."

I had heard of Dr. Pharaon before. He was highly respected and a long-time confidant of the royal family. By a strange coincidence, I had met his son, Sheik Ghaith Pharaon, in Boston before I left for Saudi Arabia, and later learned more about him when I visited Aramco.

"It always amazes me," I said, "how readily accessible the King and the royal family are. It's a good lesson in democracy."

"You can't imagine how easy it is to see the King or a prince high in the government," said Dalal. "The secretary arranges the appointments or you can go to a *majlis.* The royal family is large, and many like Prince Sultan and King Khalid are very generous."

"Now turn on your tape recorder again," said Dalal, drawing up a chair, "and we will talk like we did when we had tea in my father's room in the hospital."

I offered Jamil a chair and then turned on the tape recorder.

Dalal paused for a moment as though he were about to give a prepared speech. "Some of us believe," he said, "that the freeing of the slaves and the concubines fifteen years ago marked the beginning of a sexual revolution in this country.

"For both sexes," he added ominously. "In the old days, a man had his wives and his concubines as in the days of the Prophet Mohammed, and all sexual activity was in the home according to Moslem law. There were no whores then. Now we have many whores," he remarked unhappily.

"The situation between the men and the women is now in a bad state. Everyone is complaining but mostly the women," he concluded. "It was better before when we had concubines. Life then was more in the Islamic tradition."

"Slavery was abolished a little more than a decade ago," I said. "I can't believe that you would favor slavery in this day and age."

"It was a different kind of slavery," explained Dalal. "You see, we had sex with our concubines. They did not take money when they had sex. They were not whores. They could have children, and sometimes the men would marry them or set them free.

"The wives preferred this system because they were still in control. Now there are many whores and free whores in this country. The men are constantly running after them and the wives are very unhappy about this."

I found Dalal's repeated use of the word "whore" offensive. "What is a 'free whore'?" I asked.

"That's an immoral or easy woman with whom we can have sex but don't pay them anything," explained Jamil. "We call them 'free whores.' The 'real whores' are those who want money or expensive gifts. There are both kinds in this country.

"The real danger is that, since the men do whatever they want sexually, some of the wives feel that they have the right to do what they want, and the basic reason for this situation is the way the husbands and wives live in this country."

Dalal stood up. He appeared agitated and apparently had decided to reveal a deep and ominous secret, one over which he had agonized.

"I must tell you," he said, "that there are many women pursuing Jamil and me. Some of them are princesses."

"We both have this problem," added Jamil. "They are 'free whores' or 'easy women' who run after us for their amusement only. They do this not for money and not for love, just for sex. Many are very rich."

"I had better turn off this tape recorder," I said. "You are both on dangerous ground. You could lose your heads over this."

"No, no, leave it on," said Dalal, "we won't mention any names."

"Are these young girls?" I asked.

"Oh, no," said Jamil, "they are married or divorced. Some have children who are older than we are. They are just unhappy with their husbands and want to do the same as their husbands are doing. None of them are virgins."

"How do they contact you?" I asked.

"By telephone or by a messenger or a chauffeur whom they can trust, someone who can't read," he said.

They went on to tell me that most of these women were "modern Saudi women" who had been educated in the West and found it difficult to tolerate the philandering of their husbands. Divorce was often difficult so they compensated by having sexual dalliances with younger men.

"If a woman is found committing adultery, she can be killed for bringing dishonor upon her family," I said. "Aren't these women taking terrible risks?"

"Not if they are clever," replied Jamil. "There must be four eye-witnesses to the sex act in order to charge a woman with adultery and that would obviously be very difficult."

Occasionally, a young woman, overcome with remorse, confessed adultery voluntarily, and lost her life as a result, but that occurred very rarely, he said.

"Recently," added Jamil, "they caught a lover in the palace with one of Prince Ibrahim's wives. They beat him up but they did not kill him because he came from a prominent tribe. Moreover, his family warned the prince that 'a head is for a head.' The old prince did not dare to kill his wife's lover because he feared that one of his own children would meet the same fate.

"Both the man and the woman denied adultery," he continued, "although the man was caught in the palace bedroom. The wife was not punished because there were no witnesses to testify. There must be four witnesses present *during* the sex act, not afterward. Circumstantial evidence does not count."

"Islamic law is very rigorous in its requirements for proof," explained Dalal. "If an accusation does not hold up, the witnesses themselves are liable to get eighty lashes."

"Sounds like one of our ten commandments," I said. "Thou shalt not bear false witness."

Dalal, for some reason, kept returning to the subject of slavery and concubines. His father, he said, felt that the recent abolition of the slave and concubine system caused a moral as well as sexual upheaval in Saudi Arabia.

"When slavery was legal, Prince Ibrahim had some thirty concubines in addition to his four wives," said Dalal.

"According to the law, if the concubines had children," he added, "the prince was obliged to recognize them. The son became a prince and the daughter a princess. The mother could not be sold."

Prince Ibrahim preferred foreign women, according to Dalal. His youngest wife was from Iran. The prince bought her for two hundred pieces of gold and married her later when she bore him sons. "She was his favorite wife," he said. "When Prince Ibrahim died, two of the four wives who survived him had been former concubines. Each inherited about $1 billion."

"That's one thousand million dollars," I gasped. "Are you sure of this?"

"I am sure," said Dalal.

Jamil pointed out that, when Prince Ibrahim was a young man, some of the slaves were brought up and educated by his family and then sent to the prince as concubines when they came of age, usually between fourteen and fifteen.

"What did they do in the palace," I asked, "other than the obvious?"

"They waited on the prince, served his breakfast and ironed his clothes," said Jamil. "They had little to do except to bring him pleasure in bed. Life was easy for everyone in the palace."

"Surely for a young girl to be stolen from her family and sold as a concubine is not an easy life," I exclaimed, but he ignored me.

"When I was a boy, I remember seeing the beautiful young concubines standing about in the gardens, looking like delicate flowers. They came from everywhere in the Moslem world and were of different colors: black-skinned girls from Ethiopia, olive and brown beauties from Egypt and Iran, and fair women from Morocco and Syria.

"Prince Ibrahim was the lord of the manor. Everyone respected and feared him. The men in the village would stop and salute him when he passed them in the street.

"He was short in stature and long in discipline," he concluded. "Anyone who was not present at prayer time would be punished or banished from the palace. The gates were locked at ten o'clock. If any of his sons arrived home late, they were beaten."

Dalal took over the conversation. "The prince held on desperately to the old ways," he said. "Two years ago there were five hundred people living within the palace compound, counting all the wives and children of the various servants. He fed and clothed them all and gave them a small salary as well. His table was open to everyone. The people of the village would come for food with their plates and buckets. Everyone was expected to eat at the table of the prince. He disliked seeing a partially empty table at mealtime."

"Did he ever have a meal with his family?" I asked.

"No, he never ate with his wives and children," said Dalal. "He had his meals at the royal palace with the King or with government ministers and dignitaries at home. He usually had breakfast alone."

The prince insisted that all his wives and children have their meals together to give them a sense of family unity, according to Dalal. The prince's son, Ahmad, had told me this before.

"He was almost fanatically religious, a fundamentalist, and a champion of the austere Wahabi way of life," said Dalal. "He didn't want to travel because he felt that foreign ideologies might affect his faith and loyalty to his country.

"He was one of a kind, and his recent death marked the end of an era in Saudi Arabian history."

"It reminds me somewhat of the period after the Civil War in our country when the great plantations were broken up and the slaves were freed," I said.

"Many of the slaves preferred to stay with the prince," said Dalal, "particularly the men. They had easy lives as slaves, but the women mostly ran away."

"Perhaps the concubines didn't think they had such easy lives, with nothing to do except bring the prince pleasure in bed," I said, wondering if he realized what he had just admitted. But he merely shrugged his shoulders.

"Speaking of the women," I said, "several of Prince Ibrahim's wives were much younger than the prince. You told me about one lover. Were there others?"

There was a pause, an embarrassingly long pause.

"I am the lover of the youngest wife," said Jamil, quietly, "the Iranian slave he bought for two hundred pieces of gold. Her name is Filwa."

My first impulse was to shut off the tape recorder and terminate the discussion. This was beginning to sound like "True Confessions from Within the Seraglio." But it was a slice of Saudi Arabian life at the end of an era, which might have a bearing on the future.

Dalal immediately added coals to the fire of my imagination. "Jamil was only one of her lovers," he said. "She has had others."

"Was this affair with Filwa going on while the prince was alive?" I asked.

"Yes," said Jamil, "but remember she was thirty-five and he was almost ninety."

"Prince Ibrahim had enormous wealth and influence," I said to Jamil. "You were risking your life and hers, too."

"We were very careful," said Jamil. "We met only in my house or in Dalal's."

"Is this still going on right now?" I asked.

"Yes," said Jamil.

"And your family knows about it?"

"Yes, both our families know, Dalal's and mine," said Jamil.

"I can't imagine how this all began," I said, "considering the strict separation of the men and women."

"I will tell you," said Jamil. "Prince Ibrahim's wives were pretty bored sitting in the palace all day. Occasionally, one of them would come to visit my mother or Dalal's mother for tea.

"One day I returned home from the market," he continued, "and found Filwa there talking to my mother. I felt strange. I had not seen her for many years, since the days when we were children, like brother and sister.

"You see, Dalal and I were born on the palace grounds and we could go to the palace whenever and wherever we wished because we had blood brothers and sisters living there," said Jamil.

"I don't understand," I said.

"It is a system for protecting the royals from marrying outside the family," explained Jamil. "A princess in the palace may suckle two children of opposite sex. One is her own daughter and the other is Dalal, for example. That makes them foster brother and sister. Dalal therefore cannot marry any of Prince Ibrahim's children because he is considered a 'blood brother' even though the suckling at the royal breast occurred only once."

Jamil went over to the window and stared out into the desert. "Some time later," he continued, "Filwa came to our house. I was studying my lessons for the university. My mother had gone to the palace on an errand and my father was away on business. She made some tea and began questioning me about my love life and about sex. I was surprised and embarrassed.

"'I imagine women find you attractive,' she said.

"I told her," said Jamil, "that there were a number of women making advances to both Dalal and me, particularly older women.

"Finally, after she asked many personal questions relating to sex, I said to her, 'What do you want from me?'

"And she said, 'You know what I want from you.'

"That's how it began," concluded Jamil. "She came to my house when my parents were away or I met her in Dalal's house."

"Did the other wives know about your affair with Filwa?" I asked.

"Yes," said Jamil, "but they kept it secret because some of them also had lovers. The wives protected one another.

"Each wife," he continued, "had her own separate living quarters in the palace, with her own guards and servants who were loyal to her and protected her privacy. The clandestine visitors paid them handsomely to ensure their loyalty."

"Remember," said Jamil, "the prince was forty to fifty years older than most of his wives and, in a way, he treated them like animals. The only time he saw them was in bed, so you can imagine the situation. All he wanted was sex and sons, always more sons and more sex."

"The Saudi women were used for breeding only," said Dalal. "Today, our women have become envious of the Western women because the men in the West respect them and treat them like equals.

"The main problem is that people here can't keep up with the rapid changes that have taken place in Saudi Arabia in the past thirty years," he added. "You can't imagine it! We jumped thirteen centuries, all within thirty years. Our people's minds and morals haven't been able to adjust to it. We are going crazy, I think.

"That is why the married women are beginning to take on lovers in this country. They are suddenly facing a new and very different world."

"Speaking of lovers," said Jamil, "Filwa had many while she lived in the palace. She came as a concubine and continued to live as one even after Prince Ibrahim married her."

"We can't blame her entirely," said Dalal with compassion. "She was completely uneducated and her lessons came only from the prince. Her husband taught her to behave as a concubine and so she did. Remember, she was fifteen years old when the prince bought her. And he was seventy."

Her first lover, according to Jamil, was a very rich sheik who was in the construction business in Hofuf. He was a younger man and apparently fell in love with Filwa when she was nineteen years old. He showered her with gifts and wanted to marry her.

"Their affair went on for years," said Jamil.

"Why didn't the sheik buy Filwa from Prince Ibrahim?" I asked.

"Because he was involved with the prince in many business matters and he was afraid the prince would become suspicious," said Jamil. "Filwa, moreover, knew that the prince could not sell her because she already had given him one son and he might marry her later if she produced more. Finally, she refused to see the sheik because she felt the risk was too great."

Jamil was warming up to his story: "Two years later, Filwa had another son and the prince decided to marry her. He divorced his oldest wife to make room for Filwa, who then became his favorite wife. She had more servants than the other wives and she had her own palace. She was now the 'mother of a prince' and some called her princess.

"Prince Ibrahim was not satisfied. He wanted more sons, although he was approaching eighty. Filwa obliged him with one more son, but it was probably not the prince's, she admitted to Jamil. She had taken another lover, this time one of her husband's older sons, who was in his forties. 'It was very convenient,' she said, 'and we kept it in the family.'"

Dalal interrupted. "It is forbidden in the Koran to have sexual relations with your husband's children or with your father's children by another wife."

"We call it incest," I said. "Filwa was having an affair with her stepson."

"Filwa had one more child, this time a daughter," continued Jamil, "but daughters don't count. Filwa is not sure who the father is."

The tape recorder was still running, and Jamil had announced the name of Prince Ibrahim's son who had been Filwa's lover.

"You are very indiscreet to mention names," I said.

"It's old history," he replied. "But there was one more man who had an affair with Filwa while Prince Ibrahim was alive. He is a very famous prince."

Jamil stood up, faced me, and named the prince.

I was astounded. It was the name of a minister high in the government and well known in the Middle East.

"Thank goodness it was not the Crown Prince," I said, as I turned off the tape recorder. "I'm going to erase the last five minutes of the tape. There's no point in making trouble.

"Human beings are basically the same whether they come from Saudi Arabia, England, France, or the United States. There have been Filwas throughout history."

Several immortal French and English courtesans came immediately to mind. In a way, Filwa was more innocent than the others. After all, she had been taught to be a concubine. She was also more fortunate. She had inherited $1 billion.

"Filwa hasn't been feeling well," said Jamil. "She is coming to the clinic to see you tomorrow. I made an appointment for her. I hope you don't mind."

I awoke in the middle of the night wondering what I would do if someone left me $1 billion. There was nothing I really wanted . . . however, I do love to travel. Maybe it would be convenient to have my own plane and travel in style with friends. But then I would be burdened by the responsibilities of owning a plane, keeping the pilots happy, insurance, upkeep, and so forth. Most wealthy people complain that they are the victims of their possessions, I remembered. No, I would forget about the plane. Yachts also are a hassle, and cruising for more than a few weeks would probably be boring. I could always charter a plane or a yacht, I concluded. After all, if I invested my $1 billion at 10 percent, it would yield $100 million a year, and I could afford to splurge occasionally.

By now I was wide awake. What *would* I do with the $1 billion? I began to think back upon the wealthy and prominent people I had taken care of during my career—tycoons, giants of industry, actors, movie stars, presidents of foreign countries, and so forth. Most of them were not particularly happy people. They rarely smiled. Many of them were basically insecure, regardless of their wealth or status. But they all had one thing in common. And that was achievement. They derived satisfaction, not from their possessions, but from what they had accomplished. They were achievers!

Those who lived on inherited wealth alone and did nothing else were a disaster. I was called in consultation occasionally to treat some of these pitiful creatures in Palm Beach or in Newport. They lived in magnificent surroundings, tended to by platoons of servants, and just drank themselves to death. They were possessors, not doers.

I began to fantasize. Some people create research or charitable foundations; some create monuments to themselves like hospitals, libraries, or museums; others build industrial empires to perpetuate their names. I decided to use the $1 billion to establish centers for health care, nutrition, and food production in those areas of the world where there was the greatest need. All this was in my field of expertise. The thrust would be to help people help themselves. I couldn't think of anything that would bring me and others more happiness and satisfaction. I recalled the haunting eyes of hungry children, their bellies swollen from starvation, and the look of despair and hopelessness among people.

The depressed areas in Central and South America which I had visited on behalf of our State Department came to mind. I would begin there, perhaps in Guatemala, Honduras, San Salvador, or maybe Peru, Bolivia, or Haiti. And then there was Africa. They all needed help and $1 billion would be a start, particularly if administered efficiently by one person promoting the concept of self-help. Such programs can be contagious—and who knows where they might lead! Perhaps WHO, the World Health Organization, would become involved.

It was a happy fantasy. I fell asleep.

The next morning my wife said, "You were talking in your sleep last night. When I turned the light on, you had a silly grin on your face."

"You would grin, too, if someone gave you $1 billion," I said.

"It must have been something you ate," she said, "but in view of your newfound affluence, maybe I should buy that magnificent gold bracelet I saw on Sharah Wasir yesterday."

"Possessions don't buy happiness," I said.

After making my morning rounds in the hospital, I went to the clinic. Jamil and Filwa, accompanied by her maid, were waiting for me. Filwa was heavily veiled and wore an exotic perfume. Jamil was very attentive and introduced me immediately. As soon as we entered the examining room, Filwa regally removed her veil and black abeyya, which she handed to Jamil. He folded them carefully and placed them on a chair. She wore an elegant ankle-length colorful silk gown and smart black patent-leather shoes.

Filwa was tall and had a good figure. Her hair was hennaed reddish brown to complement her brown eyes, which were outlined heavily with kohl, a black eyeliner used in Eastern countries to beautify the eyes. Her skin was unusually fair, almost pallid. She used a red lipstick that matched her nail polish. Her perfume was almost overwhelming. This femme fatale, I thought, has come a long way: from concubine to "mother of a prince" and billionairess at the age of thirty-five! Madame du Barry hadn't done half as well.

Jamil did the translating. Filwa's main complaints were fatigue and insomnia. She said she hadn't been well since her husband died. She spoke of Prince Ibrahim with reverence.

"But I have had a hard life," she said. "I was taken away from my family in Iran when I was ten years old and went to live in the palace when I was fifteen."

Jamil explained that Prince Ibrahim's palace was sold after he died and that Filwa was still living in her own palace nearby with her children and servants. "It is an old palace," he said, "and much smaller, of course, than the one that was sold." Prince Ibrahim had given it to Filwa, his youngest and favored wife.

"All the other wives have moved away and are living in new villas of their own," he added. "They have families and sons who look after them. Filwa's sons are still quite young."

"You have no idea," said Jamil, "how Saudi men respect their mothers and take care of them. If a wife shows disrespect to her husband's mother, he might divorce her immediately."

"I have no family," said Filwa plaintively, "except for my children. I don't know anything about my parents in Iran. Twenty-five years have passed since—"

The nurse entered the room. It was time for the physical examination. Jamil and I left. Filwa's maid remained to help her mistress undress.

Outside I asked Jamil whether Filwa could remarry. "Yes," he said, "but they often don't because of their children. Some of them have lovers instead."

"I think Filwa will be an exception," I said. "She will probably marry again."

"Maybe," said Jamil quietly.

A few minutes later, I left Jamil and entered the examining room. With the help of the nurse, who also served as a translator, I was able to get a reasonably good medical history and then proceeded with the physical examination. I could find nothing abnormal except for her pallor. I told Filwa she might have a mild anemia and that I would order the usual laboratory tests and x-rays. After reassuring her that all was well, I asked her to return in two weeks for the reports.

Two weeks later they appeared at the clinic. This time Dalal came along with Jamil, Filwa, and her maid. I told them that all the tests, including the x-rays, were normal except for a mild anemia, which was very common in women her age and could be treated quite easily with medication. "Otherwise," I assured them, "Filwa is in perfect health."

There was a pause. Then Dalal spoke up. He said that Filwa wanted to go to Europe but the government would not give her a visa. He had asked a friend to intercede on her behalf with the royal family, but the King was adamant. Filwa could not leave the country.

"Are they concerned that she may take part of the $1 billion she inherited out of the country?" I asked.

"No," said Dalal, "much of that is tied up in land and real estate. I think that moral and religious issues are involved. A woman cannot leave the country unless she has a male escort who is a close member of her family. And Filwa has nobody."

"Moreover," said Jamil, "the royal family assumes a certain responsibility for her because her sons are princes. They pay Filwa 4,000 riyals a month [about $1,300 U.S.]."

That's like carrying coals to Newcastle, I thought. Filwa's royal stipend would feed about eighty of my starving children in San Salvador for a month. The fantasy of two weeks ago kept recurring.

Dalal brought me back to reality. "Could you possibly send Filwa to England for medical care?" he asked unabashedly. He knew I was very fond of him and would be more likely to oblige him.

"I don't know how I can do that without falsifying her records," I said.

It suddenly became clear that Filwa was trying to use Jamil, Dalal, and me to help her get out of Saudi Arabia. Her medical complaint was just a ruse.

"Jamil," I said, "tell Filwa that I think she is a very resourceful woman, but I cannot help her. She has had a difficult life, and I sympathize with how lonely she must feel now, but she is a survivor and I admire her for her spirit."

As Jamil told Filwa what I said she looked at me with her large brown eyes lined with kohl and smiled. We understood each other.

◊ *24* ◊

FLIGHT INTO THE FUTURE

THE TIME TO LEAVE Saudi Arabia was rapidly approaching. My contract had been extended and almost three years had passed. The pioneering days were over. The hospital and clinics were operating at full capacity and setting a standard for others to follow.

There were ninety specialist physicians on the staff, half of whom were American or English. The other half came from twenty-one different countries. We were now treating more than 100,000 patients a year. Our teaching program for interns and young resident physicians was making excellent progress, and my campaign on their behalf for a substantial increase in salary had finally succeeded. Salaries for interns had been raised to $10,000 for the first year and $15,000 for the second year following their graduation from medical school. Because free housing was included in their contracts, and a postgraduate training program was available to them in the hospital, the young physicians were very happy with the arrangement. Some of them would eventually qualify as specialists, who were in very short supply in Saudi Arabia.

Meanwhile, the cost of operating our hospital had been enormous. The total budget of Medical City was a whopping $100 million a year, of which $40 million was spent on salaries and housing for our 2,000 employees. But the investment had paid off. Over the past three years the hospital had established itself as a national resource for the care of severely ill patients from all over the kingdom and for the education and training of physicians. Plans were already underway to double the bed capacity of the hospital and to develop a research center. It was the end of one era and the beginning of another.

The graduation of the first class of Saudi doctors from the University of Riyadh Medical School was celebrated shortly before I left Saudi Arabia. It was a historic occasion. The ceremonies were held in the elegant King Faisal Hall, where the OPEC (Organization of Petroleum Exporting Countries) meetings take place. Its fourteen hundred tiered seats were upholstered in beige suède and the walls were covered with carpeting. On that landmark day there were only three hundred visitors in the audience, which accentuated the vastness of the auditorium. Printed copies of the graduation speech in Arabic and English were distributed.

His Royal Highness King Khalid sat in the center of the huge platform, looking very uncomfortable. On one side of the King was the graduating class and on the other the Minister of Health, Sir Brian Windeyer of the University of London, the principal speaker, and a number of educators and dignitaries. At the back of the platform hung a large Saudi Arabian emblem executed in gold and malachite, which added a blaze of green against the dark backdrop curtain.

The dean opened the ceremonies with the conventional *Bismillah ar-Rahman ar-Raheem* [In the name of God the most merciful, the most compassionate] and then delivered a short speech. Others followed. The final speaker, Sir Brian, sounded as though he were addressing one of the British colonies. He brought congratulations from the Queen, the Queen Mother, the Chancellor of the University of London, the Prime Minister, and almost everybody in Parliament he could think of except the Chancellor of the Exchequer. He then went on to extol the University of London and its many accomplishments in Khartoum and in Africa. Sir Brian did not really say anything, but he said it beautifully for about fifteen minutes. I congratulated him later on one sentence in his speech: "The more recent admission of women medical students was an event of real importance."

I must admit that I admire the English. They never seem to give up: they are still trying to colonize wherever and whenever possible. I felt this quite strongly while I was in Saudi Arabia. Some of them still consider the United States one of their colonies!

When the speeches were completed, the King stood up at a signal from the dean. He handed out the diplomas and a black doctor's bag to each of the seventeen graduates. I was quite disappointed that the King never smiled, never spoke a word of congratulation to these splendid young men, these Saudi Arabian pioneers who had worked hard and long overcoming language barriers and other innumerable obstacles.

When the ceremony was over I congratulated my friend Abdul Taleem, who recently had completed his apprentice internship at the hospital. We had become close friends since our desert adventure. The other graduates, most of whom I knew personally, gathered around to shake my hand. They looked upon me as one of their patrons because as chairman of the department of medicine I had helped them prepare for internships in our hospital and elsewhere. They often came to me with their personal problems as well.

I asked Abdul about the contents of the black doctor's bag. "It's filled with gold," he said, laughing, as he handed it to me. I opened the bag. It was empty except for a ten-dollar stethoscope!

They invited me to a party to celebrate their graduation. It was held in an apartment belonging to one of the graduates. About half of the doctors were married and had brought their wives. None of the women wore veils. I learned, to my surprise, that two of the Saudi wives had been educated in Germany and had graduated from medical schools there. They were working in a women's hospital nearby.

Abdul told me that there were eight women in his graduating class at the University of Riyadh, but "it would not be proper for them to appear in public." They had never been in contact with their male classmates and were taught by women doctors from Egypt and Pakistan or by men on closed-circuit television.

Several other professors of my vintage were at the party. We all sat around, drank sadiki and talked. At about ten o'clock we had dinner, Saudi style, on special carpets spread on the floor. We had the usual *kabsa*— chicken, lamb, rice, eggs, and fruit.

The sadiki flowed freely and the evening turned into an old-fashioned bull session, which went on until the early hours of the morning. We all felt comfortable with each other and everyone spoke frankly. We talked about the many changes that had taken place during the years I had been in Saudi Arabia. I told them how exciting it had been to see tall modern buildings and many thousands of homes emerging from the dust and rubble of this ancient city. Boulevards and highways had appeared almost overnight, replacing old dirt roads. The ever-changing face of Riyadh had been a constant source of wonder to me. In some other areas of the country whole new cities were being built block by block.

"In earlier times," said Abdul, "this region was a vast oasis of palm trees and was therefore named Riyadh, which means 'the gardens.' At the turn of the century it was a walled town of mud-brick houses with ten thousand inhabitants. Today the population is over a half million. It has increased seventy-five percent during the past three years."

He said that the foreign work force had increased to two million and that recently more workers were coming from Korea, the Philippines and Pakistan. There were 35,000 Americans in the country and thousands more from England, Belgium, Sweden, and West Germany.

I told them that I had arrived in Saudi Arabia during a world crisis, when the embargo by the oil-producing countries was threatening the economic stability of the industrialized world. Now, three years later, the Saudis were supplying the U.S. with 8.5 million barrels of oil daily. Although the price of oil and world-wide inflation had increased, Saudi Arabia had continued to make every effort to keep oil prices down.

"There is no question," I said, "that Crown Prince Fahd and the Saudi government are now more oriented to the West and more friendly to the United States than ever before. Many, including Prince Fahd, are sending their sons to the United States for their education. In fact, there are about 6,000 Saudis attending college in our country right now."

One of the professors remarked that the advances in education at every level had been astonishing. He said that there are one and a half million children attending public schools and that more than 40,000 students are enrolled in college, three times the number of a decade ago. New primary and secondary schools, many prefabricated, were springing up in the most remote villages, and some classes were even being held temporarily in tents.

Our host added that nearly 2,000 schools had been built throughout the country, all within a few years, a real crash program. Not many years ago 70 percent of the population were illiterate, including many of the "privileged class." Education for women was unthinkable. At one time King Faisal had threatened to call out the army to enforce the opening of a girl's school to which the religious leaders were strenuously opposed. Today one-half million girls were attending segregated schools within the framework of Islamic tradition. There were about 5,000 students in the women's college in Riyadh, and a new college for 1,200 women was under construction in Jidda.

"We have come a long way," he said with pride. "The government's second Five-year Plan, which began in 1975, allocated $144 billion for the programs 'to improve the lot of the Saudi people.' Of this enormous sum $22 billion was designated for development in the fields of health and education. This amount is second only to our budget for defense!

"There is no doubt that our government intends to provide the best education and health care to every citizen, completely free of charge. We are building several new medical schools, including a special school for women doctors. This is really impressive when you consider that there have been fewer than 150 Saudi physicians in the history of the kingdom, and all of them had to study abroad because there were no facilities at home."

"Just like me," exclaimed Nadia, one of the Saudi wives who was a physician. "I attended both college and medical school in Germany." She went on to say that the status of women had been improving and that an increasing number had been going abroad to study. Recently, however, the religious leaders had become fearful of the influence of westernization and "modern ideas." They pressed for more severe restraints and sharply curtailed the number of Saudi women attending colleges in the West. Scholarships for women to foreign universities were canceled and Saudi women were forbidden to leave the kingdom unchaperoned.

As part of this puritanical clampdown King Khalid decreed that women who did not conform to Islamic standards of dress would be punished. Even Western women had been reprimanded by the religious police for violating the strict Islamic dress code. Moreover, it was becoming increasingly difficult for Western women to visit Saudi Arabia.

"They educate us with one hand and enslave us with the other," Nadia said bitterly.

I told them that in the past year an American friend, who had lived with his wife in Saudi Arabia for more than thirty years, was unable to obtain an entry visa for her when he returned to Saudi Arabia to attend an Aramco conference!

It was two o'clock in the morning. I thanked my host for a stimulating evening and again shook hands with the young graduates. As Abdul drove me home, we recalled our experience in Chop Square last year and Abdul said that fewer hands were being amputated these days except in the case of hardened criminals. Public whipping was now the punishment for petty thievery or selling liquor.

I had seen a miserable Yemeni publicly flogged in the main square for a petty theft. The police draped a white cloth over his bare back and put a corner of it in his mouth to bite on so that he could contain his screams while forty lashes were laid on his lower back. The grimaces of pain told the story eloquently.

I also had noted that in the past two years government censorship seemed less stringent. Censorship regarding the existence of Israel, for example, had apparently been lifted in 1976, when the *International Herald Tribune* reported the raid on Entebbe which freed over a hundred hostages held by Palestinian terrorist hijackers in Uganda. In previous editions all reference to Israel had been deleted by the Saudi censors. Now the stories were reported in full. Later, in 1977, Sadat's first visit to Israel was reported in the *Arab News,* Saudi Arabia's English-language daily. This was a landmark in that it heralded a change in policy regarding the freedom of the press on foreign affairs. Censorship was otherwise unchanged, however. Pictures of women, for example, were blacked out, as always.

Abdul asked why I was leaving Saudi Arabia. I told him that changes had taken place within me, too. This had become apparent when I went home for my annual vacation. For the first time in almost three years, I felt reluctant to return to Riyadh. As I drank in the lush beauty of the New England countryside I realized that the drabness of the Arabian landscape had accentuated my thirst for harmony and color and for the sight and smell of the sea. I had become attached to the Saudi people, but I felt it was time to go home.

Abdul stopped the car in front of my villa. I had finally been promoted to the summit of the housing ladder, the elegant Princess Sara Villas, a complex of six houses with a swimming pool in a walled-off area. Each villa had a spacious veranda and a small garden with a few shrubs but no trees. At times a herd of goats wandered down the path between the houses.

I told Abdul that when I had received word that we would be moving to the Princess Sara Villas we were delighted. But the move was not without mishap. For months I had carefully hoarded in the refrigerator some caviar which my friend Dr. Bandar Akkad had brought me from Iran. While I was transferring this precious delicacy to our new home my car broke down, and in the hot sun the caviar turned to jelly.

We shook hands warmly as we parted. This had been a long and eventful day in the medical history of the new Saudi Arabia. Some of the young men and women I had been with tonight would eventually take over the health care of their country and do it well.

Time passed all too quickly. I was glad that I would still be here to help celebrate Ramadan, my favorite holiday, which began the end of August on the Gregorian calendar. Ramadan is the ninth month of the Islamic calendar and is decreed as the holy month of repentance and forgiveness for all Moslems. The observance of Ramadan is one of the five pillars of the faith. It is a bittersweet month of fasting all day and feasting all night.

Among the Saudis, there is much excitement and anticipation until the new moon is sighted and a cannon is fired to signal the beginning of Ramadan. The cannon is fired again each morning at dawn and at sunset. No food or water is allowed from sunrise to sunset during this twenty-nine-day holiday. The fasting must be absolute. Water is forbidden regardless of the heat.

The fast of Ramadan always reminded me of Prince Yusef, the first patient assigned to me when I arrived at the hospital. Although I had explained repeatedly that fasting had aggravated his ulcer condition, he smiled and viewed my remarks merely as infidel propaganda. However, the Koran excuses the ill from fasting and stipulates that those who cannot fast during Ramadan because of poor health must fast at another time.

The evenings are always festive. After the cannon is heard at sunset, the Saudi break their fast with dates and coffee before praying either at home or at the mosque. Later, the meal called *futour,* which is like a breakfast, starts with fruit juice or soup and is followed by a substantial meal. The wives make cakes and sweets rich with dried fruits, nuts, and syrup for dessert. The Saudis later prepare for the daytime fast by eating another meal, called *suhour,* around midnight or between two and three o'clock in the morning.

Visiting and conversation among families often go on until the early hours of the morning and some families stay up all night, particularly on the last day of Ramadan. Servants are not expected to work while fasting. The Moslem personnel in our hospital worked half time.

Two particular foods are popular during this holiday. One is a pastry called *sambousak,* made of a special dough in a triangular shape filled with ground meat and parsley and then deep-fried. We often bought this at the bakeries in town that also sell a popular omelet called *muttabaak,* made with chopped tomatoes, vegetables, and ground meat. To break the fast after sundown, the Saudis drink a special beverage made from condensed apricot pulp, a popular fruit juice.

"The doors of Heaven open during Ramadan," and this is the time to help the poor with gifts of food, clothing, and money. One of the reasons for observing the fast is to empathize with those who have little to eat or drink, and thereby to learn compassion.

The end of Ramadan is celebrated for three days during a special holiday of feasting and rejoicing called the Eid al Fitr. The Eid is an official holiday and a time for giving gifts, particularly to the children. It seemed that the Saudis repented and fasted all day during Ramadan, and then more than made up for it at night, especially during the Eid, when the rejoicing and feasting reached their peak.

When Princess Sultana heard that I soon would be leaving Saudi Arabia, she called me. "You must come and celebrate the Eid with us," she said. "My brother Sultan will come for you."

Sultan and Monsoor both arrived after sundown and drove me to the Daouk family complex, where we had celebrated Sultana's wedding two years ago. When we arrived, the compound was already full of cars and people. "They are all family," explained Monsoor, "cousins, aunts and uncles, and lots of children." He directed me toward Sultana's "honeymoon cottage" where I had taken the bridal couple's picture after the wedding ceremony.

Sultana was as beautiful as ever, perhaps a bit more mature. Mahmoud had gained weight and had a "settled look." They both greeted me warmly. Sultana proudly displayed her baby son as Mahmoud beamed with pride. I showed them the photographs I had taken of them in the cottage right after they were married and gave one to Sultana. Mahmoud told me he was building a large house in his father's compound "to keep the family together."

I asked him whether he was still striking oil while drilling for water, reminding him of our conversation in the hospital. They both laughed.

Later, Sultana told me that they had traveled "all over the world" on their honeymoon and that they had gone to California to visit her mother who had remarried.

"I have two questions to ask you, Sultana," I said. "Are you happy with your marriage and have you ever regretted giving up your American citizenship?"

"As you know," she said, "my marriage was prearranged and it has turned out well. Mahmoud treats me with consideration and kindness. I feel secure and protected within this huge family.

"The family," she added, "is more important than any single individual."

"What about your American citizenship?" I persisted.

"I am a princess in an old and illustrious Saudi family," she replied. "I am willing to sacrifice my freedom and certain privileges while I am in Saudi Arabia, but I intend to travel to America and Europe with Mahmoud as much as possible. And he has promised me that my son will be educated in California."

The family gathering grew larger and larger. At midnight, *suhour* was served, and several hours later I made my departure. Sultana and Mahmoud said they would call me when they next visited the United States, "maybe next year." Sultan and Monsoor drove me home.

As the word spread that I was leaving, a number of former patients came to say goodbye. Among them was Prince Yusef, who arrived at the hospital with two of his sons. He told me that he was impressed with the portrait we had given him but he still wasn't convinced that my wife had painted it. He said again with a half smile, "*You* did it!," hoping that I would admit it, but I remained firm.

"Women can do many things as well as men and sometimes better," I told him.

"Only to have babies," the prince replied.

I reminded him again that fasting on Ramadan might reactivate his bleeding ulcer. "It is in God's hands," he said.

As we parted he looked into my eyes and presented me with a beautiful set of malachite prayer beads strung on a gold chain. It was a meaningful gesture. This man was one of the few remaining great traditional princes, one of a rapidly disappearing breed of a bygone era. He was uniquely majestic. "God go with you," he said as he left.

Dr. Bandar Akkad paid me a visit at home. This young Saudi intellectual had gained an international reputation and had been quoted frequently in the American press during the past two years. We talked about many aspects of Saudi Arabian life. I told him how impressed I was with the low crime rate.

"Although the beheadings, amputation of hands, and floggings are deterrents to crime," he said, "it would be simplistic to attribute the low crime rate in our country to the severe punishments alone."

He went on to explain that originally the country consisted of nomadic Bedouins and everyone was poor. There were no extremes of wealth to breed corruption. It was a simple, egalitarian society based on faith and family. Racism did not exist. Alcohol was forbidden by the Koran and drugs were also illegal.

"Our tradition, our national characteristic, has always been to obey the law," he said. "It is part of our heritage. Survival in this harsh land was difficult enough even without crime. Any threat to the community was viewed as something to be eliminated quickly.

"We place the welfare of society before that of the individual," he said with emphasis, "and that distinguishes our culture from yours.

"In your country," he added, "you protect the rights of the individual at the expense of society. The individual comes first and society second." Bandar was of the opinion that our laws were too permissive and that human rights were not necessarily the privilege of the individual but that of society as a whole.

"Freedom is a fragile privilege or license which can be abused easily and translated into licentiousness," he said. "There is a fine line between freedom and anarchy."

As a going-away present he gave me a book of his poems written in English during his student days in California. I'll never forget this remarkable man.

It was a parting of the ways for many of us. Hugh Compton, the Medical Director, was about to leave, and Ron Lambrie's contract would be terminating in two months. He and his wife were planning to live in France. They were dear friends and we would miss them. We all exchanged addresses and telephone numbers. Some were in England, others in France, the United States, Egypt, and elsewhere. Philip Westbrook was coming back to Riyadh. He had been in London for more than a year and had a contract with a new military hospital.

I sold my beloved Pontiac to one of the doctors for $8,000, almost the same price I had paid for it originally. He considered it a great bargain. The price of automobiles had increased substantially because of inflation. The car had served me well, considering the climate and the driving conditions. I was sad to leave it and felt the same way about parting with my Sony stereophonic equipment, which also sold very quickly.

We packed my books, the ornate Arabic dagger which Abdul and I had bought in the antique *suq* near Chop Square, the exquisite rugs which we had purchased in Iran, and my favorite old desert trousers, which Ruth threatened to throw away. She called them "camel pants" and said they were not worth keeping. However, I felt that the trousers had character and evoked a sense of history. She agreed that they looked historic, and with a sigh of resignation dropped them into the trunk. The shipping department at the hospital made all the arrangements for transporting our things back to Boston.

The farewell parties were always celebrated on a Thursday night and went on until the early hours of the morning. Madeleine came with a young doctor from the hospital and told me that her affair with Prince Khalil was over. She thanked me for helping her qualify for her doctor's degree and gave me her parents' address. "If you ever want to reach me," she said, "my parents always know where I am."

Dalal brought his mother to one of the parties. We talked about Dr. Ghandour, our afternoon teas with him in the hospital and his last trip to Paris. Mrs. Ghandour brought me a book which her husband had written on Wahabism. There were tears when we parted.

Dalal told me that Filwa was still in Riyadh and was unable as yet to get a visa to leave Saudi Arabia. "Politics are involved," he said. "She is very unhappy." I felt sorry for her.

I brought a bottle of French champagne to my last party. It had been given to me by a prince and I had been saving it for a special occasion. With a flourish I wrapped a napkin about the properly chilled bottle and tried to pop the cork. Everyone gathered around with great anticipation. But nothing happened! I slowly pulled out the cork and turned the bottle bottom side up. It was completely empty. The cork apparently had dried out, even though I had stored the bottle on its side in the refrigerator all these months to keep it moist. Everyone roared with laughter. We made the toasts with sadiki.

At eleven o'clock we left for the airport and made our final farewells. This was a difficult moment. We were parting with beloved friends. Some we would never see again.

Finally, as Ruth and I sat in the inner waiting room at the airport, I began to reflect upon my years in Saudi Arabia, years which had given me an intimate glimpse into a culture which had been preserved for more than ten centuries by isolation from the outside world. I could not help but wonder whether the hectic modernization would bring an end to their traditional values and eventually destroy the integrity of the country's social fabric.

The Saudis believe their religion will protect them from all such contingencies. But man cannot serve both God and mammon. Enormous wealth was already spawning boundless greed and corruption. Psychosomatic illness and stomach ulcers, unheard of a few years ago, were now common, undoubtedly brought on by social tensions. Would Saudi Arabia succumb to the same breakdown of morality and to the epidemic of crime that had followed the feverish growth of industry and technology in our Western civilization?

Certainly their recent growth had led to an astonishing number of paradoxes and contradictions. Theatres, movies, and modern forms of public entertainment are not permitted, but there is a thriving underground trade in blue movies, which are shown at home. Many X-rated films, such as *Deep Throat,* are readily available on video cassettes. The women are heavily veiled and a Saudi man who hoards pornographic movies in his home would be mortified if his wife appeared in public with as much as a bare ankle. The women are segregated and veiled by tradition but an increasing number of Saudi men and women mix at parties. A young Saudi girl may wear a bikini at the Aramco swimming pool also open to boys, but must shroud her entire body in a black abeyya and veil when she goes to her Moslem school for girls only. Alcohol is banned but is plentiful in the homes of the rich; scotch sells on the black market for $150 a quart. Some Saudis do not drink at home but overindulge in alcohol and sex when they go abroad.

On one side are the ultra-conservative puritanical Wahabi, fighting to preserve the traditional social and religious values, and to enforce the harsh 1,400-year-old Islamic laws. On the other side are the modern, progressive young Saudis, who look upon their culture as folklore and are impatient to break with tradition. The lines of battle seem to be drawn. The government is torn between progress at all costs and the preservation of ancient doctrines. I had a premonition of an eventual head-on confrontation between the past and the present.

As more women become educated they, too, will demand emancipation and equality. Some are already on the brink of a social revolution. Debates are raging in Saudi newspapers regarding women's proper role. Many are demanding their rights while the religious leaders press harder for further restrictions, thicker veils, and longer sleeves.

Since three-quarters of all Saudis are under thirty years of age, it appears likely that the progressive element will ultimately prevail, but I remembered Prince Khalil's warning that the fundamentalists will violently oppose any sudden change in Islamic tradition and that their influence should not be underestimated. He had no way of predicting that a band of Moslem religious zealots would seize the Grand Mosque of Mecca within the year!

I had often wondered about the stability of the monarchy. "Our roots are a thousand years deep," Prince Khalil once told me. Actually, Saudi Arabia is the only country in the world which is exclusively a family enterprise. King Ibn Saud and his progeny have provided generations of kings, crown princes, governors and cabinet ministers, who run the country and keep their fingers on the pulse of the nation. The royal family is like the board of directors of a mammoth corporation and sends its elite members out into every section of the country.

Although the kingdom is dedicated to the welfare of the people and spends billions of dollars each year on education and health care, there is a growing persuasion among the newly educated middle class toward a representative form of government and greater involvement in the kingdom's affairs.

Awesome economic power is a double-edged sword. The phenomenal explosion of oil wealth has nurtured corruption and unbridled extravagance among some of the royal family. Can the monarchy, I wondered, survive the vulnerability of such enormous wealth? I thought that it probably would endure in a modified form, providing that society was ultimately the benefactor.

Just as the time of our departure drew near a man hurried toward me holding a brown paper bag. It was Nizar, the security guard who had accompanied Philip, Abdul, and me on our desert adventure a long time ago.

"I came to say goodbye," he said, "and to bring you some fresh dates from the palm tree in front of the hospital."

"That's how we first met," I reminded him, deeply touched by this gesture of friendship. I remembered him scampering up the date palm several years ago with a paper bag in one hand. "How did you get past the guard at the gate?" I asked. The room we were in was restricted to departing passengers.

"My uniform helped," he said as he handed me the bag of dates.

We shook hands. "God protect you," he said in Arabic and then he was gone.

And now I was about to fly from the Middle Ages into the Space Age. I boarded the plane with mixed feelings, sad to leave the hospital and Riyadh, but happy to return home to friends and family.

As the plane took off for London on the first leg of my trip, I tried to formulate the aspects of Saudi Arabian culture which had impressed me the most: total dedication to religion, the strong family unit, and laws which primarily protect the welfare of society. On the other side of the coin the Saudis have no constitutional government, no electoral process, no freedom of the press or right of assembly, and no women's rights.

We were soon flying over the desert, and I recalled my adventures with the Bedouins, their warm hospitality, and the remarkably intimate relationship that existed among us. Again I felt privileged to be a doctor. My profession had given me an instant entrée into a foreign culture and into the hearts and minds of the people, in all walks of life. Nobody can strip away the social and economic veneer faster than a physician, and all mankind stands naked before him. Man's mortality, the great leveler, does not distinguish between prince and pauper, or between the mighty and the downtrodden, all of whom eventually succumb alike to the same human frailties.

I had become involved with the Saudis, their lives, their loves, their thoughts, and their expectations for the future. I had grown to love these people and recalled what Hippocrates had said of the physician: "Where there is love of man, there is also love of the healing art."

The hours passed quickly. As we approached London, a shadowy female figure shrouded in black, who had been sitting in the forward part of the plane, rose and passed us on the way to the restroom. Her features were not discernible because of the thick black veil covering her head and face. In about fifteen minutes she reappeared attired in an elegant beige silk ensemble. She was a tall, strikingly beautiful woman, but what appealed to me most was her radiant smile, which seemed to illuminate the cabin as she returned to rejoin her Saudi escorts. I was reminded of the butterfly analogy on my first flight to Saudi Arabia. And like the butterfly she was now emerging from her cocoon, perhaps, symbolically to fly to the freedom of the outside world. I thought of Sultana, who chose the traditional values of the East, with the knowledge that she, too, could shed her cocoon at will to enjoy the liberty of the West.

The morning sun struck points of light on the London rooftops, studded with chimney pots and stately spires. Dominating the lush green landscape below were the glistening waters of the River Thames meandering peacefully through sleepy villages. There was something prodigal to me, at that moment, about all the green of the gardens and the foliage of the parks.

I could almost see across the Atlantic to my garden and the landmark of my home, my magnificent old copper beech tree, resplendent with a million leaves glistening in the sun like a mountain of shining new copper pennies.

GLOSSARY

The meanings of Arabic words and expressions are usually explained in the text.

abeyya   A long, black robe worn over the clothing by Saudi Arabian women.

agal   The double coil worn on top of the ghutra to hold it in place. Actually it is one ring bent into a figure of eight and is usually black.

Al Saud   The house of Saud. Al with a capital A denotes family, tribe, or clan. For example, Fahd bin Abdul-Aziz Al Saud identifies Prince Fahd as the son of King Abdul-Aziz of the House of Saud.

Arab   May be defined as anyone whose mother tongue is Arabic. The inhabitants of the Arabian peninsula are Arabs or Arabians. Iranians, however, are Persians, not Arabs, and speak a different language.

ardha   The traditional sword dance of Saudi Arabia.

Bedouins   The nomadic desert people, the original Arabs.

bilharziasis   A parasitic disease which involves the urinary tract, liver, or intestinal tract. Parasites in human waste pass into shallow, slow-moving streams where snails breed. The parasite is transformed into the infective form within the snail, then returns to the water and penetrates the skin of humans working or bathing in the infested area. The disease is common throughout Africa among the agricultural population, particularly along the Nile Delta and in the Sudan. It is endemic in Yemen and is not uncommon in Saudi Arabia.

bin (or ibn)   Son of. Sultan bin Abdul-Aziz is Sultan, the son of Abdul-Aziz.

bint   Daughter of. Hussah bint Sultan is Hussah, the daughter of Sultan.

bisht   The billowing robe worn by men over the thobe. It is usually black, brown, or cream-colored and edged with gold thread. A band of gold embroidery denotes royalty or high office. The cloak is called a *mishlah* when it is sleeveless.

Bismillah ar-Rahman ar-Raheem   "In the name of Allah, the most merciful, the most compassionate." The opening line of the Koran, which appears on all stationery in the kingdom, above every podium, and on all forms of communication.

Eid al Fitr   A special holiday of feasting to celebrate the end of the fast of Ramadan.

emir   One who commands, such as the governor of a town or province. The princes are also referred to as *emirs*.

ghutra The Saudi headdress, which is usually a checkered red and white or plain white headcloth made of cotton and worn over a skull cap.

gutwah A black veil covering the head and face of Saudi Arabian women.

hajj The pilgrimage to Mecca, one of the five pillars of Islam, required of all Moslems at least once in a lifetime. Several million Moslems come to Saudi Arabia each year for the annual pilgrimage to the holy cities of Mecca and Medina. The pilgrims are called *hajji*.

hegira The flight. The migration (or *hegira*) of Mohammed from Mecca to Medina in 622 marks the first year of the Islamic calendar. Islamic dates are designated by the abbreviation A. H. for "Anno Hegira," the year of the flight. The first day of the year 1401 A.H. for example, corresponds to November 8, 1980, on our Gregorian calendar. The Islamic calendar is based on twelve complete lunar cycles. A lunar month is the time between two successive new moons or about 29½ days. The Islamic year is, therefore, 354 days (12 × 29½), eleven days shorter than the Gregorian calendar.

hepatitis A virus infection of the liver transmitted by transfusion of contaminated blood or by infected needles. It can also be caused by the ingestion of contaminated food or water and by sexual intercourse with an infected person. Hepatitis is common in Saudi Arabia.

houris The eternally young, beautiful, and virginal nymphs in the Moslem paradise.

imam A religious leader, one who leads the prayers in a mosque.

Inshallah "God willing." A common expression in Saudi Arabia.

Islam The Moslem faith—from the Arabic meaning "submission" (to the will of God).

Kaaba Islam's holiest shrine in the Grand Mosque in Mecca toward which all Moslems face to pray. According to legend, Abraham laid the foundation for the Kaaba, which is a fifty-foot-high, cube-shaped monument draped in a specially woven black cloth. The pilgrim kisses or touches the sacred Black Stone built into the southeast corner of the Kaaba. Moslems believe that the stone was cast down by the Angel Gabriel to Ishmael, the son of Abraham, who is considered the ancestor of the Arab people. It is said that Mohammed himself later placed the Black Stone, a huge meteorite, into its new resting place in the Kaaba.

kaffiya A skull cap, usually white and embroidered, worn under the ghutra.

khanjar A curved Arabian dagger.

Koran The sacred book of Islam, containing God's revelations to the Prophet Mohammed in the form of 114 chapters, or suras.

kuttab Islamic elementary school for boys. Main assignment for students is to memorize the Koran.

La ilah illa'llah Muhammadun rasulu'llah "There is no god but God and Mohammed is His Messenger." The call to prayer and the Moslem profession of faith. These words are inscribed upon the Saudi Arabian flag.

majlis A regularly convened assembly at which a Saudi citizen may personally present a complaint or a request directly to the King, Crown Prince, or other member of the royal family. A *majlis* is also a sitting room or reception room.

maktub "It is written," expressing the Islamic belief in predestination.

matawa The religious police, sometimes called the Morals Police.

Mecca and Medina The holy cities of Islam, to which only Moslems are admitted.

muezzin The crier who calls the faithful to prayer five times daily.

qadi An Islamic judge.

Ramadan The ninth month of the Islamic calendar, the holy month of repentance and forgiveness. It is a month of fasting from dawn to sunset marked by the firing of a cannon twice daily to signal the beginning and the end of the fast.

riyal Saudi Arabian currency. The exchange until recently was about 3.3 riyals to the U.S. dollar.

Rub Al Khali The enormous desert wilderness occupying the southeast portion of Saudi Arabia. It is usually referred to as the "Empty Quarter."

sadiki "My friend." A homemade alcoholic drink tasting somewhat like vodka.

Salaat! Salaat! "Prayer! Prayer!" The cry of the Morals Police.

shamal A violent sandstorm usually caused by northwesterly winds.

Sharia "The path to follow." The Islamic law of the land, based upon the Koran. It embraces a code of Islamic justice, morals, ethics, and religious duties.

sheikh The leader or elder of a tribe or religious community; an important public figure; a person versed in the Koran and its laws.

Shiite The Shiites (from *Shiat* meaning "partisan") were originally partisans of Mohammed's son-in-law Ali. They differ from the Sunni sect in their interpretation of the Sharia laws and in the selection of Mohammed's succession. The Shiites place more emphasis on festivals and pageantry and less on fasting, prayer, and pilgrimage. There are about thirty million Shiites world-wide, considerably fewer in numbers than the Sunni Moslems. They are in the majority, however, in Iran and Iraq. In Saudi Arabia approximately 100,000 Shiites live in the Eastern Province, working as farmers, laborers, and artisans.

Sunni The orthodox sect of Islam. Its name is derived from *sunna,* meaning "tradition." The Sunni Moslems make up the overwhelming majority of the population in Saudi Arabia. About 90 percent of all Moslems throughout the world belong to this sect.

suq A native marketplace or shop.

tabeeb A doctor.

thobe A long, shirtlike garment, the national dress for Saudi men. It is made of cotton, usually white in the summer. The neckband is decorated with gold braid or is lightly embroidered. In the winter heavier material is used and the colors are darker.

trachoma A highly infectious eye disease endemic throughout Saudi Arabia and a common cause of blindness.

Ulema The body of Islamic scholars who regulate religious life in Saudi Arabia and administer justice.

wadi A rocky riverbed, usually dry except in the rainy season.

Wahabism An austere fundamentalist movement advocating an ultra-puritanical, orthodox way of life as practiced in the days of Mohammed. The Wahabi are closely identified with the House of Saud and have dominated Saudi Arabia for more than two hundred years.

zakat A small, traditional, religious tax required of all Moslems.

PRINCIPAL CHARACTERS

THE RULERS OF THE KINGDOM

King Abdul-Aziz Al Saud (1876–1953) Known as Ibn Saud, legendary founder of the present-day Kingdom of Saudi Arabia and father of all four of the kings who followed.

King Saud (1902–1969) The eldest son of Ibn Saud, ruled from 1953 to 1964; came to Boston for medical consultation in 1962.

King Faisal (1904–1975) Half-brother of King Saud; succeeded him in 1964, and sponsored the King Faisal Specialist Hospital. He was assassinated in 1975.

King Khalid. Reigned from 1975 until his death in 1982. He visited the hospital frequently, always accompanied by Crown Prince Fahd.

Crown Prince Fahd Another son of Ibn Saud, was the Crown Prince from 1975 until 1982 and became King upon Khalid's death. His half-brother Abdullah succeeded him as Crown Prince.

THE ROYAL FAMILY

Fahada Lady-in-waiting to Princess Sanwa.

Princess Fatima Attractive young wife of an influential prince in the Eastern Province.

Prince Ibrahim Al Muqrin el-Kabir The immensely wealthy and influential prince whose estate was valued at over $30 billion.

Queen Iffat Wife of King Faisal, visited Boston for medical care in 1959.

Prince Khalil The host at the memorable royal party.

Princess Lulwa Al Saud Eighty-two-year-old former wife of King Saud.

Prince Nasser One of Prince Yusef's younger sons, in charge of the family's racing stables.

Prince Salim The eldest son of Prince Yusef.

Princess Sanwa Al Saud Sought medical care while in Boston with King Saud's royal entourage.

Prince Saud bin Faisal Minister of Foreign Affairs, the son of King Faisal and Queen Iffat.

Prince Sultan The young brother of Princess Sultana.

Princess Sultana bint Musaid Al Sudairi   The Saudi Arabian princess whose mother was American.

Prince Yusef Al Saud   The eminent prince and friend of King Khalid, who was treated for massive bleeding when the hospital first opened.

OTHER SAUDI ARABIANS

Abdul Taleem   Senior medical student who acted as a guide on Chop Square and participated in the desert adventure.

Adnan Khashoggi   Billionaire businessman, head of a world-wide financial empire. Father was a physician and confidant to King Ibn Saud.

Dr. Bandar Akkad   A distinguished minister in the government.

Basama   A cousin of Wasisa, employed as a social worker by the government, and an outspoken advocate of equality for women.

Dalal   Dr. Ghandour's son.

Filwa   Widow of Prince Ibrahim.

Ghaith Pharaon   Multi-millionaire chairman of the Saudi Research and Development Corporation.

Dr. Ghandour   Physician to Prince Ibrahim el-Kabir.

Hussein Lateef   A Bedouin patient; a surprise encounter in the middle of the desert.

Jamil   A friend of Dalal, who lived in an adjoining house on the palace grounds of Prince Ibrahim.

Mahmoud Daouk   Courted and married Princess Sultana.

Marwan Al Hamad   Sixty-year-old Bedouin dying of cancer.

Monsoor   Mahmoud's brother.

Naman   The Aramco guide on the plane to Dhahran.

Nizar   The Bedouin security guard who took part in the desert adventure.

Radifa   A Saudi woman with a rare nutritional disorder; married to a Palestinian.

Rashad   A farmer in the Asir with an unusual home.

Dr. Rashad Pharaon   Father of Ghaith Pharaon; physician and close advisor to King Faisal and King Khalid.

Samira   Daughter of a Saudi merchant who attempted suicide because she wasn't permitted to return to California to complete her education.

Sattam   A young Bedouin who appeared in the clinic with a severe infection threatening blindness.

Suliman Olayan   Wealthy self-made Saudi businessman.

Wasisa   Samira's older sister who favored the Saudi traditional role for women.

HOSPITAL PERSONNEL

Laura Ball   (American) In charge of the orientation program at the hospital.

John Barrow   (American) Assistant to the executive director of the hospital and a friend of Prince Ibrahim's family.

Manda Blake   (English) Secretary of the Medical Department.

Dr. Hugh Compton   (American) Director of Medical Affairs.

Dr. Trevor Evans   (Irish) The obstetrician with an extensive repertoire of bawdy ballads.

Ann Johnson   (English) A nurse.

Kamal   (Lebanese) Male nurse in charge of Prince Yusef.

Khasna   (Iraqi) Blonde Moslem technician with a heart murmur.

Pam Lambrie   (English) Ron's wife.

Dr. Ron Lambrie   (English) Physician and good friend.

Mashur   Saudi driver in charge of transportation to and from the airport.

May-Ellen   (American) Laboratory technician who favored the Greeks on her holidays.

Moussa   An Afghan in the transportation department.

Julie Northrop   (American) The hospital admitting officer.

Nabil   (Lebanese) Male nurse and translator in the clinic.

Galal Abu Nassera   (Egyptian) Legal adviser to the hospital.

Janet Powers   (American) Dr. Compton's secretary.

Dr. George Rogers   (English) A specialist named in the lawsuit for blood money.

Frank Taylor   (American) Executive Director of the hospital.

Dr. Jonathan Warren   (English) An obstetrician who delivered Prince Khalil's first son.

Doris Westbrook   (English) Philip's wife.

Dr. Philip Westbrook   (English) Chairman of the Department of Medicine from 1975 to 1976.

Madeleine Yamine   (Belgian) Young, attractive physician who recently graduated from medical school.

OTHERS

Abdullah Al Hagri   Former Prime Minister of North Yemen, who was killed in London shortly after his visit to the hospital.

Tom Frazier   (American) In charge of personnel at Aramco.

Tricia Frazier   (American) Tom's wife.

Dr. Mel Gilbert   (Canadian) A physician at Aramco.

Mary Gilbert   (American) Mel's wife.

Colonel Ibrahim Al-Hambdi   The President of North Yemen, who was assassinated by terrorists.

Dr. Don Mason   (American) A physician at Aramco for more than twenty years.

Betty Mason   (American) Don's wife.

Edwina Parnell   (American) A nurse in Khamis Mushayt.

Dr. Stewart Randall   (American) A physician living in Khamis Mushayt.

Sam Stark   Young American in the U.S. Consulate in Riyadh.

Bill Thompson   (American) An electrical contractor from California on a business trip to Saudi Arabia.

INDEX

Abdul-Aziz Al Saud, King. *See* Ibn Saud
Abdullah, Prince, 81, 126
Abdullah Al-Hagri, Judge, 174–75, 341
Abdul Taleem, 153, 329, 339
   Chop Square and *suqs*, 136–47
   desert trip, 195, 197–211, 331
   graduation and party, 321–22, 324–25
Abeyya, 15–16, 96, 334
Ablutions, 209, 302
Abortion, 183
Abraham, 25–26, 63, 335
Abu Bakr, 26
Adultery, 33, 105–106, 188–89, 295
   four witnesses, 188, 310–311
   non-Moslem women, 301
   palace wives, 313–316
Afghanistan, 196, 289
Africa, 317, 334
Agal, 16, 334
Agents' commissions. *See* Business practices
Ahmad (Prince Ibrahim's son), 248–51, 312
Ahmed Sudairi, 104
Akkad, Bandar, Dr., 168–70, 325, 328, 339
Alcohol. *See* Drinking and drunkenness;
   Liquor; Sadiki
Ali (Mohammed's son-in-law), 336
Ali Tomeemi, 232–33
Allah, 25, 220, 282, 286
   submission to, 33, 206–207, 226, 277, 281–85
Al Saud, 334. *See also* Saud, House of
Al Sharq Hotel, 50, 84–85, 149, 163
Al Yamama Hotel, 18–19, 23, 41, 48, 84, 149, 297
Americans, 165, 169–71, 322
   at Aramco, 218–22
   in hospital, 265, 303–306
   oil exploration, 213–215
   see also United States
Amputation of hands, 189, 324, 328
Anizah Bedouin tribe, 63
Antiques *suq,* 137, 141
Arabian-American Oil Company (Aramco), 5, 49, 212–36, 330
   compound life, 216–218, 221–22, 278–79
   early years, 218–219, 225–27
   history, 213–215, 235
   Saudi workforce, 218–20, 225–26, 230
Arabian Gulf, 197, 212–213, 215
   swimming in, 235–36
Arabian Peninsula, 3–4, 26, 334
   geology of, 197–98
Arabian Sands (Thesiger, Wilfred), 3

Arabic (language), 156
Arab League, 220, 261
Arab Mind, The (Patai), 3
Arab News, 84, 324
Arabs in History, The (Lewis, Bernard), 3
Arabs, 334
   Aramco workers, 218–219, 225
   books about, 3
   culture and traditions, 219–20
   see also names, such as Bedouins;
     Egyptians; Lebanese; Saudis
Ardha, 334
Area Handbook for Saudi Arabia, 3
Artesian wells, 197–98, 201, 214, 238
Asir Mountains, 171, 176–77
Asprey, Algernon, 158
Automobiles, 138, 329
   accidents, 22–23, 151, 180, 185. *See also*
     Drivers and driving
Ayn Heet (waterhole), 198, 214

Bader, Professor, 219
Bahrain, 33, 213–214, 256
Ball, Laura, 21–24, 34, 340
Bargaining, 137, 141–42, 155
Barrow, John, 237–41, 248, 251, 340
Basama, 272–76, 339
Batha Apartments, 163, 306
Bedouins, 130, 160, 172, 198–99, 225, 238, 328
   and birth control, 127
   and camels, 4, 77–78, 81–83
   clinic patients, 57–60, 90, 207, 280–86
   daughters and Ibn Saud, 112–113
   described, 4, 63–64, 77–78, 334
   Hussein and desert picnic, 200, 203–210, 331
   intermarriage and orthodoxy, 210
   King Khalid, 38
   and *majlis,* 83, 259
   manual labor and, 218–219
   medical treatments, 59, 205–207
   pregnancies and childbirth, 207–208
   sex and virginity, 301–302
   and veils, 58–60, 90–91, 97
   visit to Prince Yusef, 61–63
   Wahabism and, 27
Bedouin women, 58–60, 90–91, 97
   and inequality, 273–74
   and male sexuality, 294
   Princess Sultana's description of, 96–97, 100, 124
   West-East transition, 15–16, 332

Beer, 217, 227
Beheadings, 140, 143–47, 174, 328
    described, 145–46
    frequency of, 186, 189
Belgium, 225, 322
Belly dancing, 130–31, 134, 162, 165
Bereavement and grief, 283–84
Berman, Shelley, 261
Bhadir, Prince, 300–301
Bilharziasis, 174–75, 334
Billfold story, 266–67
Birth control, 127, 208
Bisht, 16, 169, 334
Bismillah ar-Rahman ar-Raheem, 321, 334
Blake, Manda, 47, 81, 179–80, 340
Blindness, 74, 169, 281–82, 337
Blood brothers, 314
Blood money, 179–93, 273
Boston, 1–2, 9–14
Branding, 59, 205
British Empire, 26–27, 225. *See also*
    England; English people
Butterfly analogy, 16, 332
Burial, 250–51, 284
Business practices, 8, 15, 188, 232–35

Cabinet, Royal, 30, 67, 238, 249
"Camel pants," 329
Camels, 4, 74, 78, 200, 204–206
    marathon, 81–83
    races, 77–79
Campus Villas, 165, 265
Cancer, 57, 224, 277–79, 284–86
    and Dr. Chandour, 288–92
Capital punishment, 33, 143–47
Catholics, 260–61, 278
Caviar, 169–70, 325
Censorship, 84, 260, 324
Central American countries, 317
Champagne story, 329
Chanters and drummers, 130, 134
Chauffeurs, 98–99, 310
Chemotherapy, 286, 288
Children, 207–208, 273
    at Aramco, 229
    and divorce, 101
    see also Education
Chop Square, 137, 140, 324
Christianity, 25, 219, 228, 295
Christians, 25, 260
Christmas trees, 230–31
Circumcision, 206
Climate and temperatures, 20, 150–51, 163–65
Clothing and dress, 15–18, 334–35
    Aramco wives, 227–28
    in desert, 205

Clothing and dress *(continued)*
    foreign women, 148, 324
    hajj pilgrims, 195–96
    of royals, 16, 18, 137, 354
    Saudi women, 16, 98, 150, 324, 331
    Sultana, 95–96
    at wedding party, 132–33
Cockroaches, 149–50
Coffee, cardamom, 177, 204
Committee for the Encouragement of
    Virtue and the Elimination of Vice,
    167
Communism, 261–62
Compton, Dr. Hugh, 165, 290, 299, 328, 340
    and blood money, 180, 183–84, 187, 189–92
    and Madeleine, 296
    Prince Yusef's illness and, 28–29, 36, 39–40, 44–46
Concubines, 141, 156, 289, 295, 309–316
Connaught Hotel, 241
Construction and building, 21–22, 68–69, 234
Coronary heart disease, 279
Corruption, 233–35, 258
Courtship and marriage, 111–25, 272
Crime, 3, 138, 140, 266–67
    and punishments, 33, 142–47, 185, 189, 192–93, 328
    see also Judicial system
Customs inspection, 17, 53

Dagger. See *Khanjar*
Dalal, 289–92, 339
    and Filwa, 318–319, 329
    palace women and, 307, 310–316
    and royal stipend, 308–309
Damman, 215
Dowries, 118
Drinking and drunkenness, 109, 294
    before arrival on aircraft, 6–7
    Aramco compound and, 217
    expatriates and foreigners, 52–53, 165, 169
    punishment for, 185, 189
    royals and, 52–53, 167, 254
    after wedding party, 128
    see also Sadiki; Wine
Drivers and driving, 22–23, 125, 268–69
    Aramco wives and, 217, 227
    Philip and, 50, 56, 195, 203
Drugs, 109, 189, 328
Dysentery, 223, 279

Eastern Province, 215, 222, 238, 275
    education system, 230
    and oil, 197, 212, 213

Marriage *(continued)*
  see also Wives
Marwan Al Hamad, 285–86, 339
Mashur, 18, 340
Mason, Betty, 221–22, 224, 341
Mason, Dr. Don, 221–24, 341
Matawa (morals police), 138–39, 142, 185, 336
May-Ellen, 304–305, 340
Mecca, 1, 27, 57, 235, 284, 307, 336
  and burial, 287
  Grand Mosque, seizing of, 211, 331
  hajj pilgrimage to, 5, 33, 195, 335
  and Mohammed, 25–26, 261
Mecca Road, 53, 195, 197, 200
Medical Advisory Board, 183–84, 253, 268, 280
Medical conferences, 212. *See also* First Arabian Peninsula Medical Conference
Medical students, 136, 296, 298, 320–322, 325
Medicine, 214, 266
  American, 247, 285
Medics, 269
Medina, 25–27, 210, 261, 284, 307, 336
Men. *See* Saudi men; Saudi royals
Mezanyah (payment to royalty), 102
Mishaal bint Abdul-Aziz, Princess, 105
Mishlah, 334
Mobil Oil Company, 215
Mohammed, Prophet, 2, 28, 57, 210, 219, 252, 335
  and call to prayer, 336
  life of, 25–26, 261
Mohammed Ali, Viceroy of Egypt, 27
Mohammed Ibn Abdul Wahab, 27
Mohammed Ibn Saud, Emir, 4, 27
Monarchy, 258–59, 331
Mongolia, 196
Monsoor Daouk, 123, 125–31, 326–27, 339
  and women's wedding party, 132, 134
Morals police, 185, 324, 336
Morocco, 33, 312
Moslems, 5, 25–26, 48, 206, 251, 335
  and death, 277–278, 285–92
  degrees of faith, 284–86
  and hajj, 195–96, 335
  from Hejaz region, 306
  judicial system, 187–89
  and Koran, 33
  polygamy and adultery, 295
  see also Fatalism; Islam; Mecca; Shiite Moslems; Sunni Moslems
Mothers, 274, 318
Moussa, 43–44, 171, 266–67, 340
Movies, 52, 255–56
Muezzin, 20, 25, 336

Mulka, 119–20
Munkar (moral turpitude), 167
Murder, 33, 144, 146, 186, 189
Music, 130, 134, 162
Mutfarrajeen, 133
Muttabaak, 326

Nabil, 57–60, 280, 340
Nadia, 323
Naman, 212–214
Nassara, 267–70
Nasser, Prince, 35, 77–81, 85–89, 338
National Cancer Institute, 289
National Institutes of Health, 290
Natural gas, 212, 230
Nayef Al-Barras, 56, 81–82
Nejd region, 27, 237–38, 284, 308
Nigeria, 189
Nizar, 195, 197–211, 331–32, 339
Northrop, Julie, 280–83, 340
Northrop Corporation, 235
North Yemen, 174–75, 189, 261, 341
Novalgin, 31
Nura, 150
Nurses
  Prince Ibrahim's overdosage, 246–47
  Nassara and, 267–70
  Moslem *vs.* Western, 268
  and Saudi men, 300

Oases, 123–26, 201–202, 238
Oil, 37, 212, 230–31, 322–23
  Aramco established, 213–216
  discovery of, 5–6, 214
  Saudi Arabian economy, 5–6, 83, 331
  wealth from, 5–6, 8, 98, 109
Olayan, Suliman, 232, 339
Olayan Saudi Holding Company, 232
Oman, 189
"One billion" fantasy, 316–317
OPEC, 220
Oriental rugs, 127, 158, 160, 196

Pakistanis, 21, 189, 221, 322
Palaces, 68, 87–89, 239–41
  Royal Guest Palace, 158–59
Palace wives, 275–76, 310–316, 318–319
Palestine, 196, 262, 284
Palestinians, 261, 279, 324
Pan American Airlines, 298
Paradise, 286–87, 334
Parasitic diseases, 174, 223–24, 278–79
Parnell, Edwina, 173, 176, 341
Parties
  Eid al Fitr, 326
  hospital staff, 165–67
  Prince Khalil's celebration, 253–57

Water, 152, 197-98, 202, 214
  cost of, 121-22
  contamination and disease, 279, 335
  fasting from, 325
Watson, Cynthia, 305-306
Wealth, 98, 109, 167-68
  Bedouins and, 210-211
  business fortunes, 232-35
  Dr. Gray's one-billion fantasy, 316-317
  of Saudi Arabia, 5-6, 83, 330-31
  see also Ibrahim Al Muqrin el-Kabir,
    Prince; Yusef Al Saud, Prince
Wedding parties, 119-34
Westbrook, Doris, 50-53, 71, 81, 163, 340
Westbrook, Dr. Philip, 49-56, 64-65, 81, 84,
    163, 278, 328, 340
  desert trip, 195, 197-211, 331
  Khalil's party, 253, 258, 260, 263-64
  and Landcruiser, 50, 56, 125, 195, 203
Westernization. See Foreign influence
Western world, 75-76, 219, 274-76, 279
West Germany, 163, 322-23
Windeyer, Sir Brian, 321
Wine, 165-66, 217
Wives, 5, 28, 71, 101-102
  and concubines, 102, 289, 310
  Prince Ibrahim's, 243-44, 249-50, 291,
    312, 314, 318-319
  numbers of, 291, 295, 302
  see also Bedouin women; Saudi women;

Wives (continued)
    Women, foreign
Women, foreign, 148, 155-62, 324
  at Aramco, 217, 227-29
  hospital staff, 303-307
  married to Saudis, 93-94, 167-69
  Saudi men and sex, 294, 297-301
World Health Organization (WHO), 223,
    317
World War II, 215

Yamine, Dr. Madeleine, 296-300, 329, 340
Yemen, 141, 171, 174-75, 289, 334
Yemeni workers, 21, 163-64, 174, 186, 324
Yusef Al Saud, Prince, 77, 79, 290, 339
  background and family, 68-71, 302
  and Dr. Gray, 69-76, 327-28
  illness and hospitalization, 28-32, 34-40,
    42-46, 53, 325
  royal visits, 36-40, 45-46, 67
  Ruth's portrait of, 85-89
  wealth, 68-70

Zabbar, Dr., 181, 186
Zakat, 251, 337
Zamzam well, 25
Zeffa, 133
Zionism, 261
Zoo Road Apartments, 163